Proceedings of the Conference on Subretinal Space

W0050484

Documenta Ophthalmologica
Proceedings Series volume 25

Editor H. E. Henkes

Dr W. Junk bv Publishers The Hague-Boston-London 1981

Proceedings of the Conference on Subretinal Space, Jerusalem, October 14–19, 1979

Edited by H. Zauberman

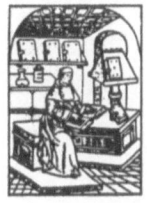

Dr W. Junk bv Publishers The Hague-Boston-London 1981

Distributors:

for the United States and Canada

Kluwer Boston, Inc.
160 Old Derby Street
Hingham, MA 02043
USA

for all other countries

Kluwer Academic Publishers Group
Distribution Center
P.O. Box 322
3300 AH Dordrecht
The Netherlands

Library of Congress Cataloging in Publication Data   ▢**IP**

Conference on Subretinal Space, Jerusalem, 1979.
    Proceedings of the Conference on Subretinal Space,
Jerusalem, October 14-19, 1979.

    (Documenta Ophthalmologica Proceedings Series; v. 25)
    1. Retina—Diseases—Congresses. 2. Retina--Congresses.
I. Zauberman, H. II. Series. III. Title: Subretinal Space.
RE551.C66   1979   617.7'3   80-20149

ISBN-13: 978-94-009-8655-8   e-ISBN-13: 978-94-009-8653-4
DOI: 10.1007/978-94-009-8653-4

Cover design: Max Velthuijs

PREFACE

The Conference on Subretinal Space, held between October 14 and 19, 1979, was organized to bring into the forefront some of the developments in basic and clinical sciences in this field. Indeed the interaction between choroid, pigment epithelium and sensory retina in terms of the physical adherence between the tissues, transport of materials and changes produced by the growth of new vessels, fluid penetration, light damage, etc. are some of the outstanding ophthalmic problems of today.

We hope that the proceedings of this Conference may be of some help in providing better understanding both of the subretinal space and of its boundaries.

HANAN ZAUBERMAN, M.D.

CONTENTS

Neovascularization of subretinal space

Retinal detachment retinopathy

Degenerations of subretinal space

Miscellaneous

X

THE RETINAL CIRCULATION:
PAST, PRESENT AND FUTURE
The Fifth Abraham Albert Ticho Lecture

PAUL HENKIND

(New York City, N.Y., U.S.A.)

This lecture is dedicated to Dr. Abraham Ticho, the renowned ophthalmologist and humanitarian. I humbly hope it does sufficient honor to his memory.

The fact that man and a number of other animals have a dual circulation which nourishes the retinal tissue is presumably of significance but the benefits of this dual blood supply remain a mystery. Many animals including birds, horses and elephants have few or no blood vessels traversing the retina and yet they have excellent visual function. The possession of retinal blood vessels in humans seems more a nuisance than anything else. They provide us with the potential for acquiring the multitude of retinopathies which can and do cause visual impairment in millions. Diabetes mellitus, hypertension, sickle cell disease, retrolental fibroplasia, Beçhet's disease and Eale's disease are but a few of the vasculopathies which can cause blindness. Leaking retinal vessels are known to be responsible for cystoid macular edema. There are many other disorders associated with derangement of the retinal circulation including the field defect seen in glaucoma as well as retinal holes which lead to detachment. While one might study the retinal circulation simply because it is so readily visible, the reality is that it attracts our attention because of the potential for vascular pathology.

It has been my good fortune, these past two decades, to be involved in studies dealing with the retinal circulation, allowing me to work with and meet so many wonderful people. In this lecture I hope to describe the status of our understanding of retinal vessels and the circulation within them. Before I talk about what retinal vessels are and what they can do, it is appropriate to briefly review the history of studies dealing with the retinal circulation.

It would seem that the anatomists of ancient Alexandria were the first to appreciate the fact that the retina contained blood vessels. They coined the term retina and suggested that the retina was a net-like structure. I imagine that the reason for this was the presence of the intraretinal vessels. With the exception of a few experimentalists in the late 18th century, no one had visualized the retinal circulation in a living creature until Helmholtz invented the ophthalmoscope. This invention revolutionized the field of ophthalmolo-

1

Docum. Ophthal. Proc. Series, Vol. 25, ed. by H. Zauberman
© 1981, Dr. W. Junk bv Publishers, The Hague

gy and, indeed, all of medicine. Within a few years of its introduction, numerous conditions affecting the retinal blood vessels had been described and illustrated. The following century can be considered, at least from the clinical standpoint, as a strictly observational time where clinicians looked at the vessels and noted if there were any gross alterations. This first one hundred years led to the production of more than one hundred atlases filled with clear, clinical description, with occasional correlation with systemic disease, but with little mention of pathogenetic mechanism. It would be incorrect to state that there was no effort to understand the properties of the retinal circulation until the mid-twentieth century but scientific studies were scarce. Significant studies of human and comparative retinal vascular anatomy were conducted by Leber and his colleagues in Germany in the latter half of the 19th century. In the mid 1920's Stewart Duke-Elder successfully cannulated retinal arteries in animals and measured directly, for the first and only time, retinal artery pressure. In the 1930's Jonas Friedenwald studied retinal pulses and Arnold Sorsby intravenously injected vital dyes, albeit not fluorescein, and examined the fundi of animals and humans with various retinal disorders.

The decade from 1940 to 1950 was outstanding due to a number of major contributions dealing with the retinal circulation. Isaac Michaelson published his superlative work on the anatomy of the human retinal vascular tree in which he described, among other things, the radial peripapillary capillaries (Michaelson & Campbell 1940). Eight years later, 1948, he published his observations on the development of retinal vessels and the significance of developmental factors in retinal disease. Most workers in the field of the retinal circulation look upon these papers and Michaelson's book, THE RETINAL CIRCULATION IN MAN AND ANIMALS (1954), as cornerstones upon which our present knowledge is founded. During that same decade, Palm (1947) demonstrated the similarity of retinal to brain vessels with regard to their impermeability to the vital dye trypan blue. This was the first clue to the existence of a blood-retinal barrier. In 1949, Friedenwald developed his PAS staining technique which permitted a unique histopathologic evaluation of the retinal vessels. This same era saw Ballantyne and Loewenstein (1943) histopathologically reconfirm the fact that diabetes mellitus produces a specific retinopathy. It was also the time in which the iatrogenic disease, retrolental fibroplasia, was first induced and soon became a leading cause of blindness in developed countries. It seems that these two diseases, diabetic retinopathy and retrolental fibroplasia (RLF) were the stimuli to a handful of individuals who were beginning to devote attention to unraveling their causes. The names of Arnall Patz and Norman Ashton immediately come to mind for they were the experimentalists who proved that excess oxygen is the cause of RLF and both have persistently examined the problem of diabetic retinopathy.

The 1950's is notable for the work of two outstanding individuals in the field of retinal vascular disorders, Robert Leishman and George Wise.

Dr. Leishman's paper entitled, THE EYE IN GENERAL VASCULAR DISEASE, HYPERTENSION AND ARTERIAL SCLEROSIS (1957), is an important treatise filled with excellent observations both clinical and histopathological. He clearly pointed out the circumstances under which human retinal vessels were likely to be reactive and why they were likely to lose their potential for reactivity. Dr. Wise devoted virtually all of his attention to the retinal circulation and attempted to bring order to a field that had a dearth of observations and often meaningless phraseology. His thesis dealing with retinal neovascularization (1956) should be read by anyone interested in fundus disease.

Our knowledge of retinal circulation would probably have remained static had it not been for two important advances in the early 1960's. One was the development of the technique of retinal digestion by Kuwabara and Cogan (1960) whereby for the first time a circulatory bed could be totally freed from its surrounding tissue, stained, examined microscopically and the details of vessel morphology readily appreciated. The other was the technique of fundus fluorescein angiography developed by two medical students, Novotny and Alvis (1961). This technique, initially cumbersome, has now been universally accepted as an indispensable diagnostic modality. Indeed, fluorescein angiography has provided the basis for much of our newer knowledge concerning the retinal circulation. It permits qualitative and quantitative assessment of this circulation in health and disease.

The 1960's was also the time when electron microscopic analysis was applied to the retinal vessels. Thus, by the mid 1960's a sophisticated armamentarium had been brought to bear on the mysteries of the retinal circulation.

I was fortunate to participate in the first experimental study utilizing all of these new techniques including Michaelson's injection methodology, fluorescein angiography, retinal digestion, histochemistry, and electron microscopy. The subject was focal retinal ischemia (Ashton et al. 1966). A very significant feature of the project was the succesful collaboration between ophthalmologists, ophthalmic pathologists, internists and physiologists, all of whom had skills to offer in approaching the important problem of acute arteriolar occlusion and its effect on surrounding structures. Upon completion of their studies the team was quite convinced that there would be little to add to their observations. As usual, this conceit of humans proved false. Within a few short years it was clear that we had created cessation of normal axoplasmic flow. In 1965 we didn't even know that such flow existed within neurons.

This is a good place to terminate the brief historical review. However for those who are historically inclined, I suggest that you compare the description of retinal vascular disease given by Sir Stewart Duke-Elder in his TEXTBOOK OF OPHTHALMOLOGY, circa 1941, with Volume 10 of his SYSTEM OF OPHTHALMOLOGY published in 1967. This will reveal the great strides

3

that were made in the understanding of the retinal circulation in the quarter century after 1940.

This narrative now turns rather personal. My exposure to ophthalmology began with George Wise who took me on as an apprentice after my first year of medical school. He was in the midst of writing his thesis on retinal neovascularization and shared with me his ideas and his clinical experience showing me, the neophyte, virtually every nuance of clinical medical problems. One of the first things he did was give me a copy of Professor Michaelson's monograph which I excitedly devoured. He encouraged me to read the works of Ashton, Patz, Leishman, among others, and to examine the many extant fundus atlases.

Following my ophthalmology residency, I had the opportunity to obtain a research position in Norman Ashton's laboratory. There, I was able to watch a remarkably gifted scientist apply the various known laboratory techniques in his quest for understanding retinal vascular disease. Fortuitously, my work with Professor Ashton coincided with studies being conceived by Colin Dollery, a physician-physiologist-pharmacologist. His interests were in the area of microcirculation and he fully appreciated Novotny and Alvis's major contribution. In a sense, I was the link between the laboratories of Ashton and Dollery. I learned from both these men and their colleagues the value of a collaborative approach to problems as complex as those of retinal vascular disease.

My first project in Professor Ashton's laboratory was to study the effects of embolization of retinal vessels with glass emboli. The work started in cats and was almost immediately successful as we were able to embolize the vascular tree and produce a host of vascular and extravascular lesions. We also induced choroidal lesions but unfortunately because of our singular purpose which was to study retinal vessels, did not pursue studies of the choroidal circulation in any sustained fashion. Shortly thereafter, we started our collaboration with Dollery and his group at Hammersmith Hospital. Our initial effort was successful beyond expectation. We had produced cotton-wool spots almost identical to those seen in humans.

An outgrowth of these embolization studies was my rediscovery of Michaelson's radial peripapillary capillaries (Henkind 1967). Analysis of the fluorescein angiograms in our young, experimental pigs revealed the presence of some hitherto unknown, thin parallel lines adjacent to the optic nerve head. Initially we felt that these might represent some sort of artifact. Using a modification of Michaelson's india ink injection technique, I examined flat mounts of normal pigs and noted the presence of very superficially placed, elongated, radially arranged, intraretinal capillaries. Examination of india ink whole mounts of kittens and cats revealed similar vessels in that species. Thus, the radial capillaries that had been described by Michaelson and Campbell in 1940 in humans and later by Kuwabara and Cogan in their digest preparations and François and Neetens in their radio-opaque dye investigations, were present in species other than man. Firmly believing that

4

every vascular bed must have a purpose, I initiated studies on the radial peripapillary capillaries. I was struck, as had been Kuwabara and Cogan, with the fact that the arrangement of the radial capillaries in man resembled a Bjerrum scotoma. This led to the development of the concept that radial capillaries played a role in the production of such scotomas in human glaucoma. Suffice it to say that my hypothesis has not been universally accepted.

As a result of my observations, Kornzweig and his colleagues (1968) were prompted to examine retinal digests of patients with uniocular glaucoma and they noted that the radial peripapillary capillaries appeared atrophied only in the eyes with glaucoma. This fit well with the observations that Alterman and I (1968) had made in felines. Even more important than the possible role of the radial. capillaries in a specific disease entity, was the finding of selective retinal capillary dropout which stimulated my thinking about the relationship of the retinal vessels to the surrounding neural and glial components.

What happens to retinal vessels when the surrounding neurons disappear and, vice versa, what happens to the neurons when the vessels disappear? Over a period of more than a decade, my colleagues and I have examined both human and experimental animal material and have come to the conclusion that retinal neuronal dropout does not lead to microvascular obliteration, but that the contrary situation of retinal vascular obliteration, particularly if acute, leads to surrounding neuronal dissolution (Henkind, Gould & Bellhorn 1975). Slow destruction of the retinal capillaries may not always cause retinal neuropil alterations, but this is a subject requiring more study.

If our observations regarding the relationship between the retinal vessels and surrounding tissue are correct, then in those situations where we find absence of the retinal vascular bed it implies that it was the vessels that were initially diseased, and not that their disappearance reflected primary neuronal disease. The application of this principle to the study of glaucoma is obvious and implicates a primary vascular involvement. In diabetic retinopathy, the picture is less clear because retinal vascular alterations take place over many months or years and it is difficult to conclude much about the actual function of the diabetic retina simply by looking at an angiogram or retinal digest preparation.

There is substantial fluorescein angiography evidence that in retinal detachments, the retinal tissue surrounding the tear is virtually avascular. Did this avascularity occur as a result of the tear, or did the retinal capillaries primarily disappear for some reason as yet unknown and thus cause an area of weakness which could no longer resist the pressures of a continually tugging vitreous? In my opinion there is great significance to this latter possibility. If one has noted a detachment in one eye of an individual then it may be appropriate to do fluorescein angiography of the contralateral eye. If one finds an area where there is absence of the retinal vascular bed that region should be closely examined and, perhaps, even treated by photocoagulation or cryotherapy. Obviously, the entire subject of retinal vascular-neuronal interrelationships requires more examination.

Another facet of the work with retinal embolization was the production of retinal collateral vessels. Following arteriolar embolization, arterio-arteriolar collateral channels developed and they were studied by ophthalmoscopy, fluorescein angiography, ink injection techniques, and retinal digestion. Quantitative analysis of these collaterals was carried out for the first time, and demonstrated beyond question the potential of retinal capillaries to turn into arterioles (Klein, Klein, Henkind & Bellhorn 1971). Previously, it had been shown that retinal capillaries were capable of becoming venules following retinal vein obstruction (Kohner et al. 1970). The retina is undoubtedly the best place to study collateral vessel formation, a fact generally overlooked by nonophthalmic investigators.

Some forays into the study of the embryologic development of the retinal circulation may be of interest to you. After my return to the United States one of Professor Ashton's star pupils, Luis d'Oliveira, elected to come to the States and work with George Wise and myself. He possessed amazing technical dexterity and our first collaboration was to reexamine the development of retinal vessels. The study of Engerman & Meyer (1965) led to conclusions contrary to those of Michaelson. They had used a modified PAS stain technique to study whole-mounted rat retinas. At the same time, Agrawal (1965) examining retinal digest preparations in rats, demonstrated that primitive cells preceded vessel ingrowth into the animal retina. Oliveira and I (1967) were able to combine ink injection with digests and conclusively demonstrate that the initial stage of vascular ingrowth is a cellular meshwork without any hint of patent vascular channels. It was from this meshwork that first primitive capillaries and later arterioles and venules developed. The following year, in collaboration with Shakib (1968), we showed by electron microscopic studies the nature of the cells that form the vascular complex and that intramural pericytes and endothelial cells arise from the same stem cell. Though our work led us to conclusions opposite to those of Michaelson, when we repeated Michaelson's methodology we reproduced his results. The point is that with the development of new methods, new observations will be made and new hypotheses formulated. Clearly, one must keep an open mind at all times and be ready to accept new advances. Subsequently we studied the development of the radial peripapillary capillaries and found that they developed differently and later than the other retinal capillaries (Henkind, Bellhorn & Poll 1973).

The impetus of the Macular Symposium held at Bath in 1975 prompted us to examine the development of the vessels of the macula. Surprisingly, no one had previously studied the subject in any detail. We found that in the fetal life of the monkey the area destined to become the macula was fully vascularized but prior to birth a remodeling process took place and vessels disappeared from the central macular area (Henkind, Bellhorn, Murphy &

Roa 1975). In the cat the situation was different and no vessels were found in the area centralis until the third week after birth. The observations of the developing macular vasculature in the rhesus monkey support the observations of Yeung *et al.* (1973) and Bird & Weale (1974). Both these groups demonstrated, by fluorescein angiography, the presence of capillaries crossing the human fovea. Obviously, such vessels are persistent remnants of the fetal vascular system which has not completely disappeared.

I think it is important to recognize that sometimes the stimulus for work comes from a request to present at a scientific meeting. One is often obliged to conduct experiments to fulfill the request. In my opinion, a well conceived symposia such as the present one, focusing on a specific topic, often generates original work.

Another stimulus for producing an original scientific paper may be a Festschrift. The request to provide an article for Sir Stewart Duke-Elder's Festschrift prompted George Wise and I to write on the subject of retinal neovascularization, collaterals and shunts (Henkind and Wise 1974). From a clinical standpoint, it was important to sort out the major retinal vascular lesions which might be mistaken for each other but which we thought had absolutely differing potentialities. We ruminated about this for more than a decade and then by a simple, albeit commanding letter were compelled to gather our evidence. Our paper described the clinical, fluorescein angiographic, and histopathological differences between retinal neovascularization, collaterals, and vascular shunts. Such was the type of work George Wise encouraged, for it made the study of retinal vascular disease meaningful and practical.

Our observations concerning remodeling of the vascular bed during embryonic and early life prompted us to consider the situation of retinal vascular aging. Until recently, there had not been a single study of this subject in normal animals and, certainly, there has never been such a study in healthy humans from early childhood to senescence. We had the opportunity to examine rats kept solely for the purpose of studying normal aging and conducted an investigation of their retinal vascular tree (Glatt and Henkind 1979). We found alterations in the retinal vessels that could be attributed to aging and not to any disease process. Some mild cellular changes were noted especially at the retinal periphery and occasional acellular capillary strands were found in aged animals. Studies such as these are necessary before one can even try to interpret the effects of specific diseases on the retinal vascular tree. Apparently the normal rat possesses a retinal vascular tree which holds up remarkably well in face of uncomplicated aging. I should like to point out that this study was conducted in collaboration with a college student who did the greater part of the work.

Many of our studies have been conducted with the assistance of college or medical students and, on occasion, high school students. The young people often bring refreshing enthusiasm and unflagging spirit to a project and I would advise investigators to tap this source of workers.

At the present time researchers in the Department of Ophthalmology at the Albert Einstein College of Medicine/Montefiore Hospital Medical Center, are conducting various studies on the retinal vascular bed and the retinal circulation. Particular attention is being paid to the permeability properties of retinal vessels in health and disease (work of Margaret Burns and Roy Bellhorn). Newer dyes and markers are being used in conjunction with ultrastructural analysis. We are also conducting indepth studies on experimentally induced intraretinal neovascularization. For example, over the past decade my colleagues and I have noted that when retinal vessels are provoked to burrow beneath their normal position in the inner nuclear layer they may, if they come in contact with the retinal pigment epithelium, change their morphology. These intraretinal new vessels instead of having normal non-fenestrated endothelial cells now have a fenestrated endothelium (Bellhorn *et al.* 1973). We postulated that this is due to the interaction of the RPE and the vessels, but must conduct more studies to confirm this. Consider the importance of this observation in a variety of subretinal neovascularization disorders. Perhaps destroying the RPE may alter the newly proliferating choroidal vessels so they will not leak!

More has been learned about the properties of the retinal circulation in the past two decades than in all preceding history yet we are far from complete understanding of this most important circulatory bed. With regard to the 'blood-retinal barrier' we know that normal retinal vessels are impermeable to fluorescein and other vital dyes, and while there is no question that certain molecules are excluded from entering into the retinal tissue, it must be recognized that many substances, including blood gasses, amino acids, lipids, and sugars, traverse the retinal capillary endothelium. The mechanisms available for the passage of such materials are not completely known, but selective transport systems are undoubtedly available in addition to paths of diffusion and pinocytosis (Henkind, Bellhorn & Schall 1980). We know from the work of Laties (1967) that the intraretinal vessels lack adrenergic innervation and yet retinal vessels can, and do, contract and dilate. How they do so is not clear. The related problem of retinal vessel autoregulation, whereby a constant flow of blood is maintained inspite of alterations in intraocular pressure or systemic blood pressure, is another subject which requires indepth analysis. We urgently need a solution to the problem of retinal neovascularization. Attacking neovascularization by destroying retinal tissue is an unsatisfactory stop-gap measure applied because we know so little about retinal neovascularization. Biochemical factors would seem to be at the root of the problem and when these factors are elucidated more appropriate therapies may be designed to eliminate unwanted new vessels.

At the outset of this lecture I suggested that it is a mystery why man and some animals possess intraretinal blood vessels. The fact is they are present and it is up to us to discover how they work and how they are affected by disease. The subject is vast but the task of unraveling the facts will prove most rewarding.

REFERENCES

Agrawal, P. K. The cellular structure and development of the retinal vessels of the rat. Orient. Arch. Ophthal. 3: 23 (1965).

Alterman, M. & P. Henkind. Radial peripapillary capillaries – 2. Possible role in Bjerrum's scotoma. Brit. J. Ophthal. 52: 26 (1968).

Ashton, N., C. T. Dollery, P. Henkind et al. Focal retinal ischemia. Brit. J. Ophtal. 50: 285 (1966).

Ballantyne, A.J. & A. Loewenstein. The pathology of diabetic retinopathy. Trans. Ophtal. Soc. U.K. 63: 95 (1943).

Bellhorn, R. W., Bellhorn, A. H. Friedman & P. Henkind. Urethan-induced retinopathy in pigmented rats. Invest. Ophth. 12: 65 (1973).

Bird, A. C. & R. A. Weale. On the retinal vasculature of the human fovea. Exp. Eye Res. 19: 409 (1974).

Engerman, R. L. & R. K. Meyer. Development of retinal vasculature in rats. Am. J. Ophthal. 60: 628 (1965).

Friedenwald, J. S. A new approach to some problems of retinal vascular disease. Amer. J. Ophthal. 32: 487 (1949).

Glatt, H. J. & P. Henkind. Aging changes in the retinal capillary bed of the rat. Microvascular Res. 18: 1 (1979).

Henkind, P. The radial peripapillary capillaries of the retina.' 1. Anatomy: Human and comparative. Brit. J. Ophthal. 51: 115 (1967).

Henkind, P., R. W. Bellhorn, M. E. Murphy & N. Roa. Development of macular vessels in monkey and cat. Brit J. Ophth. 59: 703 (1975).

Henkind, P., R. W. Bellhorn & D. Poll. Radial peripapillary capillaries. 3. Their development in the cat. Brit. J. Ophtal. 57: 595 (1973).

Henkind, P., R. W. Bellhorn & B. Schall. Retinal Edema. In: The Blood-Retinal Barriers. Edit. by I. Cunha-vaz. Plenum, New York. pp. 251-268 (1980).

Henkind, P. & L. F. de Oliveira. Development of retinal vessels in the rat. Invest. Ophthal. 6: 520 (1967).

Henkind, P., H. B. Gould & R. W. Bellhorn. Optic nerve transection in cats; effect on retinal vessels. Invest. Ophthal. 14 610 (1975).

Henkind, P. & G. N. Wise. Retinal neovascularization, collaterals, vascular shunts. Brit. J. Ophthal. 58: 413 (1974).

Klein, R., B. Klein, P. Henkind & R. Bellhorn. Retinal collateral vessel formation. Invest. Ophthal. 10: 471 (1971).

Kohner, E. M., C. T. Dollery, M. Shakib, P. Henkind et al. Experimental retinal branch vein occlusion. Amer. J. Ophthal. 69: 778 (1970).

Kornzweig, A. L., I. Eliasoph & M. Feldstein. Selective atrophy of the radial peripapillary capillaries in chronic glaucoma. Arch. Ophthal. 80: 696 (1968).

Kuwabara, T. & D. G. Cogan. Studies of retinal vascular patterns. 1. Normal architecture. Arch. Ophthal. 64: 904 (1960).

Laties, A. M. Central retinal artery innervation. Absence of adrenergic innervation to the intraocular branches. Arch. Ophthal. 77: 405 (1967).

Leishman, R. The eye in general vascular disease, hypertension and arteriosclerosis. Brit. J. Ophthal. 41: 641 (1957).

Michaelson, I. C. The mode of development of the retinal vessels and some observations of its significance in certain retinal diseases. Trans. Ophthal. Soc. U.K. 68: 137 (1948).

Michaelson, I.C. Retinal Circulation in Man and Animals. Springfield, Ill. Thomas (1954).

Michaelson, I.C. & A.C.P. Campbell. The anatomy of the finer retinal vessels. Trans. Ophthal. Soc. U.K. 60: 71 (1940).

Novotny, H.R. & D.L. Alvis. Method of photographing fluorescein in circulating blood in the human retina. Circulation 24: 82 (1961).

Palm, E. On the occurrence in the retina of conditions corresponding to the blood-brain barrier. Acta Ophthal. 25: 295 (1947).

Shakib, M., L.F. de Oliveira & P. Henkind. Development of retinal vessels. 2. Earliest stages of vessel formation. Invest. Ophthal. 7: 689 (1968).

Wise, G.N. Retinal neovascularization. Trans. Amer. Ophthal. Soc. 54: 729 (1956).

Yeung, J., G. Crock, J. Cairns et al. Macular-foveal capillaries in human retina. Austr. J. Ophthal. 1: 17 (1973).

Author's address:
Department of Ophthalmology
Albert Einstein College of Medicine
Montefiore Hospital & Medical Center
New York, N.Y.,
U.S.A.

PATHOLOGY OF THE SUB-RETINAL SPACE

MARK O. M. TSO

(*Chicago, Illinois, U.S.A.*)

The sub-retinal space is bounded externally by the retinal pigment epithelium (RPE), internally by the external limiting membrane, proximally by the intermediary tissue of Kuhnt at the peripapillary region, and distally by cell junctions between RPE and Mueller cells at the ora serrata. Each of these boundaries is distinctive structurally and reacts differently to disease conditions.

As the external boundary of the sub-retinal space, the RPE is also one of the two primary sites of the blood-retinal barrier; the other site is at the endothelium of the retinal capillary. The RPE and its zonulae occludentes prevent plasma proteins and other macromolecules of the bloodstream from reaching the sub-retinal space; however, glucose, oxygen, and other nutrients from the choroidal circulation are allowed to pass through to supply the outer layers of the retina. The transport of nutrients across the RPE is relatively inefficient when compared with the transport at the retinal capillary. Tornquist (Tornquist, Alm & Bill 1979) observed that on a single passage of blood, 35% of oxygen and 12% of glucose are extracted from the retinal circulation of the pig, while only 2% oxygen and 2% of glucose are extracted from the choroidal circulation.

The sub-retinal space is bounded internally by the external limiting membrane, which is a series of zonula adherens-like cell junctions joining adjacent Mueller cells and photoreceptor cells. These cell junctions provide a mechanical support for the outer layers of the retina. Even though the zonulae adherentes of the external limiting membrane are not tight cell junctions, they play a restrictive role in the transport of macromolecules from the sub-retinal space. In pathologic conditions that result in disruption of the blood-retinal barrier, macromolecules may pass from the choroid into the sub-retinal space but are stopped, at least temporarily, by the external limiting membrane from invading the inner layers of the retina.

The intermediary tissue of Kuhnt at the peripapillary region consists of a number of glial cells joined by a series of cell junctions (Tso, Shih & McLean

This investigation was supported in part by Public Health Service Grant EYO1903, EYO1904 and Core Grant 1P30EYO1792.

11

1975). These cell junctions are a continuation of zonulae adherentes and zonulae occludentes of the RPE.

At the ora serrata, some poorly differentiated Mueller cells and pigment epithelial cells are joined by a series of junctional complexes forming the distal boundary of the sub-retinal space. According to Pei and Smelzer (1968), these are mostly zonula adherens type cell junctions.

The sub-retinal space appears to be a closed space that is completely surrounded by cells and cell junctions. In various pathologic conditions, this closed environment is broken and serious consequences may result. In this report the pathology and repair of the RPE, the external limiting membrane, and the intermediary tissue of Kuhnt are described. Relatively little is known about the pathology of the cell junctions at the ora serrata, which will not be discussed in this report.

PATHOLOGIC CHANGES OF THE RPE ASSOCIATED WITH DISRUPTION OF THE BLOOD-RETINAL BARRIER AND THE SUB-RETINAL SPACE

Pathologic conditions of the RPE that result in disruption of the blood retinal barrier and the sub-retinal space are frequently observed in clinical ophthalmology. A well-known example is central serous retinopathy, in which the retina is serously detached and fluorescein angiography shows leakage of fluorescein through the pigment epithelium into the sub-retinal

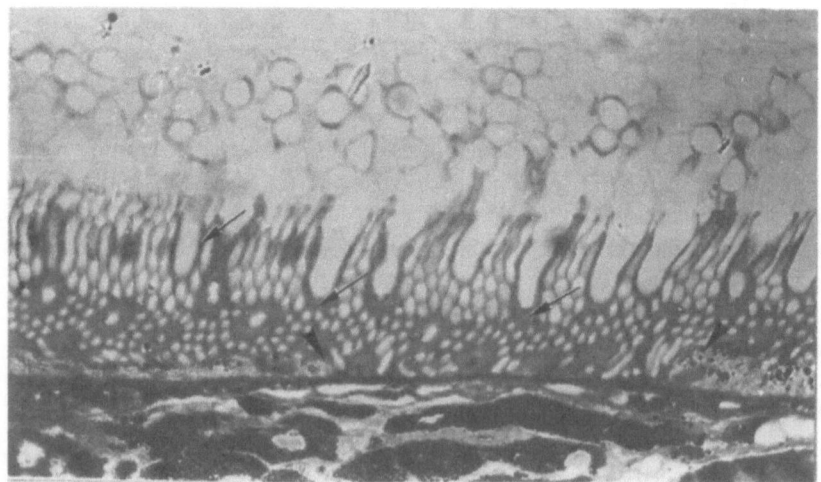

Fig. 1. The retina of a rhesus monkey whose short posterior ciliary arteries were occluded six hours before enucleation. Note the dissolution of retinal pigment epithelium (arrowheads). Horseradish peroxidase reaction products (single arrows) appear as a black stain and infiltrate the sub-retinal space. The outer segments of photoreceptor cells approximate Bruch's membrane (unstained epoxy resin section) (×400).

12

space. The closed environment of the sub-retinal space is disrupted and communicates with the interstitial space of the choroid. These pathologic conditions of the RPE may be best described in four categories.

1) *Dissolution of the RPE cells.* In certain acute and severe injuries of the RPE, dissolution of the cells may be seen within 24 hours after the insult. The RPE cells disintegrate and disappear from Bruch's membrane (Fig. 1). At the early stage macrophages are not present in the sub-retinal space, the retina appears relatively spared, and the photoreceptor outer segments approximate the bare Bruch's membrane. Fluorescein angiography shows extensive leakage of fluorescein from the choriocapillaris through Bruch's membrane into the sub-retinal space. In the same manner, when injected intravenously, tracers of larger molecular weight, such as horseradish peroxidase, pass through the choriocapillaris and Bruch's membrane and infiltrate into the sub-retinal space (Fig. 1).

This form of dissolution of RPE has been observed in acute occlusion of the short posterior ciliary artery (Tso, Kaga & Hayreh 1980) and in severe photic injury (Tso 1973).

It is interesting to note that in spite of the dissolution of the RPE cells and disruption of the blood-retinal barrier, serous detachment of the retina is not observed. So, the detachment seen in central serous retinopathy must be produced by factors other than simple disruption of the blood-retinal barrier.

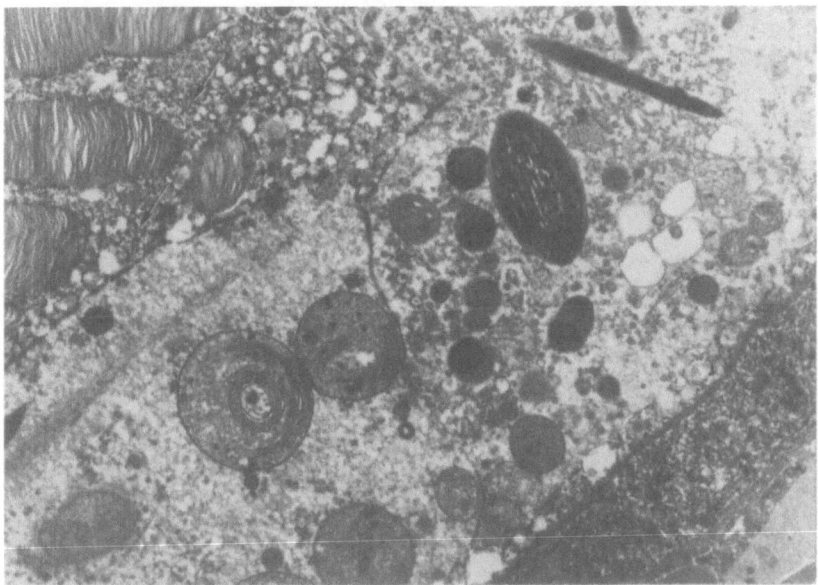

Fig. 2. Liquefactive necrosis of retinal pigment epithelium. The cells are swollen and exhibit watery cytoplasm and discontinuous plasmalemma. Reaction products of horseradish peroxidase are noted in these sub-retinal spaces (arrows) ($\times 14,410$).

2) *Necrosis of the RPE cells.* In some diseases, the retinal pigment epithelium may not be disintegrated but is necrotic. Tracer subsances, whether sodium fluorescein in fluorescein angiography or horseradish peroxidase in ultrastructural studies, pass through these necrotic cells and accumulate in the sub-retinal space. The necrotic RPE cells not only fail to serve as a barrier but are unable to retain the tracer material in the cytoplasm of the cells.

Pathologically, the RPE cells may undergo coagulative or liquefactive necrosis. Liquefactive necrosis of the RPE, as seen in acute occlusions of short posterior ciliary arteries (Tso, Kaga & Hayreh 1980) exhibits swelling of the cells. The cytoplasm becomes watery, the plasmalemma is discontinuous,

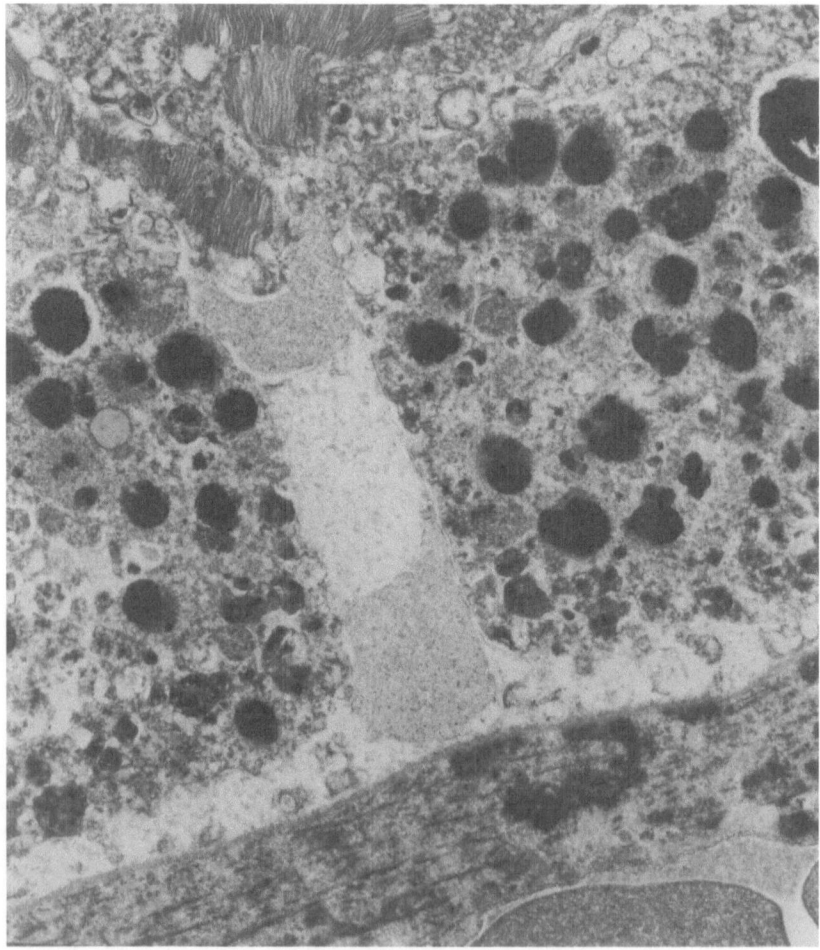

Fig. 3. Coagulative necrosis of retinal pigment epithelium. The cells are shrunken, the cytoplasm appears granular, and the outer segments are disorganized ($\times 13,500$).

14

and the mitochondria appear as lamellar bodies (Fig. 2). On the other hand, in coagulative necrosis, as produced by photocoagulation (Tso 1973), the RPE cells are shrunken, the plasmalemma appears discontinuous, and the cytoplasm becomes dense and granular (Fig. 3). The necrotic cells attract macrophages, which quickly disintegrate and remove the debris.

3) *Decompensation of the RPE cells.* In some pathologic conditions the RPE cells are decompensated, but no necrosis is seen. These decompensated cells have continuous plasmalemma but tend to have dilated endoplasmic reticulum and thus allow passage of tracers such as horseradish peroxidase and sodium fluorescein into the cytoplasm (Fig. 4). These tracers may or may not reach the sub-retinal space through the apex of these cells. Given time, some of these decompensated cells may recover and regain the barrier function.

Such decompensation of cells may be seen in the retinal edema (Tso & Shih 1977) following lens extraction with vitreous loss or in eyes with ocular hypotony secondary to cyclocryotherapy (Tso & Shih 1976).

4) *Disruption of cell junctions.* Disruption of the zonula adherens and zonula occludens of the RPE as an isolated pathologic alteration is uncommon. In most disease conditions, the RPE plasmalemma and cytoplasm appear to be

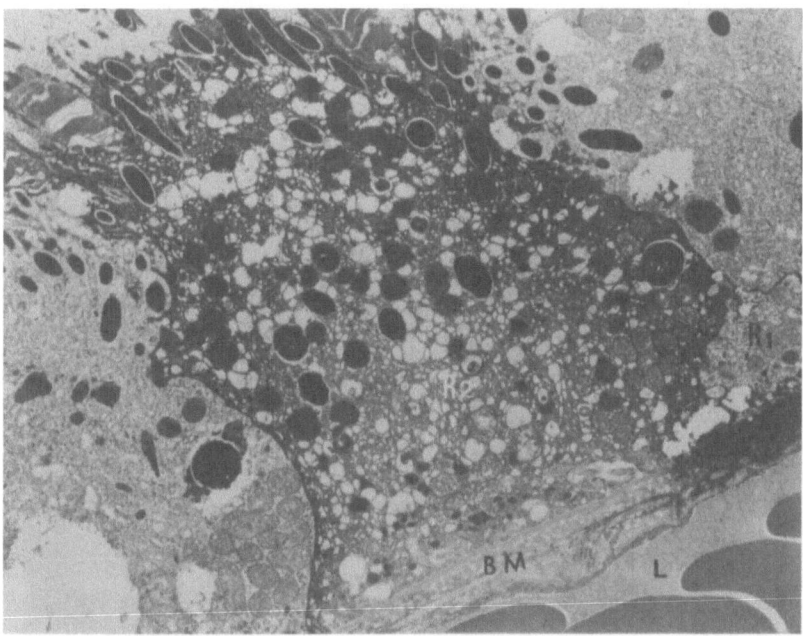

Fig. 4. Decompensation of retinal pigment epithelium in the eye of a rhesus monkey that had ocular hypotony after cryocyclotherapy. Horseradish peroxidase diffusely infiltrates in the cytoplasm of the cell R_2. The neighboring cells (R_1), However, appear to be intact ($\times 12,400$).

more susceptible to injury than the cell junctions. Necrosis of cells is observed without dissolution of the cell junctions. However, in a study of malignant melanoma of choroid associated with papillary proliferation of the RPE (Wallow & Tso 1972), we have observed the dissociation of cell junctions of the RPE cells.

REPAIR OF THE RPE

While RPE cells do not proliferate in a normal state, they have a great capacity for regeneration and proliferation in pathologic states, resulting in re-formation of the blood-retinal barrier and preservation of the closed environment of the sub-retinal space. The reparative processes of the RPE may best be described in four categories.

1) *Simple proliferation and regeneration of RPE.* When a small, localized necrotic RPE lesion is inflicted, macrophages from the bloodstream migrate into the sub-retinal space and remove the necrotic tissue. The normal pigment epithelial cells surrounding the lesion flatten and slide over to reline Bruch's membrane (Fig. 5) (Tso, Wallow, Powell & Zimmerman 1972).

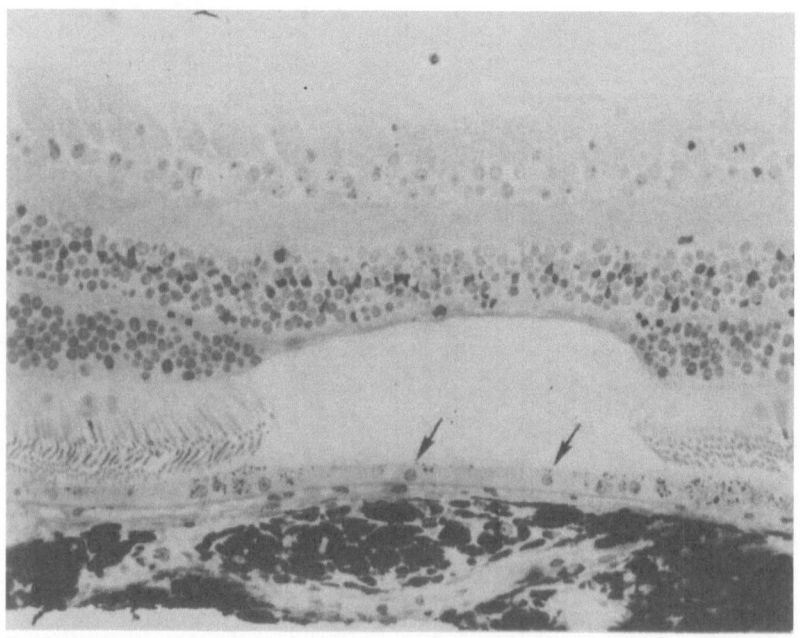

Fig. 5. Simple regeneration of retinal pigment epithelial cells in a photocoagulation lesion of the retina. Regenerated pigment epithelial cells (arrows) proliferate and reline Bruch's membrane. The regenerative cells are amelanotic. The damaged photoreceptor cells have been removed from the sub-retinal space ($\times 245$).

16

Mitotic figures have been observed in the pigment epithelium around these lesions. Zonula occludens and zonula adherens develop between the newly formed RPE cells. Frequently, these cells remain amelanotic and may even appear thin and atrophic, but their function as blood-retinal barrier is re-established.

2) *Placoid proliferation of RPE.* In more severe injury, the reparative proliferation of the pigment epithelium is excessive and many layers of the pigment epithelial cells are formed (Tso 1973; Tso, Fine & Zimmerman 1972). The cells in the innermost layer assume a cuboidal shape and restore a normal relationship with the outer segments of the photoreceptor cells (Fig. 6). The proliferated RPE cells in the other layers assume a spindle shape, produce abundant basement membrane-like material, and form scattered cell junctions. These proliferated RPE cells are frequently described in the literature as 'fibrous metaplasia'. In fact, these cells retain most of their epithelial characteristics. Re-formation of the blood-retinal barrier may be delayed over a prolonged period of time in areas showing placoid proliferation.

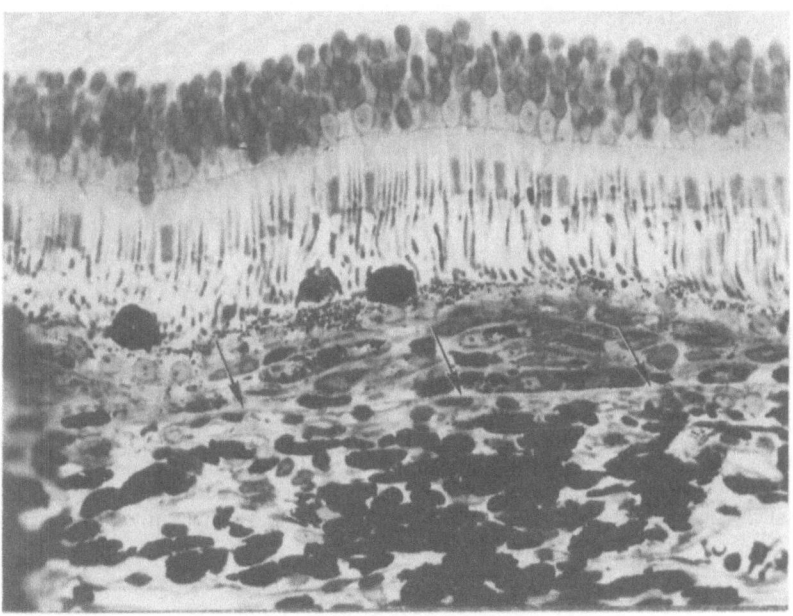

Fig. 6. Placoid proliferation of retinal pigment epithelium of the retina of a rhesus monkey that had been exposed to the light of an indirect ophthalmoscope. Excessive proliferation of retinal pigment epithelial cells form a placoid lesion on Bruch's membrane (arrows). The cells of the inner layer of the plaque assume a cuboidal shape and re-establish a normal relationship with the regenerated outer segments of photoreceptor cells (×350).

3) *Failure of regeneration of pigment epithelium.* In certain diseases, when the RPE lesion is extensive or generalized, the adjacent pigment epithelium fail to proliferate to cover the entire lesion. Mueller cells and glial cells from the overlying retina grow toward Bruch's membrane and form a chorioretinal scar (Wallow & Tso 1973). The blood-retinal barrier may never be re-formed.

4) *Chronic decompensation of the RPE.* In still other diseases, the RPE cells remain chronically decompensated by a persistent generalized disease process, yet they are not necrotic. Without necrosis, proliferation of the adjacent pigment epithelial cells does not take place. Decompensation of these cells may last for many months (Fig. 7), resulting in retinal edema and decompensation of the photoreceptor cells (Tso & Yoneya 1980).

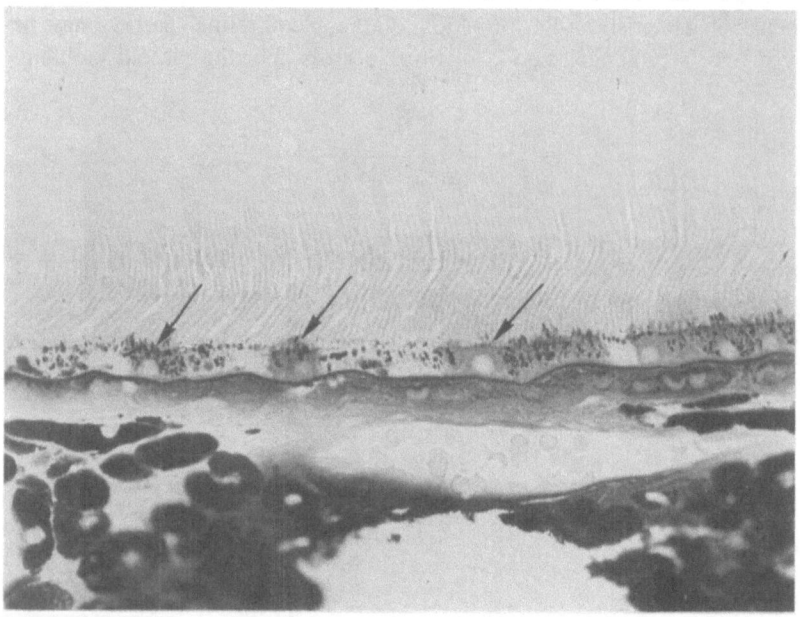

Fig. 7. Chronic decompensation of retinal pigment epithelium in the retina of a rhesus monkey that had been exposed to the light of an indirect ophthalmoscope 18 months prior to enucleation. Scattered retinal pigment epithelial cells (arrows) remain decompensated, and horseradish peroxidase infiltrates into the cytoplasm of these cells (×395).

PATHOLOGIC CHANGES OF THE
EXTERNAL LIMITING MEMBRANE

The sub-retinal space is bounded internally by the external limiting membrane of the retina, which consists of a series of cell junctions of the zonula adherens type, joining adjacent photoreceptor cells and Mueller cells. In various diseases affecting the photoreceptor cells or Mueller cells, the external limiting membrane is disrupted and the sub-retinal space is in direct communication with the interstitial space of the retina. An example of disruption of the external limiting membrane is seen in moderate photocoagulation lesions of the retina (Wallow & Tso 1973). In these lesions, damage is inflicted in the outer layers of retina, resulting in necrosis of photoreceptor cells and some of the cell processes of the Mueller cells, but not the inner nuclear layer, where the nuclei and perikarya of the Mueller cells remain unharmed. The necrotic photoreceptor cells are quickly removed by macrophages, and the remaining Mueller cell processes expand and are joined with the adjacent Mueller cells. A new external limiting membrane is re-formed consisting only of Mueller cell processes without intervening photoreceptor cells (Fig. 8) (Wallow & Tso 1973).

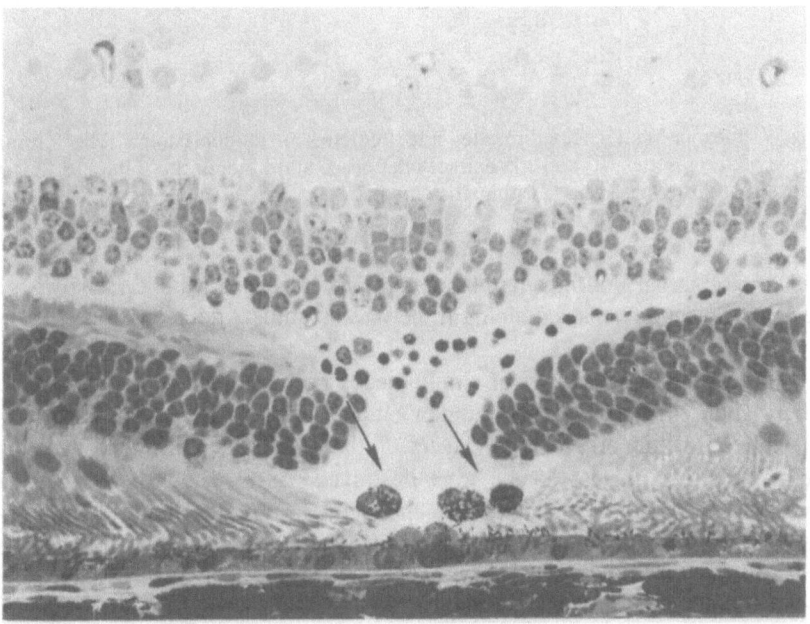

Fig. 8. Re-formation of the external limiting membrane (arrows) in a photocoagulation lesion of a rhesus monkey. The Mueller cell processes expand and re-form an external limiting membrane consisting only of Mueller cells (×350).

Similarly, in retinitis pigmentosa, a gradual but extensive loss of photoreceptor cells takes place, and the environment of the subretinal space is altered drastically. An external limiting membrane, however, frequently persists. As the photoreceptor cells are dropped out, the external limiting membrane is re-formed by Mueller cell processes joining with each other. The

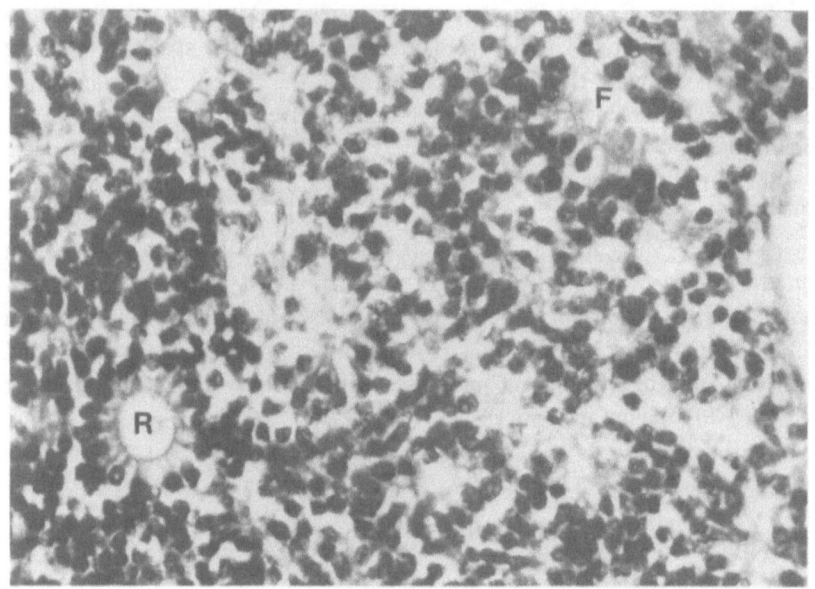

Fig. 9. Flexner-Wintersteiner rosettes and fluorettes in retinoblastoma. The luminal space of the rosettes (R) and the extracellular space surrounding the fluorettes (F) are minature sub-retinal spaces, within the tumor.

resulting external limiting membrane consists largely of Mueller cells with a few photoreceptor cells remaining in between (Santos-Anderson, Tso & Fishman 1980).

In an experimental study of simultaneous occlusion of the central retinal artery and vein in the rhesus monkey (Juarez, Tso, Van Heuven, Hayreh & Hayreh 1978), all of the inner layers of the retina, including the ganglion cells and inner nuclear layers, were destroyed. As a result, the cell bodies and processes of the Mueller cell degenerated. On the other hand, the photoreceptor cells, mainly nourished by the choroidal circulation, survived. As the Mueller cell processes degenerated, the photoreceptor cells joined with each other by zonulae adherentes and an external limiting membrane, consisting entirely of photoreceptor cells, was formed.

In retinal dysplasia, abnormal proliferation of photoreceptor cells takes place, resulting in rosette formation. This creates minature sub-retinal spaces within the retina. These sub-retinal spaces are surrounded by external limiting membrane on all sides.

Similarly, in neoplastic proliferation of retinoblastoma cells, the sub-retinal space may be created within the retina. The lumen of the Flexner-Wintersteiner rosettes (Tso, Fine & Zimmerman 1969) is an example (Fig. 9). The luminal membrane of the rosette consists of a series of zonulae adherentes simulating the external limiting membrane. Within this space, mucopoly-

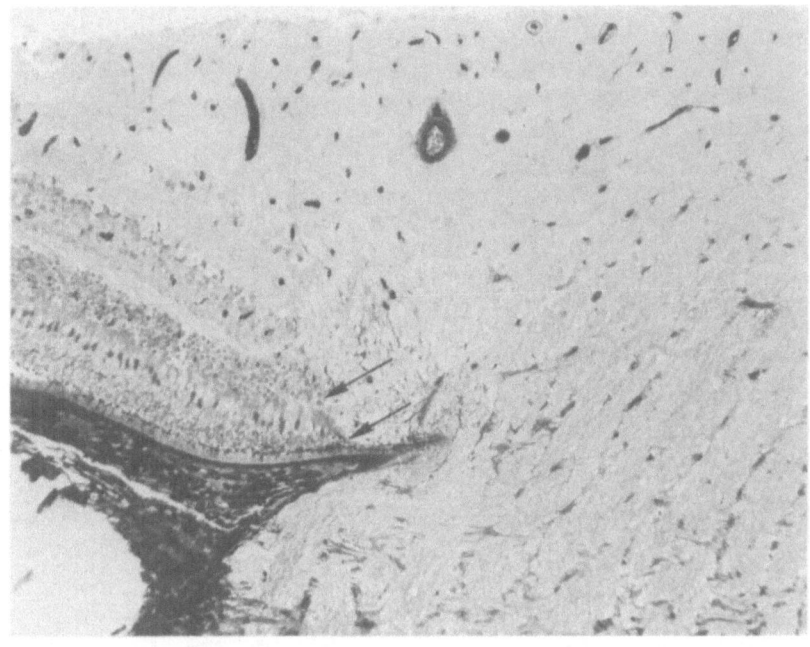

Fig. 10. The optic nervehead of a rhesus monkey with papilledema secondary to raised intracranial pressure. The intermediary tissue of Kuhnt (arrows) is stretched as the peripapillary retina is displaced laterally (×110).

sacchride partially sensitive to hyaluronidase is found. Cell processes resembling inner segments, cilia, and outer segments of photoreceptor cells protrude from the neoplastic cells into the lumen of the rosettes. Similarly, the interstitial space around the fluerettes of retinoblastoma is a minature subretinal space.

PATHOLOGIC CHANGES OF THE
INTERMEDIARY TISSUE OF KUHNT

The sub-retinal space is bounded proximally at the peripapillary region by a series of cell junctions between glial cells that form the intermediary tissue of Kuhnt. In the normal optic nervehead, horseradish peroxidase tracer in the interstitial space of the optic nervehead may not pass through these cell junctions into the subretinal space (Tso, Shih & McLean 1975). However, in papilledema (Tso & Hayreh 1977), axonal swelling at the optic nervehead displaces the peripapillary retina laterally (Figs. 10 and 11), and the tight cell junctions between the glial cells of the intermediary tissue of Kuhnt may be broken. The sub-retinal space may then be open to the interstitial space of

21

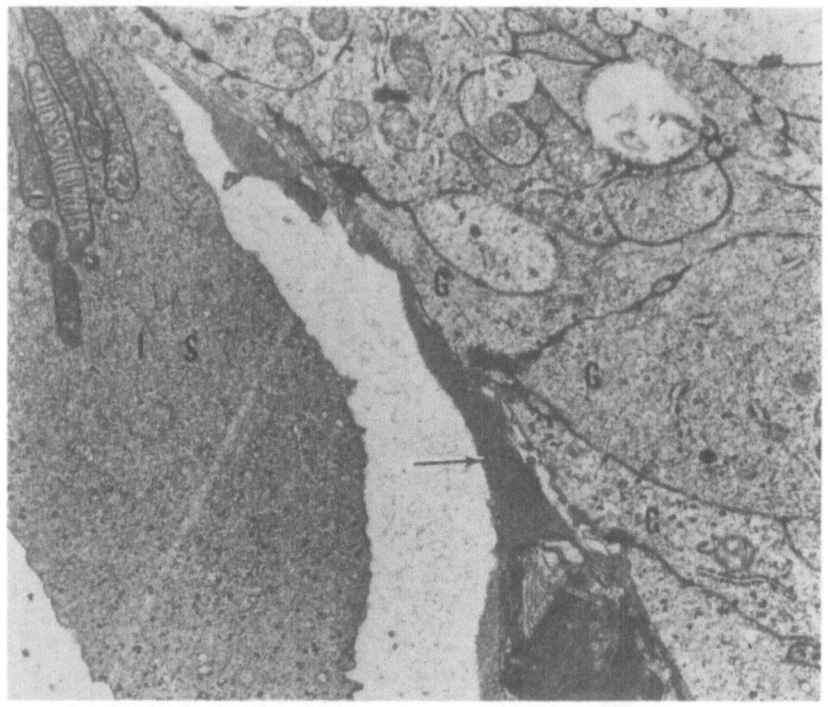

Fig. 11. Disruption of intermediary tissue of Kuhnt in a case of papilledema. Horseradish peroxidase extends from the interstitial space of the optic nerve through the glial cells (G) of the intermediary tissue of Kuhnt into the sub-retinal space (arrow). IS, inner segment of retina (×14,000).

the optic nervehead, and sub-retinal fluid may accumulate in the peripapillary region. As papilledema subsides, the intermediary tissue of Kuhnt may be re-formed.

CONCLUSION

As indicated, the sub-retinal space enjoys a closed environment bounded on all sides by cells or cell junctions. In various pathologic processes, the cell or cell junctions of the boundaries result in cellular damage, necrosis, or disruption of cell junctions. The closed environment of the sub-retinal space is then open to direct communication with the interstitial space of the choroid, retina, or optic nerve. In our pathologic studies, a rapid reparative process is frequently observed, and the closed environment of the sub-retinal space is once again established by the regeneration of the RPE or re-formation of the external limiting membrane or intermediary tissue of Kuhnt. The body apparently realizes the importance of the closed environment of the sub-retinal space. On the other hand, why a closed environment must be maintained in the sub-retinal space remains a puzzle and requires further research.

REFERENCES

Juarez, C.P., M.O.M. Tso, R.A.J. Van Heuven, M.S. Hayreh & S.S. Hayreh. An ultrastructural study of retinal ischemia. Read before the Association for Research in Vision and Ophthalmology annual meeting, Sarasota, Florida (1978).

Pei, Y F. & G.K. Smelser. Some fine structural features of the ora serrata region in primate eyes. Invest. Ophthalmol. 7: 672 (1968).

Santos-Anderson, R., M.O.M. Tso & G. Fishman. A light and electron microscopic study of retinitis pigmentosa. In preparation.

Tornquist, P.A., A. Alm & A. Bill. Studies on ocular blood flow and retinal capillary permeability to sodium in pigs. Physiol. Scand. 1979, in press.

Tso, M.O.M. Photic maculopathy in rhesus monkey: A light and electron microscopic study. Invest. Ophthalmol. 12: 17 (1973).

Tso, M.O.M., B.S. Fine & L.E. Zimmerman. The Flexner-Wintersteiner rosettes in retinoblastoma. Arch. Pathol. 88: 664 (1969).

Tso, M.O.M., B.S. Fine & L.E. Zimmerman. Photic maculopathy produced by indirect ophthalmoscope: A clinical and histopathologic study. Amer. J. Ophthalmol. 73: 686 (1972).

Tso, M.O.M. & S.S. Hayreh. Optic disc edema in raised intracranial pressure. III. A Pathologic study of experimental papilledema. Arch. Ophthalmol. 95: 1448 (1977).

Tso, M.O.M., N. Kaga & S.S. Hayreh. A histopathologic study of occlusion in short posterior ciliary artery. In preparation.

Tso, M.O.M. & C.Y. Shih. Disruption of the blood-retinal barrier in ocular hypotony: A preliminary report. Exp. Eye Res. 23: 209 (1976).

Tso, M.O.M. & C.Y. Shih. Experimental macular edema after lens extraction. Invest. Ophthalmol. 16: 381 (1977).

Tso, M.O.M., C.Y. Shih & I. McLean. Is there a blood-brain barrier at the optic nervehead. Arch. Ophthalmol. 93: 815 (1975).

Tso, M.O.M., I.H.L. Wallow, J.O. Powell & L.E. Zimmerman. Recovery of the rod and cone after photic injury. Trans. Amer. Acad. Ophthalmol. Otolaryngol. 76: 12: 47 (1972).

Tso, M.O.M. & S. Yoneya. The Blood-retinal barrier in photic maculopathy. Read before the Association for Research in Vision and Ophthalmology annual Meeting, Orlando, Florida (1980).

Wallow, I.H.L. & M.O.M. Tso. Proliferation of the retinal pigment epithelium over malignant choroidal tumors: A light and electron microscopic study. Amer J. Ophthalmol. 73: 914 (1972).

Wallow, I.H.L., & M.O.M. Tso. Retinal repair after xenon arc photocoagulation: III. The evaluation of retinal lesions in the rhesus monkey. Amer. J. Ophthalmol. 79: 951 (1973).

Author's Address:
Department of Ophthalmology
University of Illinois
Eye and Ear Infirmary
1855 West Taylor Street
Chicago, IL, 60612
U.S.A.

PROTEINS OF THE BOVINE INTERPHOTORECEPTOR MATRIX

ALICE J. ADLER & KATHERINE M. SEVERIN

(*Boston, MA, U.S.A.*)

ABSTRACT

Soluble material from the interphotoreceptor matrix of adult bovine eyes was isolated by washing of the retina and of the apical pigment epithelium (PE) surface. The macromolecules present in this layer consisted of 98% proteins, 2% glycosaminoglycans and <0.1% nucleic acids. Preliminary characterization of the matrix proteins was performed with respect to their molecular weights, tissues of origin, and ability to augment cellular adhesion. SDS-polyacrylamide gel electrophoresis of dithiothreitol-reduced bovine interphotoreceptor matrix revealed a major Coomassie blue-staining band at 140,000 MW plus several between 20,000 and 65,000 with a prominent protein at 47,000. This pattern was completely different from those of serum, vitreous or pathological human subretinal fluid – even serum albumin was totally absent from the matrix – and from tissue homogenates of retina or PE. However, most of the matrix proteins could be accounted for as products of either the retina or PE, as seen by their resemblance to proteins retrieved from the culture media when bovine retinas or PE cells (obtained by trypsin treatment of the eyecup) were incubated overnight. Subretinal fluid contained none of these product proteins. The principal matrix glycoprotein, as shown by PAS staining of gels, had MW 140,000 and was isolated by means of concanavalin A-Sepharose chromatography. Bovine interphotoreceptor matrix was tested in short-term, slowly rotating suspension cultures containing dissociated PE cells and/or rod outer segments, as a model system for retinal adhesion. Although matrix did not enhance adhesion between PE and outer segments in mixed cultures, PE reaggregation itself appeared to be augmented.

INTRODUCTION

The interphotoreceptor matrix (IPM) is the material normally present in the subretinal space. This extracellular matrix is bounded posteriorly by the pigment epithelium (PE) apical surface and anteriorly by the external limiting membrane. Photoreceptor inner and outer segments project into the matrix but do not fill the space; there are gaps of up to 3 microns between human receptors (Hogan *et al.* 1971). The volume of IPM in a human eye, calculated from electron photomicrographs, is approximately 0.01–0.02 ml. The IPM is not to be confused with subretinal fluid, which is the result of an abnormal condition (retinal detachment), and which can expand the subretinal space to 1–2 ml.

25

The finding of glycosaminoglycans (GAGs, also known as mucopolysac-charides) in the IPM, on the basis of histological examination (Zimmerman & Eastham 1959) stimulated the chemical fractionation and characterization (Berman & Bach 1968; Bach & Berman 1971a, b) of these matrix compo-nents. However, no attention has been devoted to other constituents of the matrix, including the proteins, although analysis shows that there is about 50 times more protein present (by weight) than GAG. Therefore, this study was undertaken to begin to examine the proteins of the IPM, employing bovine eyes as a readily available source. One specific goal was to investigate which tissues are responsible for synthesis of the matrix proteins. Another aim was to compare these proteins with the ones found in pathological human sub-retinal fluid, in order to probe the physiological state of retina and PE during retinal detachment.

Recent studies have shown that some cell surface glycoproteins are responsible for specific cell adhesion processes, and can be shed into extra-cellular media. Examples are fibronectin in fibroblasts and some other cells (Yamada & Olden 1978), and retina-specific adhesion protein(s) in embryonic chick retina (Hausman & Moscona 1975; Rutishauser et al. 1976). Therefore, we wished to see whether any proteins in the IPM might play a role in maintaining adhesion between the retina and PE. For this purpose interpho-toreceptor matrix was tested in a model cell aggregation assay system con-taining isolated PE cells and receptor outer segments.

MATERIALS AND METHODS

Tissue preparations. Adult bovine eyes were brought on ice from a local meat dealer, and used within 3 hours of death:

Interphotoreceptor matrix, defined as the soluble material between the retina and PE, was isolated by a modification of the Berman and Bach (1968) method: Eyes were cut 2 mm posterior to the ora serrata. The vitreous was removed carefully, without causing a retinal or choroidal detachment. Final traces of vitreous were removed by washing the retinal surface with 0.9% NaCl and 5 mM sodium phosphate, pH 7.4 (PBS). Retinas were excised, pooled in PBS (2 ml/eye), slowly stirred at 4 degrees, and filtered through plastic mesh (0.8 mm pore size). The filtrate was saved, and the stirring procedure was repeated on the residual retinas. The anterior (apical) surface of the PE, still in the eyecup, was extracted by rinsing with PBS (1–2 ml/eye). This wash was added to the retina filtrate, and clarified by centrifuga-tion (1 hr. at 27000 xg). (PE cells were not brushed out of the eyecup before washing because of possible leakage of the basal PE surface; Saari et al. 1977.) Yield was about 8 mg IPM protein per eye.

Pigment epithelium (PE) cells were prepared by trypsin treatment of the rinsed eyecup (Edwards 1977 and private communication), not by a brush-ing-out procedure. Best results were obtained with 0.12% Difco trypsin for

1.5–2 hours at 37 degrees under sterile conditions with slow shaking. Cell count after washing was 1–2×10^6 cells/eye, 80% viability, no visible contamination except for occasional free pigment granules.

Conditioned culture media, containing products synthesized by PE cells or retina, were obtained by incubating these tissues, separately, in F-10 (Ham) medium (Gibco) containing 0.5% glucose, antibiotics, and 5% CO_2 gas. No serum was added. Rotating suspension culture conditions (Moscona 1961) were employed, swirling 60 rpm at 37 degrees for 18 hours. Occasionally radioactive precursors (30 μCi/ml tritiated leucine or glucosamine) were added. The incubation supernatants remaining after centrifugation (to remove tissue) are referred to as PI in the case of cultured PE, and RI for retina.

Crude photoreceptor *outer segments* (OS) were prepared from beef retinas by the method of Chader *et al.* (1974) with minor modifications. Density gradients were not used and solutions were kept sterile.

Subretinal fluid (SRF) samples were obtained from Dr. Tatsuo Hirose shortly after he performed retina re-attachment surgery with scleral buckling. Sample 1 was from a detachment of 1 week duration and contained 10 mg/ml protein; sample 2 was of 6 months duration, 17 mg/ml protein. Neither sample contained significant blood serum contamination; the number of red blood cells counted in each sample was used to calculate the concentration of serum protein, which accounted for <1% of the total protein in each case.

Soluble preparations (IPM, SRF, PI, RI, serum) were often concentrated (usually 10-fold) by passage through B-15 macrosolute concentrators (Amicon).

Chemical assays. Protein concentration was determined by the method of Lowry *et al.* (1951); DNA by diphenylamine (Burton 1956).

Sugar analyses were conducted colorimetrically: Neutral sugars by the anthrone method (Roe 1955), modified to do assays in the 2–200 μg range, and corrected for tryptophan interference of the protein. Amino sugars by the Elson-Morgan reaction (Mazlen *et al.* 1970) after the hydrolysate was run through a cation exchange column to remove neutral sugar. Uronic acids by the carbazole assay (Bitter & Muir 1962) 1–50 μg range. The extinction coefficients of Berman & Bach (1968) were employed to correct for interference among types of sugar.

Fractionation procedures. All chromatographic fractionations of IPM employed about 200 mg of matrix protein and a column bed 0.9 cm diameter by 25 cm high. Flow rate was 2 ml/min, fraction size about 1 ml.

For concanavalin A-Sepharose fractionation, the sample was introduced in 10 mM tris, pH $7.0 + 0.14$ M NaCl: the run-off peak was coded as CA. The column was then eluted with 50 mM α-methyl-D-mannoside in the same buffer, and the pooled fractions eluted with the sugar were called CB.

When a diethylaminoethyl-Sephadex column was used, the initial solvent was 5 mM tris, pH 7.0 (wash-out fraction DA). When the column was then subjected to a linear salt gradient (0–1 M NaCl in 5 mM tris) two peaks were obtained: DB (at 0.15 M NaCl) and DC (at 0.35 M).

For sulfopropyl-Sephadex fractionation, the IPM was introduced in 20 mM sodium citrate, pH 5.4. The run-off peak was called SA. (The remainder of the protein, SB, was retrieved in 50 mM sodium phosphate, pH 8.1 + 2 M NaCl.) The SA fraction, containing proteoglycans, was freed of nucleic acids by treatment with 10% trichloroacetic acid, dialyzed against water, lyophilized and purified by precipitation with 5 volumes of ethanol.

Polyacrylamide gel electrophoresis. SDS (1%) gel electrophoresis was carried out in polyacrylamide (5%) tube gels (0.5 × 13 cm) by the method of Fairbanks *et al.* (1971). Samples were prepared in 20 mM tris, pH 7.0 + 2 mM EDTA + 50 mM dithiothreitol, and heated (100 degrees for 5 min) prior to electrophoresis. Gels were stained either for protein (Coomassie blue stain, Fairbanks *et al.* 1971) or for carbohydrate (PAS method, Glossmann and Neville 1971). Radioactive gels were frozen, sliced (1.6 mm thickness), solubilized in 30% H_2O_2, and counted in Aquasol.

Disc gels (Davis 1964) were run in the same equipment at pH 8.6 without SDS.

Cell aggregation studies. PE cells were suspended in MEM medium (no Ca^{+2}) and set in spinner culture (Brackenbury *et al.* 1977) for 17 hours at about 225 rpm (stir bar speed) at 37 degrees. The cells (6×10^6 per culture, mainly single cells) were resuspended in 3 ml F-10 medium containing antibiotics and 10% sucrose. For different experiments the assay mixture also contained receptor outer segments (3×10^7) and/or IPM protein (3 mg). The flasks were set up as rotary suspension cultures (Moscona 1961) at 60 rpm, 37 degrees, for 0.5 to 20 hours. Cultures were examined periodically by phase contrast microscopy.

RESULTS

Interphotoreceptor proteins matrix: molecular weights. When a mixture of proteins is subjected to gel electrophoresis in the presence of SDS, each protein migrates solely according to its molecular weight. Fig. 1a shows the molecular weight distribution of proteins in the IPM, which has bands at 140,000 and several between 20,000 and 65,000 with a prominent protein at 47,000. Collagen and fibronectin were not present. Gels from homogenates of neighboring tissues are presented for comparison. The matrix is seen to have no bands in common with retina or PE homogenates. However, several proteins, including the 47,000 band, are shared by IPM and PI (the incubation medium from cultured PE cells). Most of the other IPM proteins (except for the 140,000 band) are found in RI (not shown), the comparable conditioned medium from retina. The gel results are listed in Table 1.

28

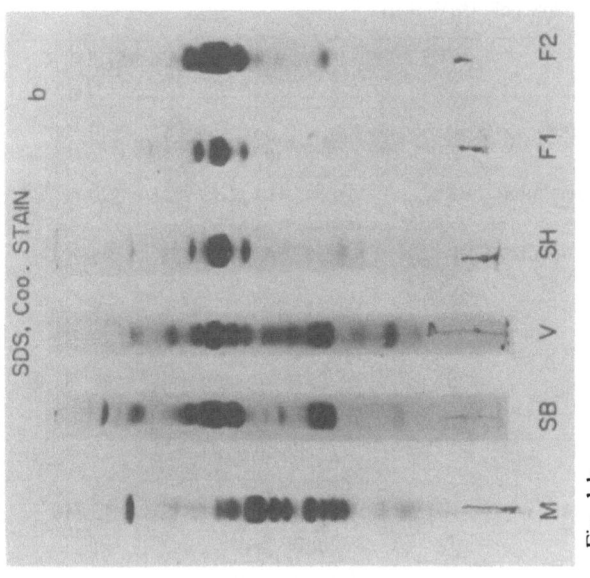

Fig. 1.a.

Fig. 1.b.

Fig. 1. Polyacrylamide gel electrophoresis in the presence of SDS and DTT. Gels stained for protein with Coomassie blue. Direction of migration is from top to bottom; O is origin, TD is position of tracking dye.

(a) M = bovine interphotoreceptor matrix, PI = culture medium after overnight incubation of bovine pigment epithelium cells in suspension culture, PE = homogenate of bovine pigment epithelium cells, R = homogenate of bovine retina, OS = homogenate of bovine photoreceptor outer segments, ST = protein standards (bovine serum albumin, MW 68,000; bovine gamma-globulin subunits 52,000 and 23,000; ovalbumin 43,000; cytochrome c, 12,000), CB = concanavalin A-binding glycoprotein fraction of IPM.

(b) SB = bovine serum, V = bovine vitreous, SH = human serum, F1 = human subretinal fluid (sample 1, duration of detachment 1 week), F2 = subretinal fluid (sample 2, 6 months).

29

Table 1. Major proteins on SDS gels ($MW \times 10^{-3}$)

Tissue or fraction [a]	Code	Coomassie blue stain	PAS stain
interphotoreceptor matrix, IPM	M	140, 90, 64, 55, 47, 41, 38, 29, 27, 24, 21	140, 90
culture medium after retina incubation	RI	90, 55, 41, 37, 29, 27, 24, 21	90
culture medium after PE incubation	PI	47, 38, 34, 27, 15-12	47, 12
retina homogenate	R	25, 11, 8	12
PE homogenate	PE	51, 40, 35, 19, 11, 8	12
photoreceptor outer segments	OS	55, 35	37, 8
vitreous	V	SB+100, 60, 14	
serum: bovine and human	SB, SH	150, 80, 67, 51, 40, 23	43, 40
subretinal fluid: samples 1 and 2	F1, F2	80, 67, 51, 23	43, 40
IPM, not reduced with DTT	MO.	M minus 64	
IPM fractions:	CA	M minus 140	
Con A [b] eluted with buffer	CB	140	140
eluted with mannoside			
DEAE [c] eluted with 0.15 M NaCl	DB	55, 20	
SP [d] purified GAG fraction	SA	160, 70, 25	
incubated [e] precipitate	MP	140, 47	140, 90, 8
supernatant	MS	M	

[a] All samples are bovine except for SH, F1 and F2 (human).
[b] Fractionated on concanavalin A-Sepharose column.
[c] Diethylaminoethyl-Sephadex column.
[d] Fractionated on sulfopropyl-Sephadex column, followed by purification of glycosaminoglycan or proteoglycan fraction (from dilute buffer elution) by trichloroacetic acid treatment and ethanol precipitation.
[e] Incubated overnight in rotary suspension culture.

Comparison to serum and subretinal fluid. The molecular weight distribution of IPM proteins is compared to that of sera, vitreous and subretinal fluid samples in Fig. 1b. No serum proteins, not even albumin (MW 68,000) appear in the matrix. (This was true even for gels purposely overloaded with protein and overexposed photographically to reveal trace bands.) Bovine vitreous includes all the serum proteins plus a few tissue-specific ones (at 100, 60, and 14×10^3).

Two typical subretinal fluid samples are shown (F1 and F2). They are comprised completely of serum proteins, with prominent bands at the positions of transferrin (MW 80,000), serum albumin and gamma-globulin subunits; no IPM proteins are present. Furthermore, the subretinal fluid sam-

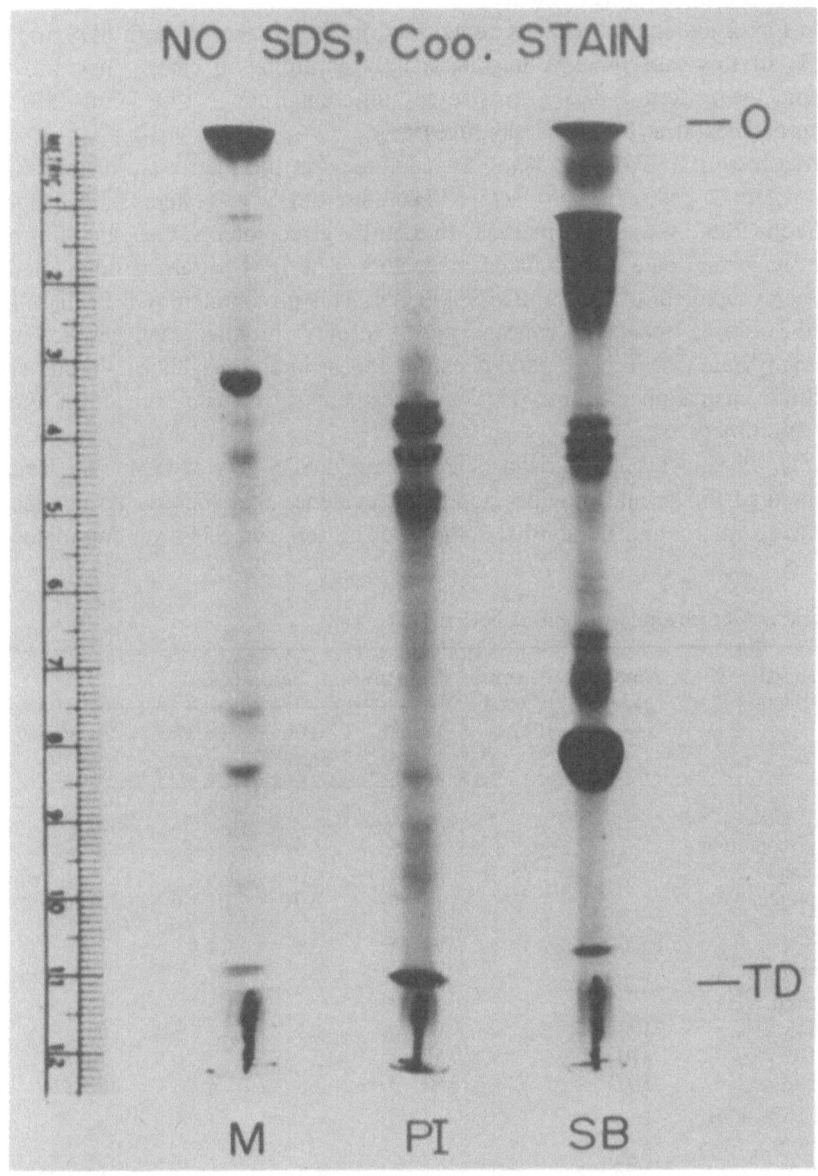

Fig. 2. Disc gel electrophoresis in the absence of SDS. Coomassie blue stain. Code letters as defined in Fig. 1.

ples do not contain proteins from PE or retina cells (PE and R) or proteins synthesized by them (PI and RI).

In Fig. 2 are shown gels electrophoresed in the absence of both SDS and DTT. In this case proteins migrate mainly according to charge, not size. Again, the pattern of IPM (M) is totally different from that of serum (SB). (The dark band at 8.1 cm is albumin.)

Glycoproteins in IPM and tissues. Glycoproteins in the matrix are of interest as potential cell adhesion factors. Therefore, SDS gels were stained for carbohydrate by the PAS method, to identify glycoproteins. Gels are shown in Fig. 3, and data are tabulated in Table 1. The IPM pattern is dominated by a glycoprotein of apparent MW 140,000. This glycoprotein (CB in Figs. 1 and 3) can be isolated by concanavalin A affinity chromatography, is rich in carbohydrate (See Table 2), and does not appear in any neighboring tissue or culture incubation medium. The outer segment gel contains rhodopsin and its multimers.

Fig. 3b shows a comparison of PAS-stained SDS gels of IPM, sera, and subretinal fluids, and provides additional evidence that there is no overlap between matrix and these other samples. (The sera and SRFs are dominated

Table 2. Carbohydrate content of bovine IPM

Material or fraction	Amount (μg/eye)	Percent of total IPM	Composition: Percentage of			
			Protein	Neutral sugar	Amino sugar	Uronic acid
Typical glycoprotein			85-95	3–10	2–8	0
Typical proteoglycan			10–20	2–10	15–40	15–40
IPM	8300		93	2.8	2.6	1.0
IPM fractions from DEAE:						
DA [a]	7100		97	1.3		0.4
DB	410	5	82	12		1.0
DC	580	7	80	2.8	6	8.1
IPM fractions from Con A:						
CA	7500		95	1.8		1.1
CB	220	2.7	74	16	9	0.4
IPM fraction from SP:						
SA (purified GAG)	180	2.2	17	8	36	33

[a] Abbreviations and code letters are the same as in Table 1. In addition, DA = fraction eluted from DEAE-Sephadex in dilute buffer; DC = fraction eluted at 0.35 *M* NaCl.

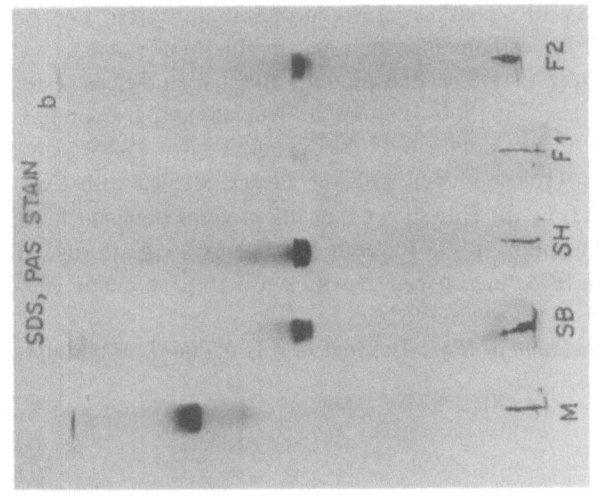

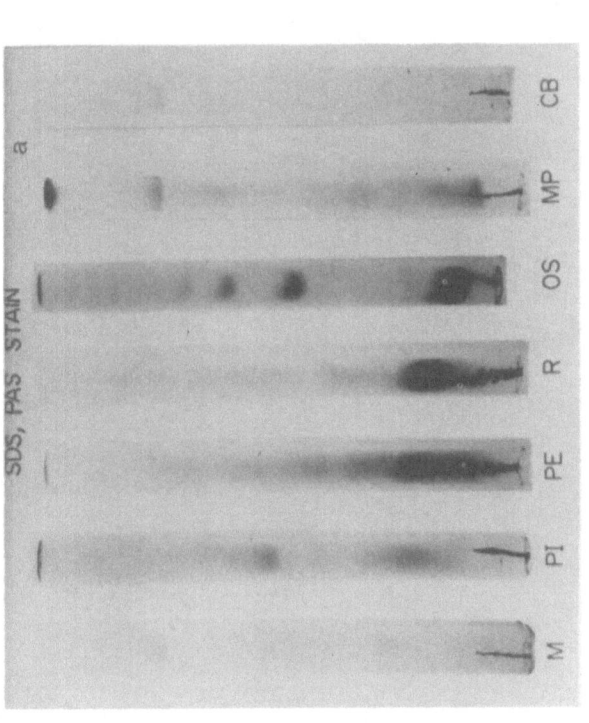

Fig. 3. Gel electrophoresis in the presence of SDS. Gels stained for carbohydrate with periodic acid-Schiff reagent (PAS). Molecular weight scale is the same as in Fig. 1. Code letters as defined in Fig. 1. In addition, MP = material precipitating from solution upon overnight incubation of IPM at 37 degrees.

by bands at 40 and 43×10^3, possibly orosomucoid, α-antitrypsin and/or haptoglobin β-chain; all are carbohydrate-rich and in this MW range.)

Fig. 4 shows the pattern of radioactive proteins in PI after PE cells are cultured with labelled precursors. Both the protein (leucine) and glycoprotein (glucosamine) profiles are dominated by bands at 45–49 and 12–14×10^3 MW, which correspond well with the PI gels stained with Coomassie (Fig. 1) and PAS (Fig. 3). This shows that the proteins obtained from the conditioned culture medium (PI) of PE cells, which correspond to several of the bands found in IPM, are indeed newly synthesized proteins (not degradation products).

Composition and fractionation of IPM. The matrix was fractionated chroma-

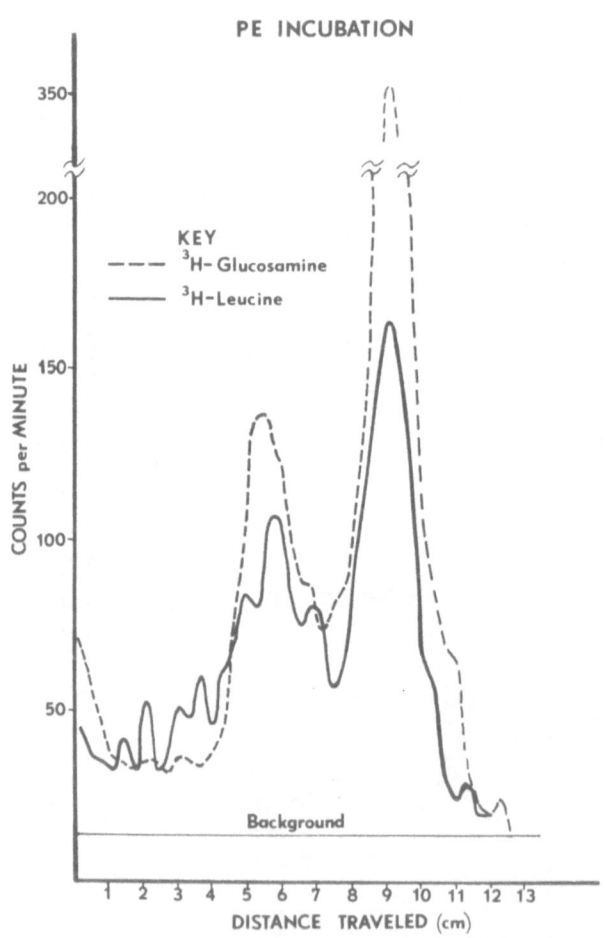

Fig. 4. SDS polyacrylamide gel electrophoretic pattern of labelled proteins in PI. PE cells were incubated overnight in suspension culture in the presence of 90 μCi of tritiated glucosamine or leucine. The conditioned culture medium (PI) was electrophoresed, and 1.6-mm gel slices were solubilized and counted.

tographically by several methods, and carbohydrate composition was assayed to yield information on glycoprotein components.

Unfractionated IPM and the small proteoglycan (or GAG) component from IPM yielded compositional data (Table 2) that agree well with Berman and Bach (1968). The proteoglycan fraction is seen to comprise only about 2% of the macromolecular components of the matrix. DNA accounts for less than another 0.1%. The remainder consists of proteins, some of which are glycoproteins. The average sugar (neutral plus amino) content of the protein is about 4%.

IPM was fractionated on DEAE-Sephadex in order to isolate glycoproteins which, because of their increased negative charge, would be expected to be eluted at higher salt concentration (in a gradient) than would the bulk of the proteins (fraction DA). Berman & Bach (1968) had previously used this chromatographic method to isolate GAGs from IPM, but discarded the protein and glycoprotein fractions. Peak DB, eluting at 0.15 M NaCl, is enriched in neutral sugar, showing the presence of glycoprotein, and will be examined further. Fraction DC (0.35 M salt) appears to be largely proteoglycan.

Concanavalin A is a lectin which specifically binds mannose. Affinity chromatography of IPM on con A-Sepharose resulted in a small fraction (CB) which bound to con A and is very rich in carbohydrate. This fraction appears to be a pure glycoprotein of MW 140,000 (Figs. 1 and 3).

Aggregation studies. Bovine PE cells were obtained by trypsin treatment and were allowed to replenish their cell surface as single cells in spinner culture (Brackenbury *et al.* 1977). They were then put into rotary suspension culture (Moscona 1961), where they aggregated rapidly, as shown in Fig. 5. The clumps formed by 20 hours can be several mm in diameter (Fig. 5d).

Photoreceptor outer segments (OS) exhibit no tendency to interact with each other (Fig. 6a) or with PE cells (not shown) in rotary culture, even after 18 hours. We were interested in testing interphotoreceptor matrix in such an aggregation assay, as a model to see whether IPM would aid (or hinder) PE-OS interaction in retinal adhesion.

When IPM alone was incubated under rotary culture conditions, strands and clumps of material (MP fraction) precipitated out of solution (Fig. 6b). (Upon SDS electrophoresis, Table 1, this fraction exhibited the major proteins of IPM.) When IPM was added to the culture medium with PE cells, the cells aggregated, at somewhat faster than their normal rate, selectively onto the precipitated material (not shown). OS did not interact with matrix.

When PE cells, outer segments and IPM were all cultured together, the aggregated PE cells adhered to the matrix precipitate (Fig. 6c), but the OS were not selectively included into the aggregate. This is shown more clearly in Fig. 6d, the edge of a large PE-IPM clump, where the outer segments are seen free, in solution, with no tendency to adhere to PE cells.

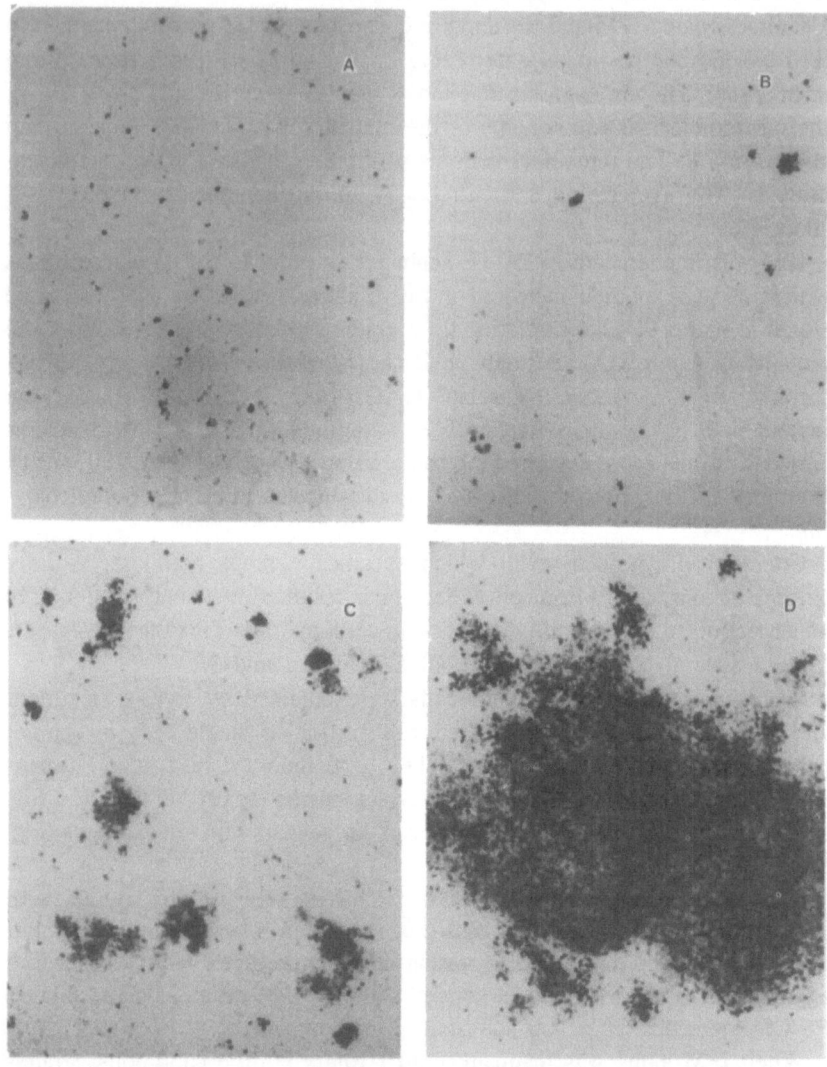

Fig. 5. Aggregation of bovine pigment epithelium cells in rotary suspension culture.
(a) Time = 0 (cells taken directly out of spinner culture).
(b) Time = 0.5 hour.
(c) Time = 3 hours.
(d) Time = 20 hours.
Original magnifications ×50.

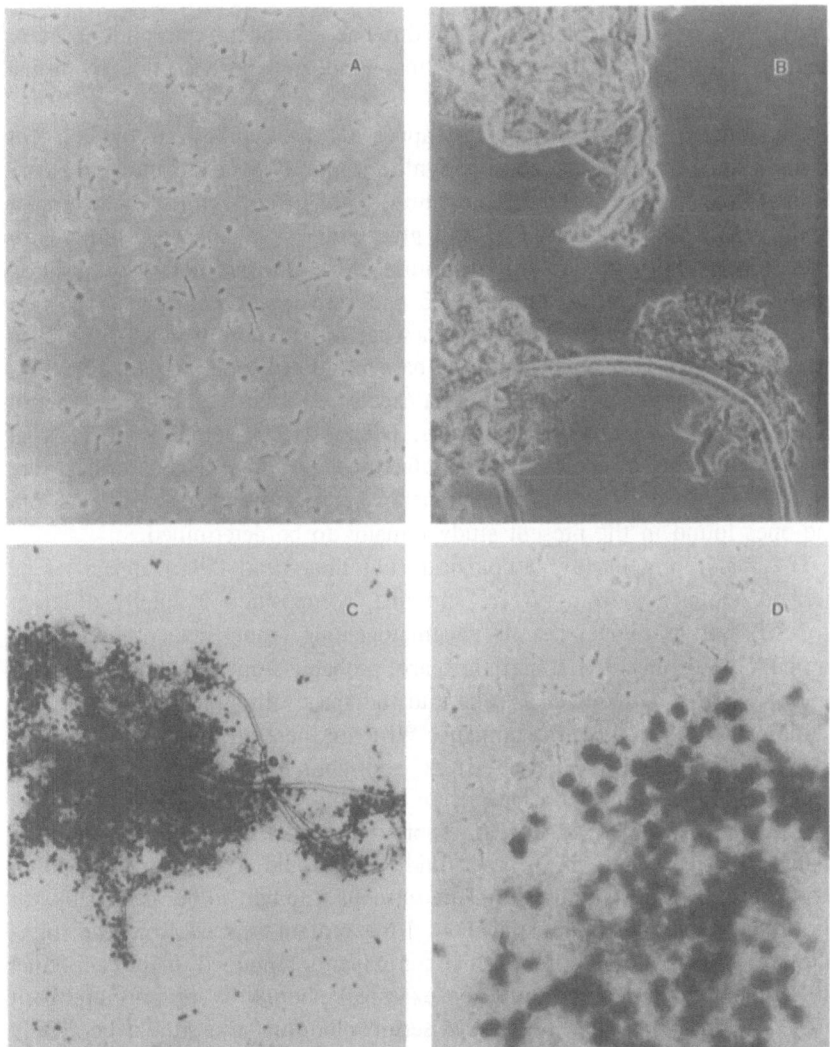

Fig. 6. Effect of bovine interphotoreceptor matrix (IPM) upon aggregation of PE cells and photoreceptor outer segments. All preparations were incubated in rotary suspension culture for 3 hours.

(a) outer segments (OS) alone.

(b) IPM alone. Note strands and clumps of precipitated material.

(c) PE cells, OS and IPM taken together. (OS are out of focus.)

(d) same mixed culture as in (c), showing edge of a large PE-IPM aggregate. Phase contrast microscopy.

Magnifications ×200, except ×50 for (c).

37

DISCUSSION

The data in this report help to clarify three aspects of the interphotoreceptor matrix: its origins, relation to subretinal fluid, and possible role in retinal adhesion.

The proteins found in the IPM appear to be synthesized by adjacent tissues; some are products actively synthesized and given off into the extracellular space by the pigment epithelium, most by the retina. Of the major IPM proteins, only the 140,000 MW glycoprotein remains unaccounted for with respect to origin. The proteins found in the IPM are not decomposition products, released from damaged PE and retina, nor do they arise from serum infusion. This situation is somewhat different from that of the IPM glycosaminoglycans, which appear to be synthesized totally by the PE (Berman 1964; Edwards 1978), with retina capable of producing a different set of GAGs (Morris *et al.* 1977). However, Feeney (1973) found that cell coat fucose-containing glycoproteins, manufactured by both PE and retina, were then shed into the IPM. The relationship between those glycoproteins and the ones found in the present study remains to be determined.

The major proteins of pathological subretinal fluid (SRF) appear to be derived completely from serum, and SRF composition is totally different from IPM. It is known that in rhegmatogenous retinal detachment serum proteins diffuse into the subretinal space, probably from the choroidal circulation, and that vitreous also leaks into the space (through the break in the retina). However, a dilemma remains: Why are there no traces of matrix (for example 47,000 MW) and tissue-specific vitreous (e.g., 100,000) proteins in subretinal fluid? Consider a fairly large detachment involving half the retinal surface, and accompanied by 1 ml subretinal fluid. As part of the approximately 10 mg of protein in the fluid, one would expect to find about 0.5–1 mg protein originating from the vitreous (thought to be responsible for the initial subretinal fluid) and about 1 mg protein washed from the interphotoreceptor matrix. If these initial components remained in the subretinal fluid, the 47,000 IPM protein (for example) should be present at about 0.05–0.1 times the concentration of serum albumin, and should be clearly visible on SDS gels of subretinal fluid (SRF). However, neither this band nor the less prominent IPM and tissue-specific vitreous proteins are present in SRF. Perhaps there exists a dynamic equilibrium during a retinal detachment, such that serum proteins are constantly diffusing into the SRF, and all components are able to diffuse out.

Another finding relevant to the state of the adjacent tissues in retinal detachment, is the absence of proteins synthesized and secreted by pigment epithelium (PI) or retina (RI) in the SRF. This may be an indication that these tissues are not metabolically active during a detachment. On the other hand, neither are the PE and retina cells decaying, as shown by the lack of cell homogenate proteins (PE and R) in the SRF; there is no tissue leakage. This evidence of intact cell structure confirms Berman's (this conference) finding that the retinol-binding protein occurring in SRF arises only from serum, not from injured PE cells.

The cell aggregation studies reported here provide no evidence that any component of the interphotoreceptor matrix is involved in maintenance of retinal adhesion, either as a viscous GAG glue (Zauberman et al. 1972) or as a specific glycoprotein recognition factor (Hausman and Moscona 1975). Several reasons may be considered for this negative result: Perhaps interaction between isolated PE cells and outer segments is too simplified a model for retina – PE attachment. Perhaps, if specific recognition glycoproteins exist in this system, they do so only in the embryonic developmental stage (Moscona 1962), or maybe such proteins remain on those cell surfaces in close apposition (outer segment tips and PE apical villi) and are never released into the bulk IPM. Finally, it is possible that cell-membrane metabolic fluid pumps will be found to be solely responsible for retinal adhesion, without the necessity of involving more specific mechanisms.

ACKNOWLEDGMENT

This work was supported, in part, by Research to Prevent Blindness and an Academic Investigator Award (1-K07-EY-00134) from the National Eye Institute to A. J. A.

REFERENCES

Bach, G. & E. R. Berman. Amino sugar-containing compounds of the retina. I. Isolation and identification. Biochim. Biophys. Acta 252: 453-461 (1971a).

Bach, G. & E. R. Berman. Amino sugar-containing compounds of the retina II. Structural studies. Biochim. Biophys. Acta 252: 461-471 (1971b).

Berman, E. R. The biosynthesis of mucopolysaccharides and glycoproteins in pigment epithelial cells of bovine retina. Biochim. Biophys. Acta 83: 371-373 (1964).

Berman, E. R. & G. Bach. The acid mucopolysaccharides of cattle retina. Biochem. J. 108: 75-88 (1968).

Bitter, T. & H. M. Muir. A modified uronic acid carbazole reaction. Analyt. Biochem. 4: 330-334 (1962).

Brackenbury, R., J.-P. Thiery, U. Rutishauser & G. M. Edelman. Adhesion among neural cells of the chick embryo. I. An immunological assay for molecules involved in cell-cell binding. J. Biol. Chem. 252: 6835-6840 (1977).

Burton, K. A study of the conditions and mechanism of the diphenylamine reaction for the colorimetric estimation of DNA. Biochem. J. 62: 315-323 (1956).

Chader, G., M. Johnson, R. Fletcher & R. Bensinger. Cyclic nucleotide phosphodiesterase of the bovine retina. J. Neurochem. 22: 93-99 (1974).

Davis, B. J. Disc electrophoresis. II. Method and application to human serum proteins. Annals N.Y. Acad. Sci. 121: 404-427 (1964).

Edwards, R. B. Culture of rat retinal pigment epithelium In Vitro. 13: 301-304 (1977).

Edwards, R. B. Synthesis of glycosaminoglycans by cultured human retinal pigment epithelium. Invest. Ophthalmol. (ARVO supplement) 17: 124 (1978).

Fairbanks, G., T.L. Steck & D.F.H. Wallach. Electrophoretic analysis of the major polypeptides of the human erythrocyte membrane. Biochem. 10: 2606-2617 (1971).

Feeney, L. Synthesis of interphotoreceptor matrix. I. Autoradiography of ^{3}H-fucose incorporation. Invest. Ophthalmol. 12: 739-751 (1973).

Glossmann, H. & D.M. Neville. Glycoproteins of cell surfaces. J. Biol. Chem. 246: 6339-6346 (1971).

Hausman, R.E. &·A.A. Moscona. Purification and characterization of the retina-specific cell-aggregating factor. Proc. Nat. Acad. Sci U.S.A. 72: 916-920 (1975).

Hogan, M.J., J.A. Alvarado & J.E. Weddell. 'Histology of the Human Eye', W.B. Saunders Co., Phila., pp. 404-409 (1971).

Lowry, O.H., N.J. Rosebrough, A.L. Farr & R.J. Randall. Protein measurement with the Folin phenol reagent. J. Biol Chem 193: 265-275 (1951).

Mazlen, R.G., C.G. Muellenberg & P.J. O'Brien. L-glutamine D-fructose-6-phosphate amidotransferase from bovine retina. Exptl. Eye Res. 9: 1-11 (1970).

Morris, J.E., J.J. Hopwood & A. Dorfman. Biosynthesis of glycosaminoglycans in the developing retina. Devel. Biol. 58: 313-327 (1977).

Moscona, A.A. Rotation-mediated histogenic aggregation of dissociated cells. Exptl. Cell Res. 22: 455-475 (1961).

Moscona, A.A. Analysis of cell recombinations in experimental synthesis of tissues *in vitro*. J. Cell Comp. Physiol. 60 (suppl. 1): 65-80 (1962).

Roe, J H. The determination of sugar in blood and spinal fluid with anthrone reagent. J. Biol. Chem. 212: 335-343 (1955).

Rutishauser, U., J.-P. Thiery, R. Brackenbury, B.-A. Sela & G.M. Edelman. Mechanisms of adhesion among cells from neural tissues of the chick embryo. Proc. Nat. Acad. Sci U.S.A. 73: 577-581 (1976).

Saari, J.C., A.H. Bunt, S. Futterman & E.R. Berman. Localization of cellular retinol-binding protein in bovine retina and retinal pigment epithelium, with a consideration of the pigment epithelium isolation technique. Invest. Ophthalmol. 16: 797-806 (1977).

Yamada, K.M. & K. Olden. Fibronectins – adhesive glycoproteins of cell surface and blood. Nature 275: 179-184 (1978).

Zauberman, H., H. de Guillebon & F.J. Holly. Retinal traction in vitro. Invest. Ophthalmol. 11: 46-55 (1972).

Zimmerman, L.E. & A.B. Eastham. Acid mucopolysaccharide in the retinal pigment epithelium and visual cell layer of the developing mouse eye. Amer. J. Ophthalmol. 47: 488-498 (1959).

Authors' address:
Eye Research Institute of Retina Foundation
20 Staniford St.
Boston, MA 02114
U.S.A.

PIGMENT EPITHELIUM, RETINA JUNCTION AND PHOTORECEPTOR DISTRIBUTION IN MAN AND IN THE HORSE
Histological, ultrastructural and electrophysiological study

J. FRANÇOIS, V. VICTORIA-TRONCOSO, A. DE ROUCK,
L. WOUTERS & A. VAN GERVEN
(*Ghent, Belgium*)

ABSTRACT

Although there is both a morphological resemblance of the photoreceptors and an electroretinographic similarity, in man and in the horse, in the latter there is no proper macula. Moreover, over the whole of the retina of the horse, the rods predominate over the cones.

INTRODUCTION

To our knowledge, the distribution of the photoreceptors and the junction between the retinal pigment epithelium and the external segment of the photoreceptors, which is essential for the perception of light stimuli, are unknown in horses. The objective of this research is three-fold:

1. A morphological study of the junction zone between the pigment epithelium and the photoreceptors.
2. A morphometric study of the distribution of the cones and rods in the several topographical regions of the retina of the horse and its comparison with that of man.
3. A study of the relation between the distribution of the photoreceptors and the electrophysiological response.

EQUIPMENT AND METHODS

Electrophysiological technique

We examined horses of ages from two to four years. After premedication with promazine (Prazine Wyeth), narcosis was obtained by intubation with a mixture of halothane (Fluothane ICI, Destelbergen, Belgium), oxygen and

41

nitrous oxide in a semi-closed system. The orbicular muscle was paralysed by local anaesthesia of the auriculo-palpebral nerve. The oxygen concentration was rigorously monitored by means of an oxygen analyser (O_2-Sendor 100 Drägerwerk AG, Lübeck, Germany), in order to avoid any hypoxaemia. At the place of the neutral electrode (canthus medialis) and at that of the earth-electrode (ipsilateral ear), the skin was first of all shaved and then coated with a conducting paste (Mingograph electrode cream Siemens Elema, Brussels). The active corneal electrode consisted of a scleral contact lens, provided with a lateral tube containing a chlorinated silver electrode in the form of a spiral, holding a wad of cotton-wool soaked in serum. The photostimulator (van Ahrend-van Gogh, Amsterdam, Netherlands) was set up at 200 mm from the eye. The intensity variations were obtained by interposing neutral filters (neutral-density filters Agfa-Gevaert, Antwerp, Belgium). The recordings were made by means of a CP8 encephalograph (van Ahrend-van Gogh, Amsterdam). The pupils were dilated by 4% atropine sulphate.

When the horse had been anaesthetised, it was adapted to darkness for five minutes and then adapted to light at various levels of illuminance for two minutes each, to conclude with adaptation to darkness for thirty minutes.

For the histological and ultrastructural examination, the eyes were washed immediately after the horse had been slaughtered. The cornea, iris, lens, and vitreous having been removed, the eyes were prefixed for forty-eight hours in 3% glutaraldehyde. Next, the retina and the choroid were detached from the sclera at the level of the posterior pole and cut up into small pieces. Finally, they were fixed in osmium tetroxide before being treated according to Spurr's method (1969).

The regions studied are indicated on the diagram of Fig. 1. The counting was carried out on the photographs of thick sections stained with toluidine blue (Fig. 2).

RESULTS

1. *Junction between the pigment epithelium and the photoreceptors in man at the electron-microscope*

a. *Macular region*

I. *Apical extremity of the pigment epithelium cells (François and Victoria-Troncoso 1977).* At the transmission *electron-microscope*, the pigment epithelium displayed a hexagonal and very regular cell mosaic. These cells were more pigmented at the level of the macular region. They measured 14 μm × 10–14 μm (Salzmann 1912; Ts'o & Friedman 1967). Their apical part was shrouded in a membrane which developed numerous microvillosi-

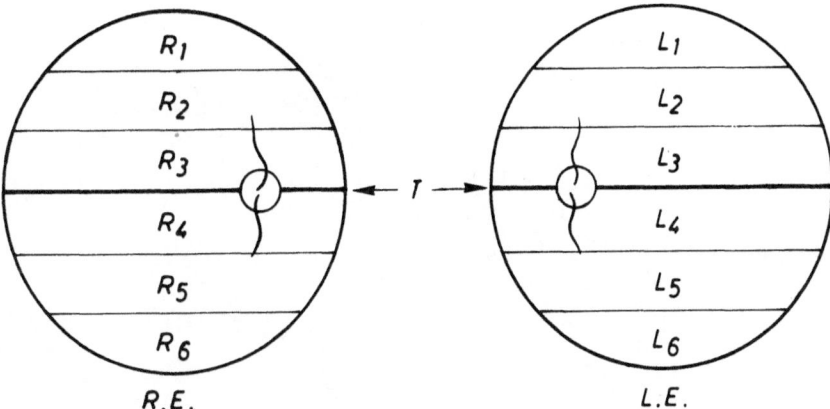

Fig. 1. Schema showing the retinal regions examined in the horse. T = tapetum lucidum. R = right eye and L = left eye. The subdivisions R_1, R_2 ---, L_1, L_2 --- indicate the different zones below and above the tapetum lucidum.

ties; these were arranged as excrescences in the shape of 'glove fingers' which projected forward. Three types of them could be distinguished (Figs. 1 and 2):

1. Long microvilli 6 µm long, which insinuated themselves between the external segments of the photoreceptors, as far as a third of their length.

2. Microvilli of medium length, having wide and irregular bases and lengths from 3 to 6 µm; they touched the extremities of the photoreceptors, but did not insinuate themselves between them.

3. Short microvilli 1 to 3 µm long, which probably represented microvillosities in the course of formation and which did not reach the photoreceptors.

The apical cytoplasm of the cells was filled with pigment granules which, in adults, were tyrosinase-negative (Miyamoto & Fitzpatrick 1957) and with a number of rounded particles, which were enclosed in membranes and contained a substance of a velvet-like appearance. Morphologically, these particles were lysosomes.

There were also inclusions, in some cases voluminous, above all at the bases of the widest microvillosities; there were several types of them, but all were enclosed in membranes:

1. Some of them had the same appearance and the same regularity as the external segments of the photoreceptors. Their membranes were well-defined and displayed the characteristic structure of a 'stack of disks'.

2. In others, the space between the membranes was enlarged and filled with a substance having a homogeneous grey electron-density. In many places, the membranes were fused together.

3. Finally, there were homogeneous masses of moderate electron-density, where parallel striations were to be seen here and there.

43

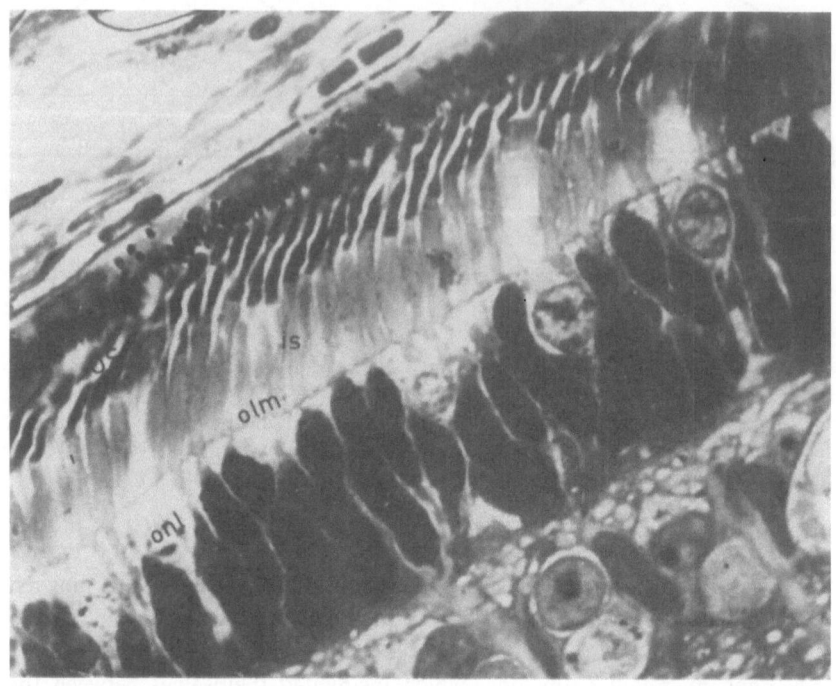

Fig. 2. Thick section of the horse's retina (as the one utilized for counting), stained with toluidine blue. It shows the cellular layers from the choriocapillaris to the internal nuclear layer. OS = external segments of the photoreceptors. I.S. = internal segments of the photoreceptors. The cones with their clear nucleus are easily differentiated from the rods with their dark nucleus in the external nuclear layer (onl). Clear field microscopy (×400).

The membrane that surrounded these structures was fairly often double: an internal membrane, which was the cell membrane of the photoreceptor, and an external membrane, which was formed by the invagination of the cell membrane of the pigment cells.

All the particles which we have just described represented phagosomes at different stages of digestion.

II. *External segment of the photoreceptors (François & Victoria-Troncoso 1977).* At the level of the macula, there were elongated cones, resembling rods. At the transmission *electron-microscope,* it was seen that the external segments at the level of the fovea consisted of about 1200 membranous disks. Each disk comprised a membrane 50 Å thick, the intradiscal space being 40 Å, and the interdiscal space being 180 Å (Spitznas 1970). The intradiscal space, which was filled with lipids, was thus wider than in the case of rods. Moreover, the cones did not display any lateral slots. In reality, all the disks, which were arranged perpendicularly to the axis of the cones, were formed of two parallel and continuous membranes which were folded laterally. The cell membrane surrounded the external segment, without there being any connections between it and the membranes of the disks. These floated in an amorphous medium containing glycoproteins. Only the external third of the external segment of the photoreceptor was surrounded by the microvilli of the pigment epithelium. There were in some cases cytoplasmic prolongations originating in the internal segment. All of these structures were held together by a mucoid substance.

III. *Substance separating the apical segments of the pigment cells from the external segments of the photoreceptors.* At the transmission *electron-microscope* the space that separated the external segments of the photoreceptors from the microvilli of the pigment epithelium was very irregular. It measured from 0 to 5 μm, and it was filled with a homogeneous substance of low electron density.

Its histochemical characteristics are summarised in Table 1. It was a mucopolysaccharide which was partially sulphated and partially sensitive to hyaluronidase.

Table 1.

Method	Substance separating the photoreceptors from the pigment epithelium
Pas	+
Alcian Blue pH 1	+ +
Alcian Blue pH 2,5	+ +
Colloidal iron	−
Hyaluronidase test	+ or − depending on the sections

b. *Perimacular and peripheral regions*

The human retina contains between 110 and 125 million rods and between 6 and 7 million cones. The density of the cones diminishes rather suddenly from 147,000 per square millimetre at the level of the fovea, to 100 per square millimetre at the extreme periphery. There are 5000 of them per square millimetre at the level of the equator. Although there are no rods at the level of the fovea, there are 160,000 of them per square millimetre at a distance of $2\frac{1}{2}$ mm from it. That number then falls off, to arrive at about 30,000 at the periphery.

A rod disk measures 150 Å, of which 20 Å correspond to the intradiscal space, which itself measures 150 Å.

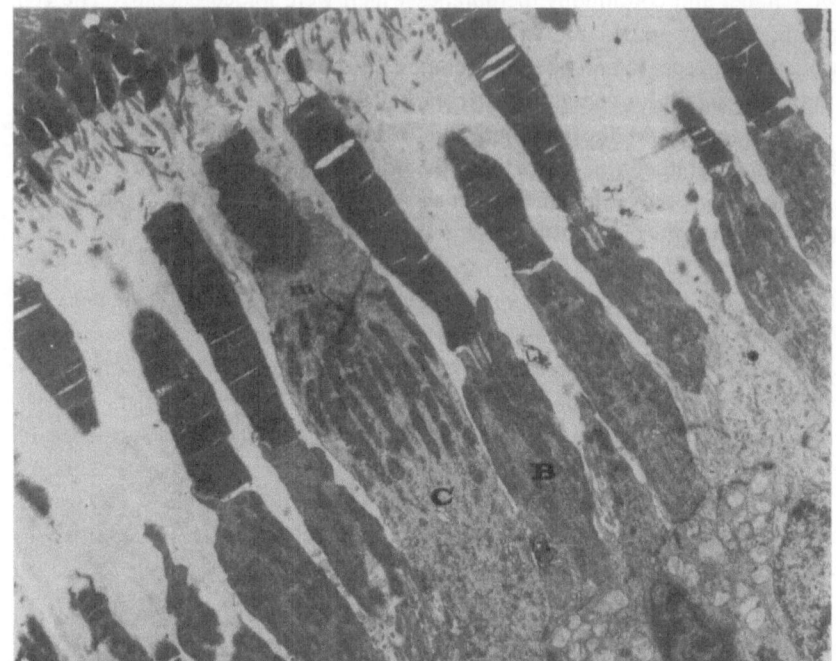

Fig. 3.

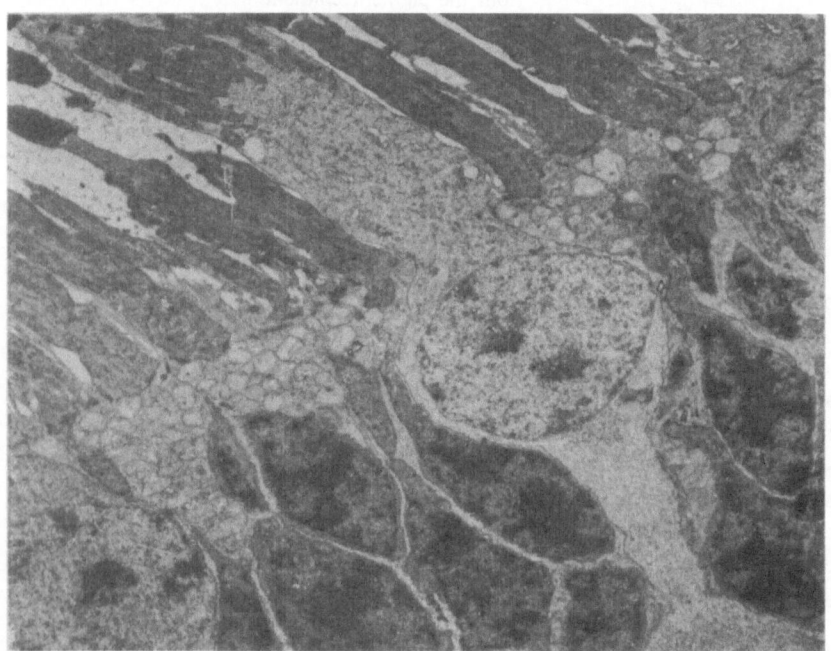

Fig. 4.

46

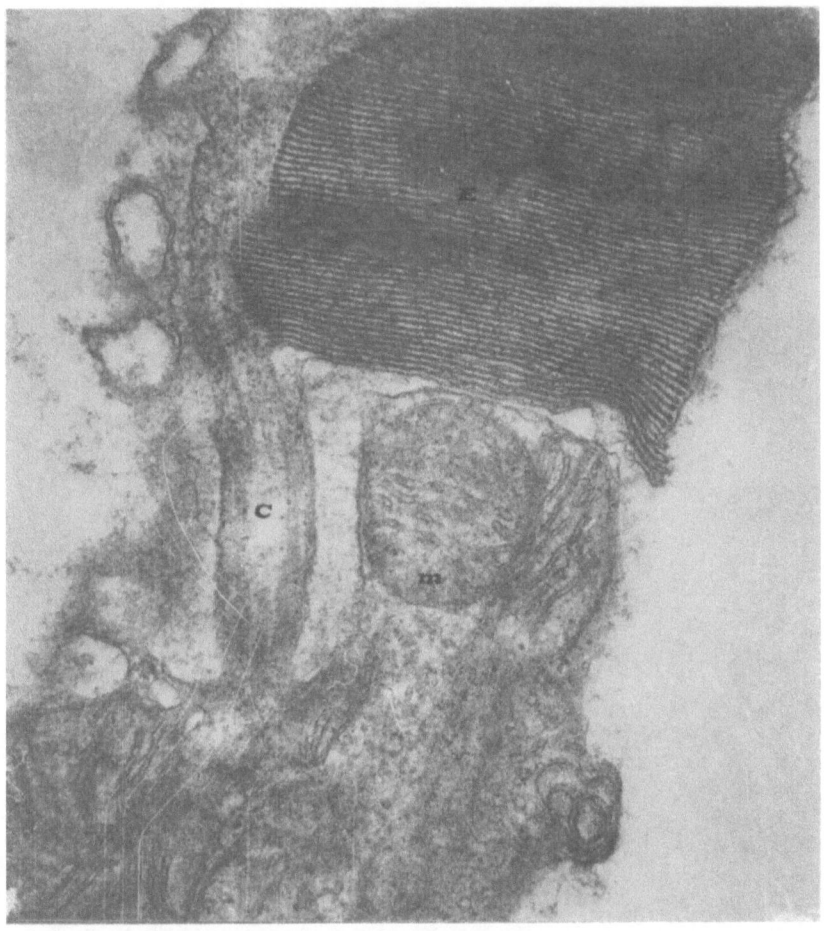

Fig. 5. Part of a rod with its external segment (E), its connecting filament (c) and its mitochondria (m). Electron microscopy (×22,400).

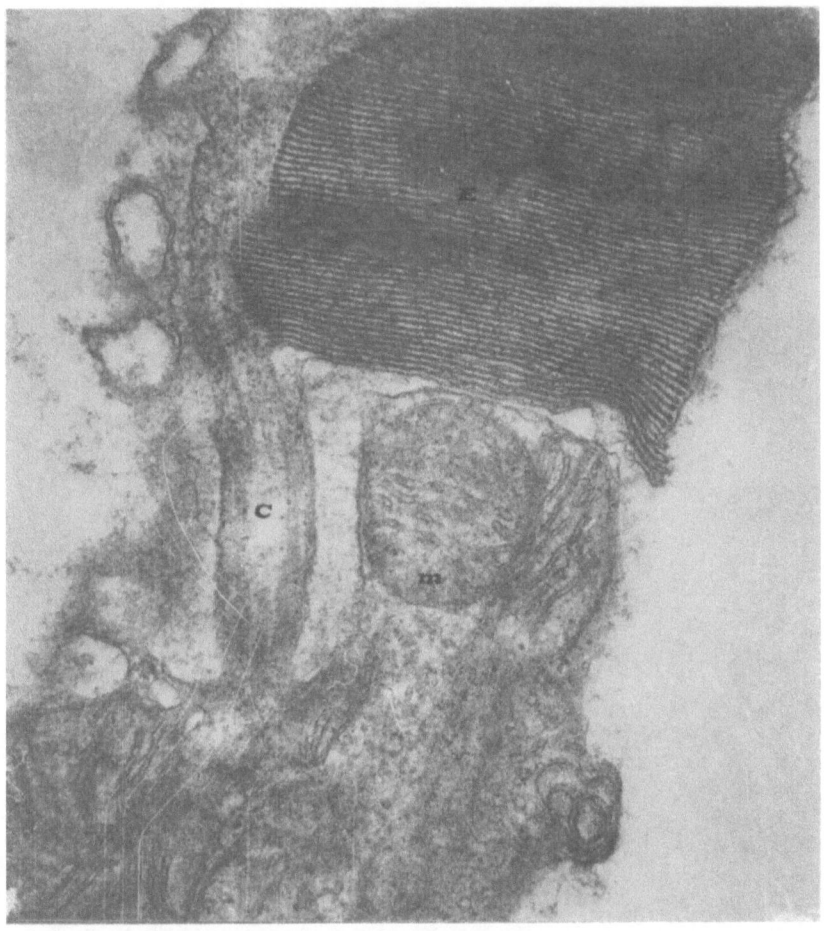

Fig. 3. Junction between the pigment epithelium and the photoreceptors at low magnification. The cones (C) and the rods (B) contain numerous elongated mitochondria (m). The microvilli (v) encompass the external segments of the photoreceptors in order to phagocyte them. Electron microscopy (×22,400).

Fig. 4. Photoreceptors at the level of the external nuclear layer. The chromatine is obviously less dense in the cones than in the rods. Electron microscopy (×4000).

47

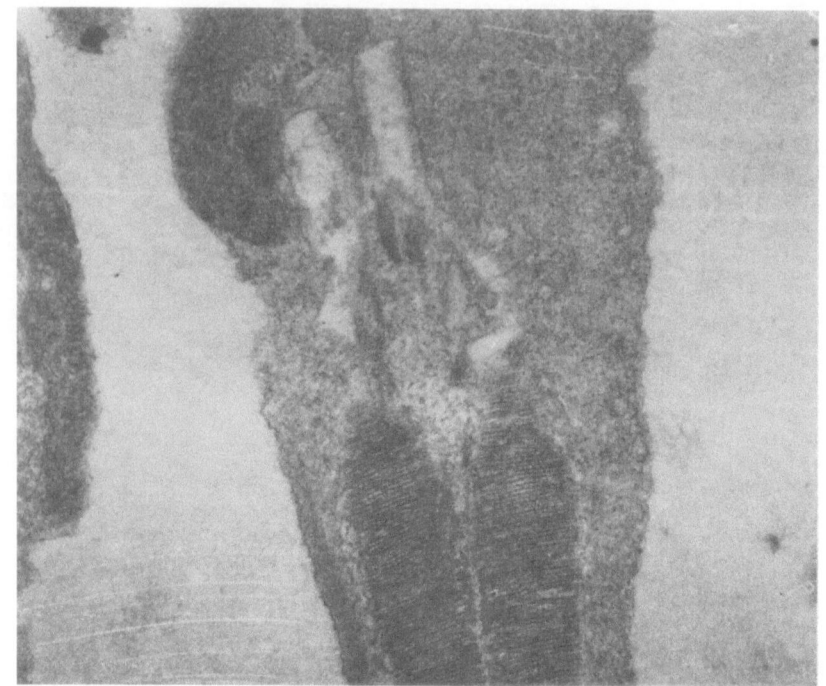

Fig. 6.

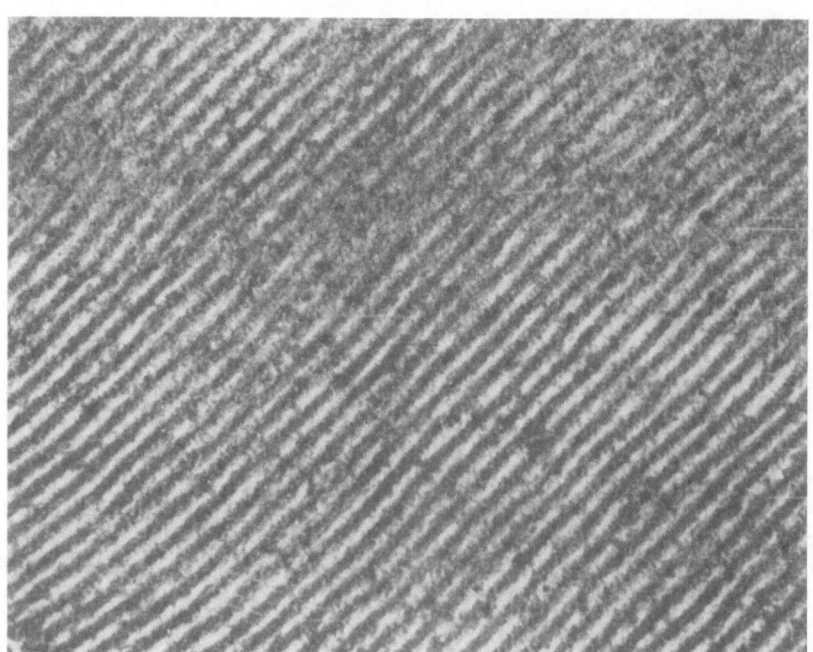

Fig. 7.

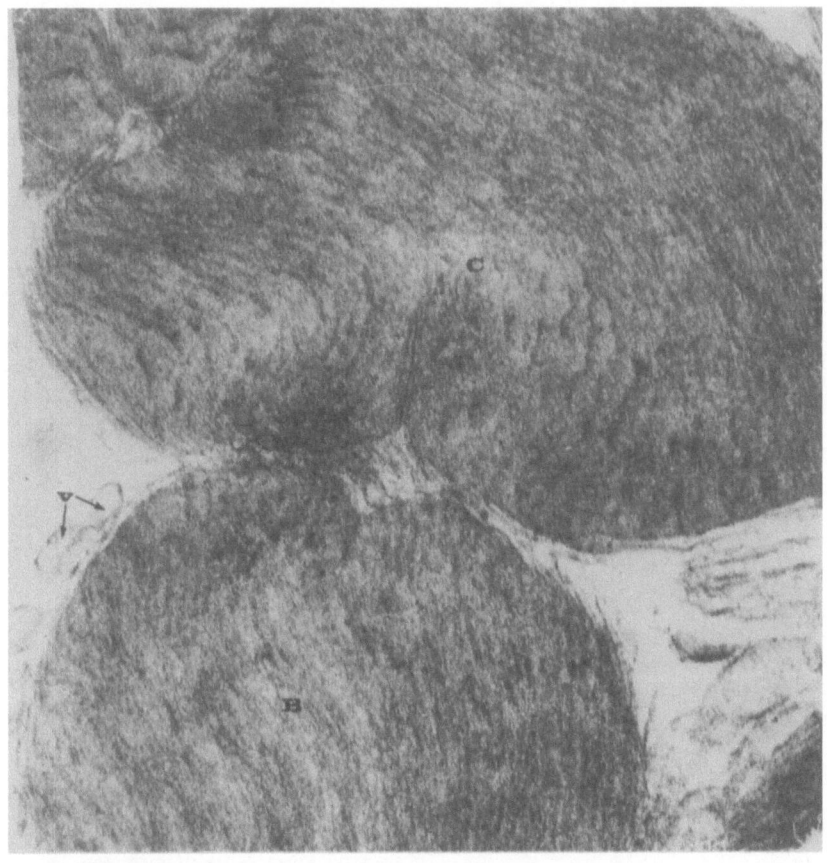

Fig. 8. Transversal section of a cone (C) and of a rod (B) near their external extremity. Transversal section of some microvillosities of the pigment epithelium (v). Electron microscopy ($\times 28,000$).

Fig. 6. Some rods show a bilobate external segment. Electron microscopy ($\times 12,600$).

Fig. 7. Disks and interdiscal spaces at the level of the external segment of a rod. Electron microscopy ($\times 77,000$).

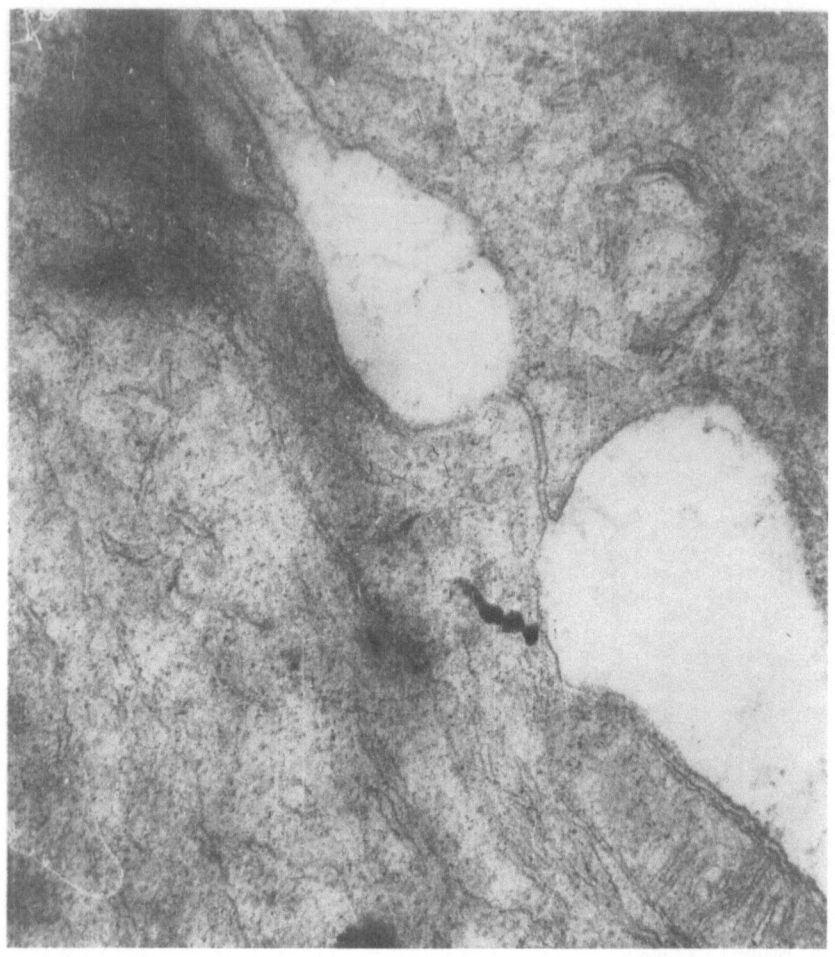

Fig. 9. Connexion between two photoreceptors at the level of their internal segment. Electron microscopy (×22,400).

2. *Junction between the pigment epithelium and* *the photoreceptors in the horse at the electron-microscope*

The structure, both of the cells of the pigment epithelium and of the photoreceptors, was essentially identical in the horse and in man (Figs. 3 to 13).

In the horse, the pigment epithelium (Figs. 10 to 12) was highly developed. Its cells contained numerous mitochondria which displayed a large number of crests and many vacuoles of pinocytosis, several particles of the

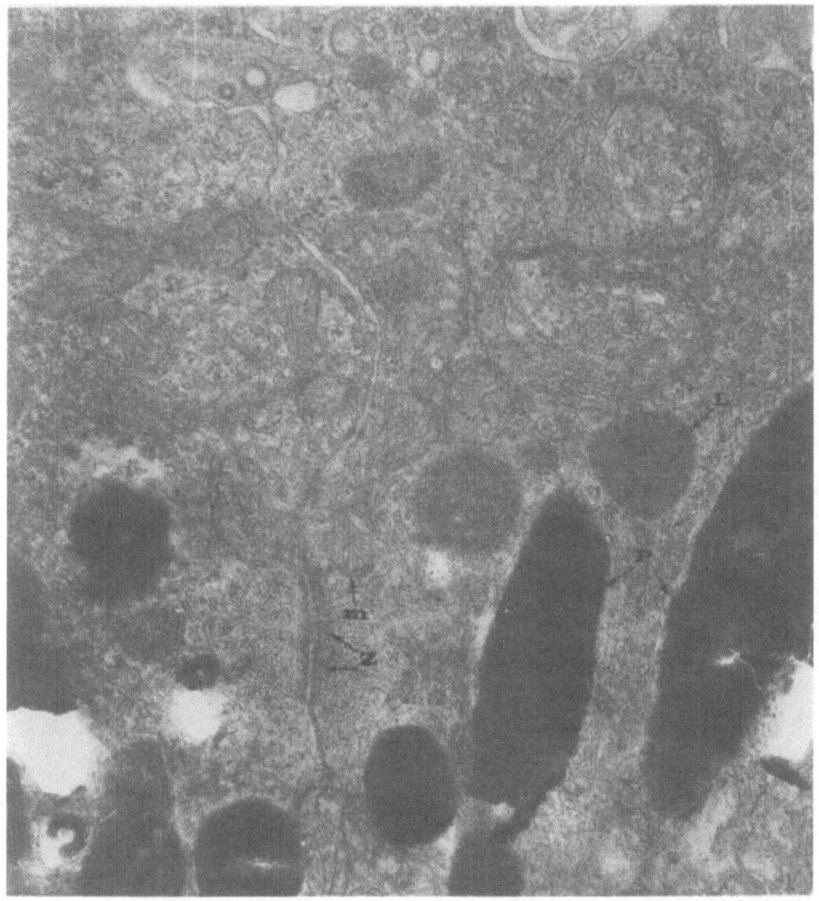

Fig. 10. Two cells of the pigment epithelium at high magnification. P = pigment granules. L = lysosomes. m = mitochondria. Z = zonula occludens. Electron microscopy (×17,600).

lysosomal type having a velvet-like content, as well as an endoplasmic reticulum. These cells were attached one to another by zonulae occludentes (Fig. 10), which were wider than in man. There were also some phagosomes (Figs. 11 to 13), which were in some cases plurilobular and still displayed striations, remnants of the disks of the external segments of the photoreceptors.

The photoreceptors, also, were similar to those in man. It was easy to distinguish the bulbous appearance of the external segments of the cones (Figs. 3 and 4) and the finer structure of the external segments of the rods.

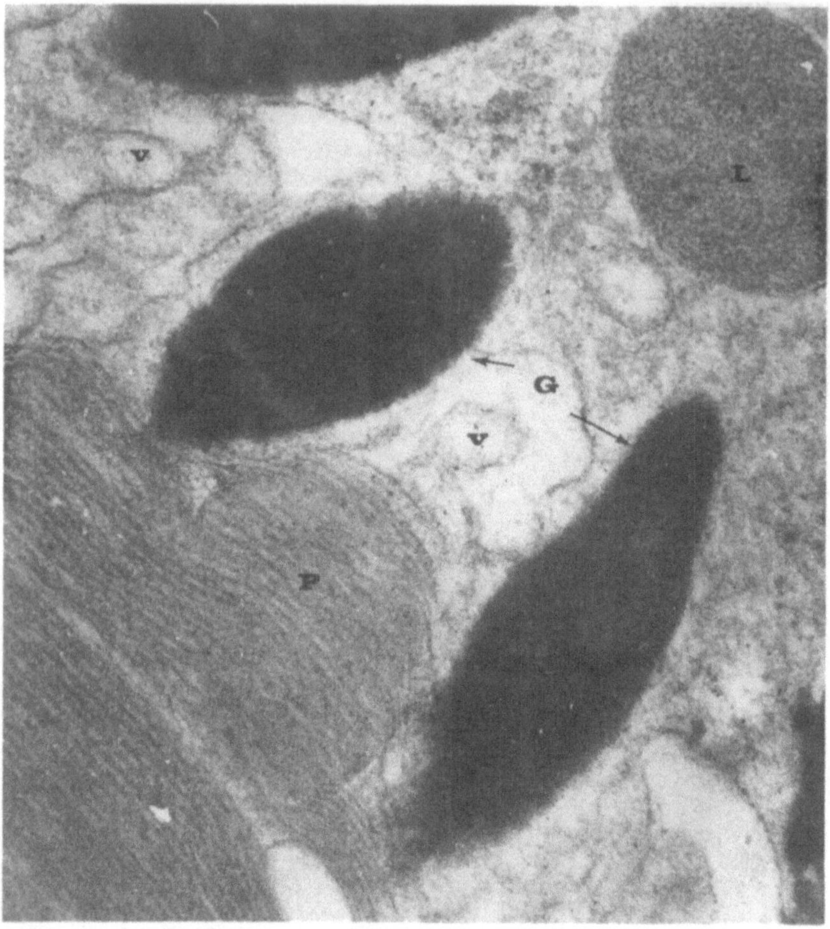

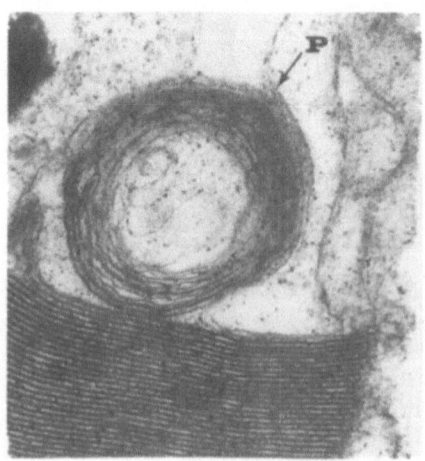

Fig. 11.

Fig. 12.

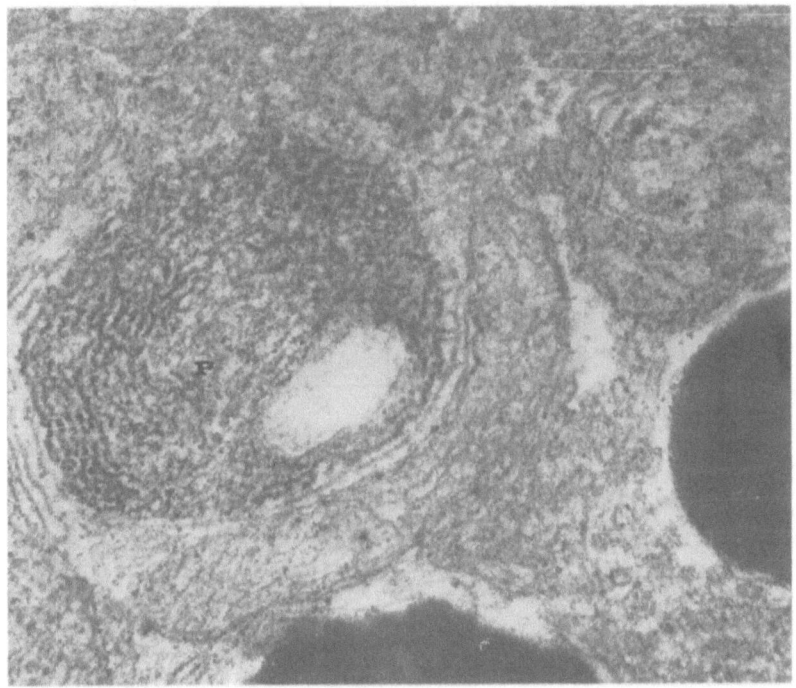

Fig. 13. Phagosome (P) at high magnification in a cell of the pigment epithelium, surrounded by membranous structures and small vesicles. Electron microscopy (×42,000).

By both optical and low-magnification electron-microscopy, we were able to distinguish between the nuclei of the rods and those of the cones, which made it possible to count the number of cells of both types (Fig. 2). The nuclei of the rods were packed very close together in the external nuclear layer. The chromatin of the rods was more dense than that of the cones. The cell membrane of the rods was less visible than this of the cones, which took on the appearance of a fine line.

The *morphometrical study* by counting the cells in the several zones of the horse retina is sketched in Fig. 1.

Fig. 14 indicates the percentage of the cones relative to the rods. There was no significant difference between the tapetum lucidum and the tapetum

←

Fig. 11. External segment of a photoreceptor, a part of which (P) is phagocyted at the level of the microvillosities (v) of the pigment epithelium in order to form a phagosome. L = lysosome, which is responsible for the digestion. Electron microscopy (×35,000).

Fig. 12. At a later stage, a part of the disks are detached in order to form the phagosome (P). Electron microscopy (×45,000).

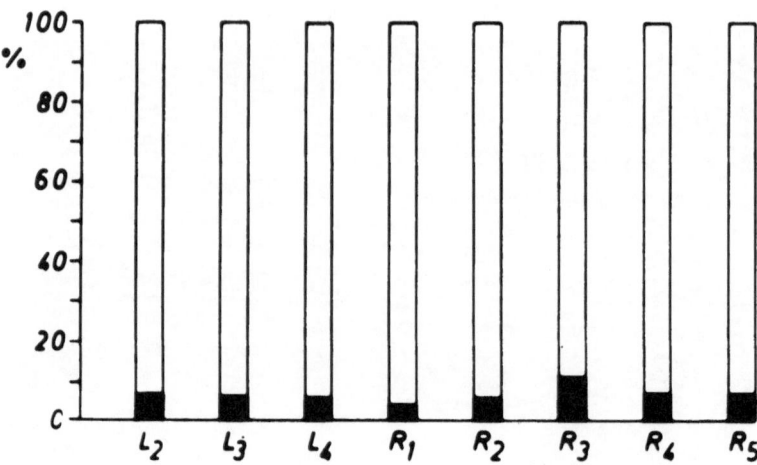

Fig. 14. Percentage of horse's cones and rods in the various topographic zones, indicated in Fig. 1. The distribution is rather homogeneous. The higher percentage of cones at the level of R_3 is not statistically significant.

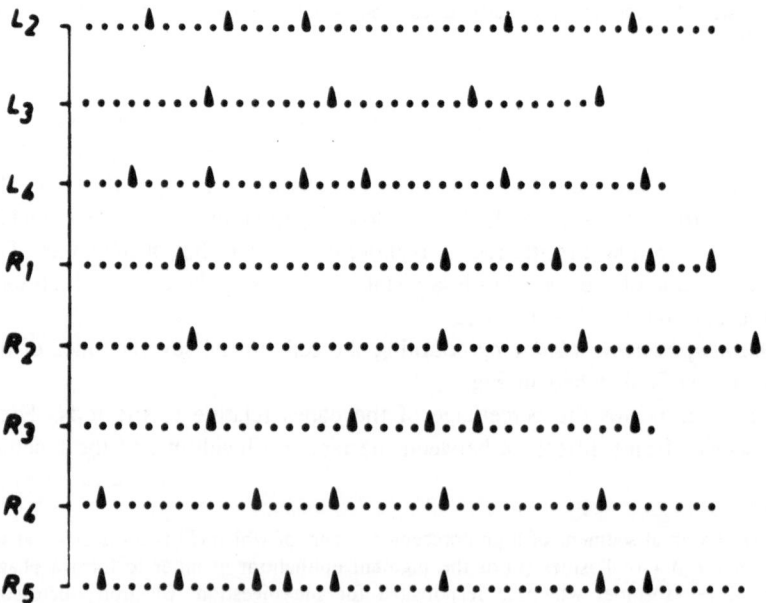

Fig. 15. Example of counting of cones (▲) and rods (●) in the horse in the various topographic zones indicated in Fig. 1. The distribution is rather homogeneous in each zone.

nigrum, nor between the several topographical zones. The L_3 region (the central part of the posterior pole) contained only a slightly larger number of cones than the other regions (about 17%); the difference was not statistically significant.

Fig. 15 shows the numbers of cones and rods in sections taken at random. Thus, from eight to fifteen rods were found between two cones in the R_2 region, and from one to nine rods between two cones in the R_5 region. No statistically significant difference was evident between the different regions, be they central or peripheral.

The retina of the horse did not display anywhere any concentration of cones, such as is found at the level of the macula in man. In the horse, the cones were homogeneously distributed and in rather small numbers over the whole extent of the retina, notwithstanding that their density may be slightly higher at the level of the posterior pole (Figs. 14 and 15).

The plurilobular external segments were much more frequently observed in the horse than in man. There were weak connections by zonulae occludentes between the cytoplasmic extensions of the photoreceptors.

ELECTROPHYSIOLOGICAL STUDY

In man, the electroretinograms show parallel and probably independent activities, one of them corresponding to the cones and the other to the rods. The two systems of receptors respond to impulses of illumination by complex electric discharges resulting from the interaction of several components, the origin of which is located at well-defined levels of the retina. These responses are similar for both types of receptors, but their temporal characteristics are very different. Their relative importance depends upon the conditions of adaptation of the retina, the nature of the light stimulation and the physical characteristics of the recording equipment used.

The interaction of the two systems has the effect that the electroretinogram is a response with multiple components, of which the most often clinically investigated are the cornea-negative initial *a*-wave, the cornea-positive *b*-wave and the oscillatory potential. Notwithstanding that the *b*-wave is merely an epiphenomenon resulting from the depolarisation of the Müller's cells, it is nevertheless thanks to it that it is possible to demonstrate the duality of the retina. The *b*-wave produced by the activity of the cones is spiked and rapid; it does not develop in the course of dark adaptation. The *b*-wave produced by the rods is lower and more rounded; it develops slowly during dark adaptation toward a terminal amplitude, which depends upon the conditions of the investigation, the time necessary for attaining that response depending upon the pre-adaptation adopted.

The response of the cones can be isolated, either by their stimulation by red light or by recording the responses with an illuminance such that the

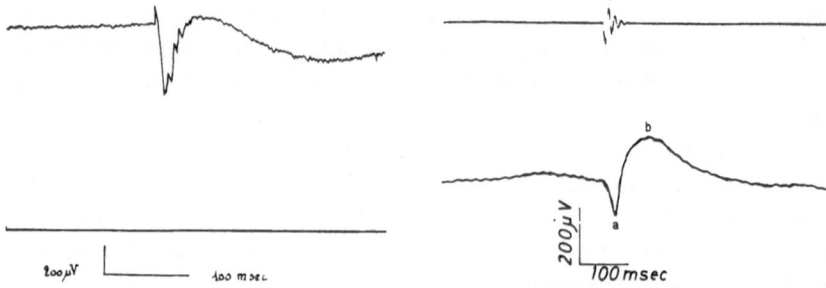

Fig. 16. Scotopic electroretinogram in response to a xenon flash (maximum intensity). The speeds and the amplifications have been modified in order to obtain similar curves. At the left, scotopic ERG in man, at the right scotopic ERG in the horse. In the horse, the duration of the *b*-wave, which is of about 300 msec, the absence of oscillatory potential and the predominance of the *b*-wave have to be noted.

activity of the rods is suppressed completely. The response of the rods can be isolated by adopting stimulation by blue light of low intensity.

The determination of the critical fusion frequency as a function of the stimulation intensity also makes it possible to distinguish the cones from the rods. By that method one obtains a biphasic curve whose first segment corresponds to the fusion of the rods and the second to that of the cones.

Moreover, the relative importance of the two systems of receptors can be determined by comparing the amplitude curves of the *b*-waves under two different levels of illuminance, for example, in darkness and with an illuminance of 300 lux. The amplitude of the scotopic response is, indeed, determined by the activity of the rods, which completely obscures the activity of the cones, which is too rapid and too slight.

In the horse, the duality of the retina was again found, but there was, nonetheless, a marked predominance of the activity of the rods (Figs. 16 and 19). The electroretinograms showed very large and rounded *b*-waves, which progressively increased in amplitude during dark adaptation. Even after moderate pre-adaptation, the terminal amplitude of the *b*-wave was reached only very slowly, compared with the results obtained in man. After pre-adaptation at 80 lux, the scotopic *b*-wave, in the horse, reached its maximum amplitude only after about thirty minutes, whereas in man only ten minutes are required. Furthermore, in the horse, the terminal scotopic electroretinogram was much less complex than in man under similar conditions. The *a*-wave was smaller and there was no oscillatory potential. Altogether, the response was reminiscent of that of monochromates (Fig. 16).

However, that fact does not signify that the cones do not contribute to the production of the response, as is demonstrated by the curve of the fusion frequency as a function of the stimulation intensity. Exactly as in man, this curve shows that, in the horse, there are two segments (Fig. 17). The critical fusion frequency for the cone segment amounted, in the horse, to 60 Hz,

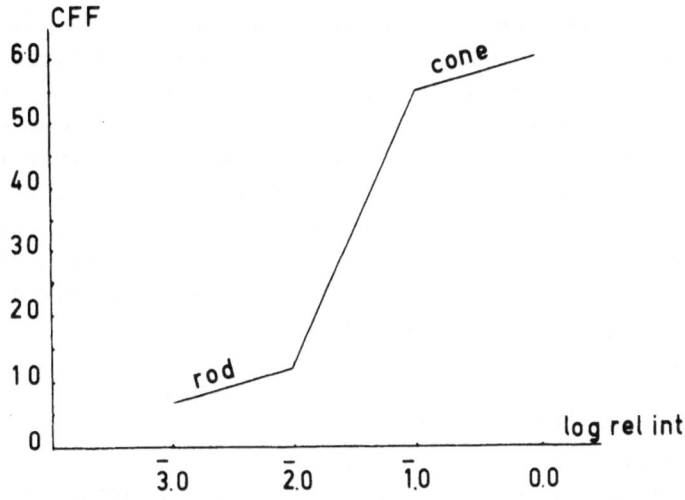

Fig. 17. Curve of electroretinographical fusioń frequency in function of the stimulation intensity (xenon flash).

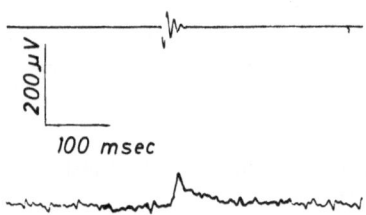

Fig. 18. Photopic electroretinogram of the horse. Pupillary illuminance of 700 lux during 5 min. Xenon flash. Maximum intensity. Response of the cones. The *b*-wave is smaller, sharper and more rapid than that of the rods. Culmination time 34 msec.

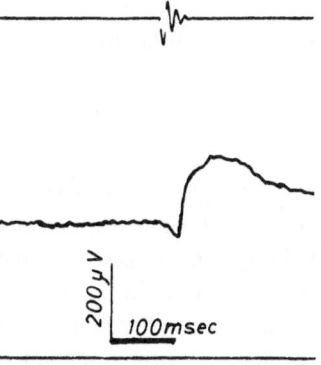

Fig. 19. Scotopic electroretinogram of the horse (poney of 3 years). Response of the rods in blue light (Kodak wratten blue) after a dark adaptation of 30 min. The culmination time of the *b*-wave corresponds to that of the rods.

which is very comparable with the values obtained in man. It was more difficult to obtain in the horse a response of the cones with isolated stimulation. With red light, it was even impossible to demonstrate, in the horse, any response at all with the available stimulation intensities, whereas, in man, we obtained clear responses of amplitudes of 100 μV or more, under the same conditions. With white light, an illuminance of 700 lux at the level of the pupil was necessary, in the horse, in order to obtain a response displaying the characteristics of cones (Fig. 18), whereas, in man, an illuminance of 300 lux is already adequate to eliminate all the rod components and to show up the optimum response of the cones. In man, the ratio

$$\frac{\text{maximum amplitude, } b\text{-wave, cones}}{\text{maximum amplitude, } b\text{-wave, rods}} = 0.33 \pm 0.08,$$

whereas in the horse it is less than 0.25.

All the electroretinographic characteristics of man and of the horse are summarised in Table 2.

Table 2. Electroretinographic characteristics

Electroretinogram	Man	Horse
Light adaptation: illuminance necessary to obtain a cone response	300 lux	700 lux
Dark adaptation: duration necessary to obtain a maximum response	short adaptation	long adaptation
Electroretinographic morphology in darkness	complex, *a*-wave very ample, oscillatory potential evident	relatively simple, *a*-wave less ample, oscillatory potential absent
Response in red light	evident	absent
Curve of critical fusion frequency	biphasic	biphasic
Ratio amplitude of the cone *b*-wave: amplitude of the rod *b*-wave	0,33 ± 0,08	0,25

In conclusion, it may be said that the electroretinogram of the horse, just like that of man, shows the duality of the retina, but that the contribution of the rods is predominant. Although the response of the cones in the horse may be morphologically similar to that in man, it is nevertheless more difficult to demonstrate it, and its amplitude is smaller. The lesser part played by the cones in the scotopic electroretinogram of the horse is represented by a smoother *a*-wave and by the absence of oscillatory potential. Furthermore, the results of the electrophysiological study in the horse correspond perfectly with the distribution of the photoreceptors in the retina.

CONCLUSIONS

There is a morphological resemblance between the photoreceptors in man and those in the horse.

Although there seems to be, in the horse, a greater density of the cones at the level of the posterior pole, there is strictly speaking no macula. The electroretinographic study confirms, on this point, the histological examination. It confirms the duality of the retina, but shows that the contribution of the rods is clearly preponderant. The lesser role played by the cones, in the scotopic electroretinogram in the horse, is indicated by a less pronounced *a*-wave and by the absence of an oscillatory potential. This explains the poor vision of the horse, particularly under photopic conditions.

There exists, in the horse, interconnections between the photoreceptors (Fig. 9). However, Davanger (1979) was able to show by scanning electron-microscopy that there exist, in man also, cytoplasmic extensions.

We have already described the junction between the pigment epithelium and the photoreceptors in man (François & Victoria-Troncoso 1977). In the horse, the structure of this junction is similar. The greatest difference between man and the horse is represented by the cone: rod ratio in the several zones of the retina.

The phenomena of renewal of the photoreceptors after phagocytosis of the external segments by the pigment epithelium are identical in the horse and man (François & Victoria-Troncoso 1977).

REFERENCES

Bairaitti, A. Jr. & N. Orzalesi. The ultrastructure of the pigment epithelium and of the photoreceptor-pigment epithelium junction in the human retina. J. Ultrastruct. Res. 9: 484-489 (1963).

Berman, E.R. & J. Bach. The acid mucupolysaccharides of cattle retina. Biochem. J. 108: 75-79 (1968).

Davanger M. Some recent observations by SEM in the retina. La microscopie électronique à balayage en ophtalmologie. Symposium; Brest, June (1979).

François J. & V. Victoria-Troncoso. La Jonction entre l'épithélium pigmentaire et les photorécepteurs au niveau de la macula. Ann. Oculistique (Paris) 210: 203-211 (1977).

Miyamoto, M. & T.B. Fitzpatrick. On the nature of the pigment in retinal pigment epithelium. Science 126: 449-450 (1957).

Salzmann M. The anatomy and histology of the human eyeball. Chicago, Denticke (1912).

Schmidt W J. Doppelbrechung, Dichroismus und Feinbau des Aussengliedes der Sehzellen von Frosch. Z. Zellforsch. 22: 485 (1935).

Spitznas M. Zur Feinstruktur der sog. Membrana limitans externa der menschlichen Retina. Graefes Arch. Ophthal. 180: 44 (1970).

Spitznas M. & M.J. Hogan. Interrelationship of outer segments of photoreceptors and the retinal pigment epithelium. Interrelationship in the human eye. Arch Ophthal. 84: 810 (1970).

Spurr A. A low viscosity epoxy resin embedding medium for electron microscopy. J. Ultrastruct. Res. 26: 41-43 (1969).

Ts'o, M.O.M. & E. Friedman. The retinal pigment epithelium. I. Comparative histology. Arch. Ophthal. 78: 641-650 (1967).

Young, R.W. The renewal of photoreceptor cell outer segment. J. Cell Biol. 33: 61-71 (1967).

Zimmerman, L.E. Applications of histochemical methods for the demonstration of acid mucopolysaccharides to ophthalmic pathology. Trans. Amer. Acad. Ophthal. Otolaryng. 62: 697 (1958).

Authors' address:
Ophthalmological Clinic
University of Ghent
135 De Pintelaan
B–9000 Ghent
Belgium

RETINAL RE-ATTACHMENT FORCES CREATED BY ABSORPTION OF SUBRETINAL FLUID

(Columbia, S.C., U.S.A.)

ABSTRACT

Retinal breaks up to 3 mm above the crest of a scleral buckle will reliably lead to retinal re-attachment. Evidence suggesting retinal pigment epithelial and/or choroidal absorption of subretinal fluid (SRF) is given. Physical forces contributing to retinal detachment are discussed. Absorption of SRF induces a 'lift' force which tends to reapproximate the retina to the scleral buckle. A mathematical expression for the reapproximating lift force is derived. An order of magnitude calculation of the lift force is made. An estimate of the order of magnitude of residual detachment forces is 10^{-5} dynes.

INTRODUCTION

Scleral buckling procedures for repair of retinal detachment without drainage of subretinal fluid have become increasingly popular. Certain selected cases of retinal detachment are known to be unsuitable for the non-drainage procedure. Lincoff & Kreissig (1972) have shown that detachments with giant tears, severe vitreous traction, old detachments with inferior tears and senile choroidopathy, staphylomatous eyes, closure of the central retinal artery, and uncertain localization are indications for drainage of subretinal fluid.

RE-ATTACHMENT WITHOUT CLOSURE OF THE BREAK

Additionally O'Connor (1973) has shown that if the retinal break was more than 3 mm. above a circumferential or large radial buckle or if the retinal break could not be completely surrounded with one or more applications of a firmly placed cryosurgical probe, then drainage of subretinal fluid (SRF) should be considered. Strikingly, 51% of the retinal tears were open but within 3 mm. of the buckle at the end of the procedure in O'Connors series of 200 non-drained cases. All of his cases in this category were successfully re-attached, although two cases with the breaks posterior to the equator

61

required post-operative photocoagulation to 'affect a functional closure of the hole.'

The process involved in subsequent post-operative closure of the retinal break is variously thought to be due to buckle intrusion and chorioretinal exudation, settling of the retina on the buckle, and increased buckle height due to elasticity of the buckle and further hypotony of the globe (O'Connor 1976; Escoffery et al. 1976; Lincoff et al. 1972).

DELAYED ABSORPTION OF SUBRETINAL FLUID

The persistence of fluid in the immediate post-operative period is frequently seen. In the majority of cases, absorption of SRF is complete in 24–48 hours (O'Connor 1973). O'Connor stated that either a defect in the absorptive mechanism or of the operative procedure was present if all SRF had not been absorbed by the fifth post-operative day. Defective absorption due to senile choroidopathy was seen in 8% of O'Connors Custodis re-attachment procedures. The defect probably resulted from degenerative changes in Bruch's membrane and the choriocapillaris. In these patients, the peripheral fundus of the fellow eye had a 'generalized yellow appearance with retinal pigment epithelial atrophy and lacy accumulation of pigment in the equatorial zone.'

Robertson (1979) found that SRF persisted longer than six weeks in 39 (6.8%) of 575 cases which ultimately re-attached. Subretinal precipitates were present pre-operatively in 25% of the patients with absorption delayed greater than six weeks, but in only 12% of all patients with detachment. Long standing peripheral detachments typically sparing the macula were also associated with delayed absorption. SRF was analyzed for protein content when intraoperative drainage was performed. In the cases of delayed absorption, there was a significantly greater protein concentration in the pre-operatively longer standing cases. In the patients with delayed absorption, he found no correlation with age, size of the largest break, number of cryopexy lesions, number of quadrants of detached retina, presence or absence of aphakia and presence or absence of uveitis.

Leaver (1976) noted persistence of SRF at least one week in 25% of the patients treated with non-drainage procedures. He found a positive correlation with duration of the retinal detachment. He found no correlation between the absorption rate and the age of the patient, severe myopia, or volume of SRF.

Escoffery (1976) states that delayed absorption can be expected in senility and myopia due to an atrophic choroid.

EXPERIMENTAL EVIDENCE FOR ABSORPTION OF SRF
AND OTHER ATTACHMENT FORCES

Adhesive forces between the *in vitro* retinal pigment epithelium (RPE) and the photoreception layer of the retina can be explained on the basis of rheologic properties of a cementing substance (Zauberman *et al.* 1972). The cementing substance is probably the matrix seen between the RPE and sensory retina which histochemically is a mucopolysaccharide (Zimmerman & Eastham 1959).

Adhesive forces of this kind are governed only by the rate of separation, but have no absolute force opposing separation:

$$F t = \frac{3 \pi a^4 N}{4} \left(\frac{1}{h_1^2} - \frac{1}{h_2^2} \right)$$

F = applied force
t = duration of force
N = viscosity of adhesive
a = radius of specimen
h_1 & h_2 are the initial and final thickness of the adhesive (Zauberman *et al.* 1972).

Traction detachments created *in vivo* remain relatively small in rabbits (Zauberman & de Guillebron 1972). Shortly after death, the detachment obtained is three to eight times larger. The small size of the detachment surrounding the traction retinal breaks *in vivo* indicates undiminished retinal adhesion in the vicinity of the retinal breaks. This finding lends support to the theory that there is removal of fluid from the potential subretinal space by an active pump in the pigment epithelium rather than by a passive mechanism such as flow conductivity of the retina (Fatt & Shantinath 1971).

Experiments in which the subretinal space was cannulated, failed to show lower pressure there than in the anterior chamber (Maurice *et al.* 1971). This result was interpreted as showing (1) Hydrostatic factors could exert only a small influence in retinal adhesion and (2) the RPE is probably much more impermeable to fluid flow than the sensory retina.

The SRF in experimental traction detachments appears to be from the vitreous percolating through the retina since there was no diffusion of sulphan blue dye from the choroid into the subretinal space (Zauberman & de Guillebron 1972). Ascorbate concentrations in human SRF resemble the ascorbate concentrations in the aqueous humor of the posterior chamber (Van Heuvel & Larn 1978). This finding has led van Heuven to postulate that the aqueous humor contributes to formation of the SRF. He also notes that the relative hypotony of patients with rhegmatogenous retinal detachments may be accounted for by the additional absorption of aqueous through the choroid exposed by the detachment.

The transport of water across the RPE may be related to a metabolically activated ion pump. Perhaps a mechanism similar to the carbonic anhydrase dependent aqueous formation in the ciliary body is present in the retinal RPE. Histo-chemical studies have shown carbonic anhydrase at the basal parts of the ciliary pigment epithelium in rabbits (Kolker & Hetherington 1970).

DETACHMENT FORCES

Any weakening of the attachment forces will contribute to detachment and/or delayed absorption of SRF. Nevertheless, certain specific mechanisms appear to contribute more directly to detachments.

Exudative retinal detachments appear to represent a failure of the normal absorptive properties of the RPE to keep up with the production of SRF. Thus, the absorptive ability of the RPE may be normal or decreased. In some localized tumors the fluid can readily shift to a dependent position relatively distant from the lesion. This would suggest that although the RPE is relatively normal, its absorptive capacities are being exceeded by the exudative capacity of the tumor. In idiopathic central serous detachment an RPE detachment or break is occasionally seen to be leaking fluorescein stained fluid into the subretinal space. This is presumably due to direct passage of serous exudate from the choriocapillaris through devitalized pigment epithelium into the subretinal space (Gass 1977). In inflammatory exudative detachments, (e.g. Harada's disease, herpes zoster, and uveitis) the devitalized areas of the RPE are thought to be the source of exudative fluid. Vitreoretinal traction bands can cause traction retinal detachment, traction retinal schisis, and retinal breaks. Continued vitreous traction around the edges of a retinal break are particularly predisposing to progressive retinal detachment (Teng & Chi 1957). Pre-retinal, subretinal and intraretinal fibrosis lead to star-fold formation, equatorial ridges, and fixed radial folds which foreshorten the retina. This gives rise to a net traction away from the RPE in the unbuckled eye. In Rachal's series of 1088 retinal repairs, the cause of primary failure in 259 cases was due to massive periretinal retraction in 26.6% and to a pre-retinal membrane in 32.8% (Rachel & Burton 1979).

Rhegmatogenous detachments may arise from rotary vitreous currents induced by eye movements in the presence of a retinal break. Rosengren (1976) demonstrated elevation of a latex membrane with a small hole in it on the inner surface of a glass bottle filled with water when rotary movements were produced by torsion of the container. The rapid peripheral currents resulting from to and fro rotary movements were seen to cause dissection of water beneath the membrane. Rosengren (1950) has noted rapid settling of a detachment often within 30 minutes when the patient is immobilized. Redetachment occurs as soon as eye movements are resumed.

Increased viscosity markedly subdued the detaching peripheral currents in Rosengren's model. He reasoned that since the viscosity of the vitreous increases with the concentration of hyaluronic acid, the low hyaluronic acid concentrations found in the vitreous of aphakes and myopes might account for their vulnerability to detachment.

The pattern of progressive fluid accumulation in rhegmatogenous detachments often suggests the location of the retinal break (Lincoff & Gieser 1971). Fluid accumulates around the original break, then dissects toward the ora and the disc and then spreads dependently as if under the influence of gravity (O'Connor 1976). This pattern suggests that the SRF has a greater density or specific gravity than the fluid cavity overlying the retinal detachment. The protein concentration of the SRF was found to be highest in long standing retinal detachments and in cases undergoing re-operations (Robertson 1979). There was no relationship between protein concentration and the following factors: patient's age, the duration of the detachment, the number of quadrants involved, the presence or absence of aphakia, demarcation lines and subretinal precipitate, the interval between surgery and the resorption of fluid, the size of the largest break.

Laminar convection can be observed in some cases of idiopathic central serous detachment by the leakage of dye through a break in the RPE on fluorescein angiography. Convection would undoubtably be a small force if it plays any part at all in other types of retinal detachment.

A MODEL FOR RE-ATTACHMENT FORCES CREATED
BY ABSORPTION OF SUBRETINAL FLUID

The following model attempts to describe mathematically the force resulting from absorption of SRF by the RPE when a break in the retina remains elevated above the scleral buckle at the end of the procedure. Although the underlying hydrodynamic principles are intuitively obvious, the mathematical description can become very complex unless simplifying assumptions are made at the outset.

The initial and most basic assumption is that the RPE in combination with the underlying choroid, actively removes SRF from the subretinal space to the choroid. This process is assumed to occur at a fixed rate in a given eye. The RPE is also assumed to be relatively impermeable to the diffusion of fluid back from the choroid to the subretinal space.

In this particular model we will assume that there are no exudative processes, and that any vitreoretinal traction would be relaxed if the retina were resting on the buckle. The detachment forces induced by rapid peripheral currents upon eye motion as noted by Rosengren, will not be considered at this time. Convective forces in the subretinal fluid, as well as the gravitational effects of the SRF being denser than the overlying vitreous will be considered negligible. The SRF will be considered a Newtonian fluid.

Schematically, an unbuckled bullous rhegmatogenous detachment may be represented like this:

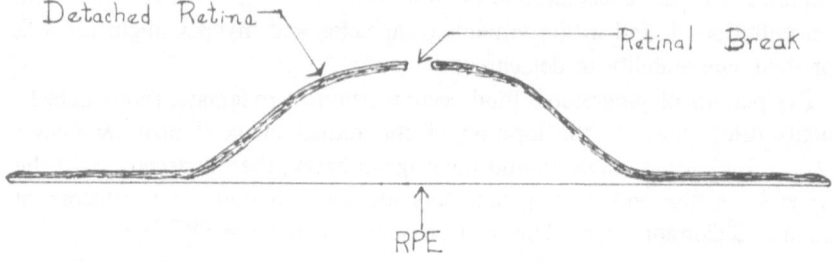

Fig. 1

A wide buckle around a relatively small, but unclosed hole may be schematically represented like this:

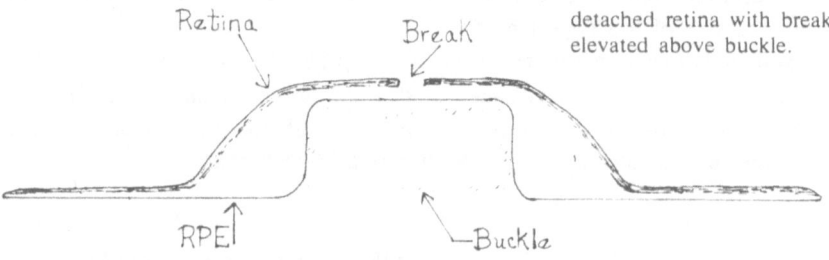

detached retina with break elevated above buckle.

Fig. 2

The relationship between the RPE on the crest of the buckle and the overlying retinal break and detached retina may be represented ideally as two plates with a hole in the center of the upper one:

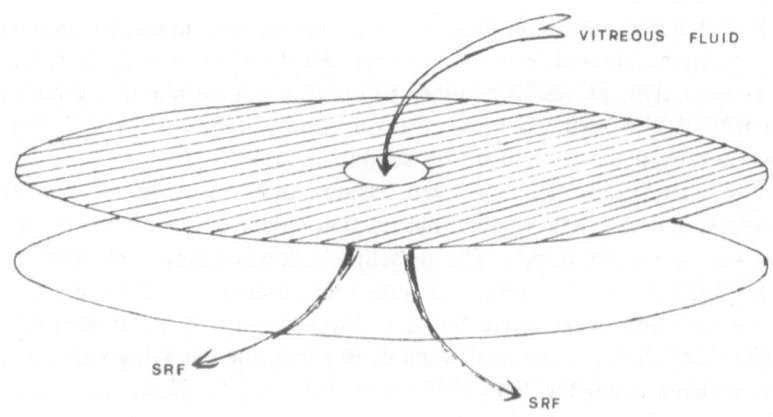

Fig. 3

The absorption of SRF by the RPE then induces a flow of fluid from the vitreous through the retinal break and between the RPE and detached retina overlying the crest of the buckle. Due to resistance to flow between these two plates there is a pressure drop between the plates downstream from the retinal break. The pressure in the vitreous overlying the retinal detachment is the same at the retinal break and downstream from it. This induces a 'lift' force which tends to push the detached retina towards the RPE. This can be represented schematically like this:

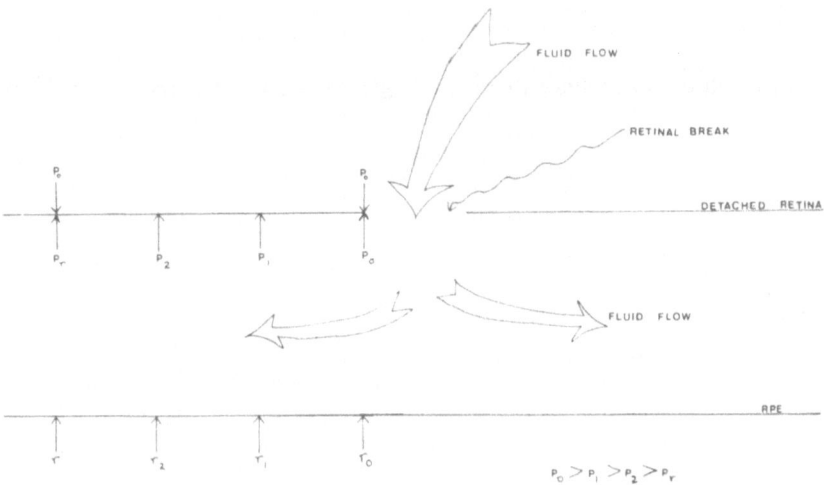

Fig.4

Since $P_0 > P_2$ the retina will be pushed towards the RPE at r_2 by a pressure equal to $P_0 - P_2$.

The mean velocity (U_m) for two dimensional flow through a straight channel at a section far from its ends is (Goldstein, 1965):

$$U_m = \frac{-h^2}{3\mu} \frac{\partial p}{\partial r}$$

where $h = \frac{1}{2}$ the width of the channel,
μ = a measure of viscosity, and
δp = the partial derivate describing the change in the pressure (δP) as we go downstream (δr). Here we ignore the complexities of two dimensional flow in the inlet length.

In our particular situation, all the fluid must flow through the retinal break and will be assigned the velocity U_0 at that point. As the fluid flows through the retinal break $U_0 = U_m$. As the fluid spreads out between the plates its

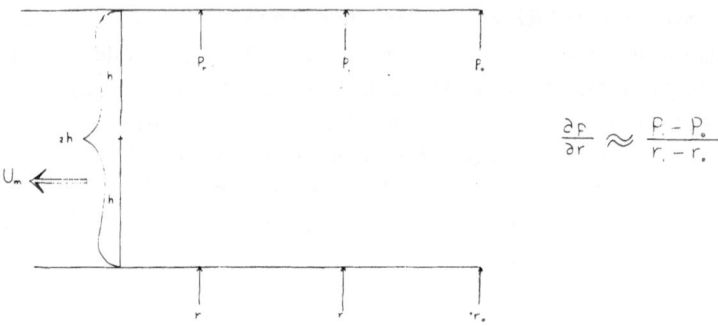

$$\frac{\partial P}{\partial r} \approx \frac{P_r - P_o}{r_r - r_o}$$

Fig. 5

velocity will diminish since there is a larger cross-sectional area for the fluid to flow through:

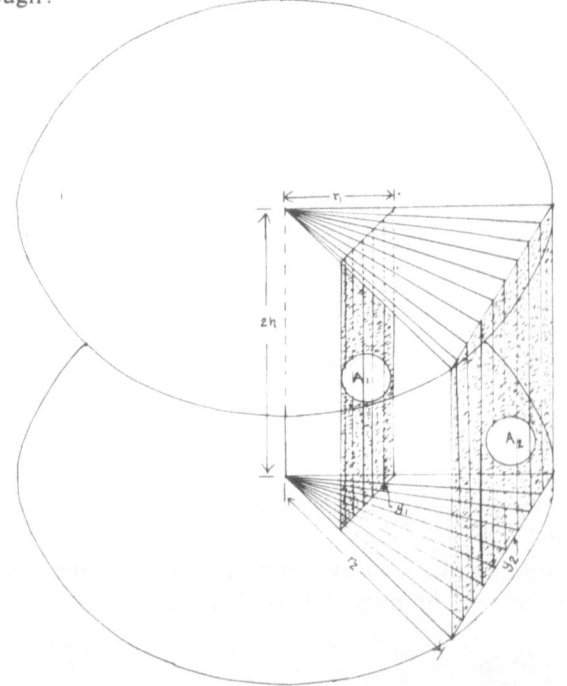

Fig. 6

cross sectional area 1 = A_1 = 2h y_1
cross-sectional area 2 = A_2 = 2h y_2

From the law of similar triangles, we can see the $\dfrac{r_1}{r_2} = \dfrac{y_1}{y_2}$. Since 2 h is constant

$\dfrac{A_2}{A_1} = \dfrac{r_2}{r_1}$. Since the fluids velocity will decrease by the amount it has to spread out we have:

$$\frac{U_2}{U_1} = \frac{A_1}{A_2} = \frac{r_1}{r_2}$$

68

Thus U_m is a function of r described by:

$$U_m = \frac{U_0 r_0}{r} \text{ as long as } r > 0$$

We thus have:

$$\frac{U_0 r_0}{r} = \frac{-h^2}{3\mu} \frac{\partial P}{\partial r}$$

Integrating:

$$\int_{P_0}^{P_r} d_P = \int_{r_0}^{r} - \frac{U_0 r_0}{r} \frac{3\mu}{h^2} d_r$$

We obtain:

$$P_r - P_0 = \frac{3\mu U_0 r_0}{h^2} \log\left(\frac{r_0}{r}\right)$$

We may replace U_0 by the volume flow rate (Q) throw the cylindrical cross sectional area at the edge of the hole:

$$U_0 = \frac{Q}{2\pi r_0} (2\,h)$$

Later it will be useful to replace Q by the choroidal resorption rate per unit area (C) times the area of the choroid or RPE (A) exposed by the detached retina.

$$\text{Thus } Q = CA, \text{ and } U_0 = \frac{CA}{4\pi r_0 h}$$

$$\text{Thus: } P_r - P_0 = \frac{3\mu CA}{4\pi h^3} \log\left(\frac{r}{r_0}\right)$$

For a cylindrical buckle of radius R we can obtain the reattachment force (F) over the crest of the buckle by integrating over the area:

$$F = \int (P_r - P_0)\, dA = \frac{3\mu CA}{4\pi h^3} \int_{r_0}^{R} \log\left(\frac{r}{r_0}\right) d\,(\pi r^2)$$

The reattachment force over the crest of the buckle is then:

$$F = \frac{3\mu CA\, r_0^2}{4h^3} \left\{ \frac{R^2}{r_0^2}\left(\log\frac{R}{r_0} - \frac{1}{2}\right) + \frac{1}{2} \right\}$$

69

If the detachment is much larger than the crest of the buckle, the reattachment force over the whole detachment will be substantially greater. Nevertheless, the reapproximating force over the crest of the buckle is the clinically important quantity, since we know that if the hole is flat on the crest of the buckle the remaining subretinal fluid will eventually be reabsorbed.

A number of interesting observations arise from the expression for reattachment force. (1) Since the lift force is proportioned to $1/h^3$, halving the distance between the retina and the buckle will increase the reapproximating lift force by a factor of 8. (2) The lift force is directly proportional to the viscosity (μ), the choroidal absorption rate per unit area (C), and the area under the detachment (A). Doubling μ, C, or A will double the reapproximating force. (3) The relationship between the lift force and the radius of the buckle (R) and the radius of the hole (r_0) is more complex. Basically the reapproximating force increases very rapidly as R increases and as r_0 decreases as long as the buckle is larger than the hole ($R > r_0$).

Graphically this may be represented:

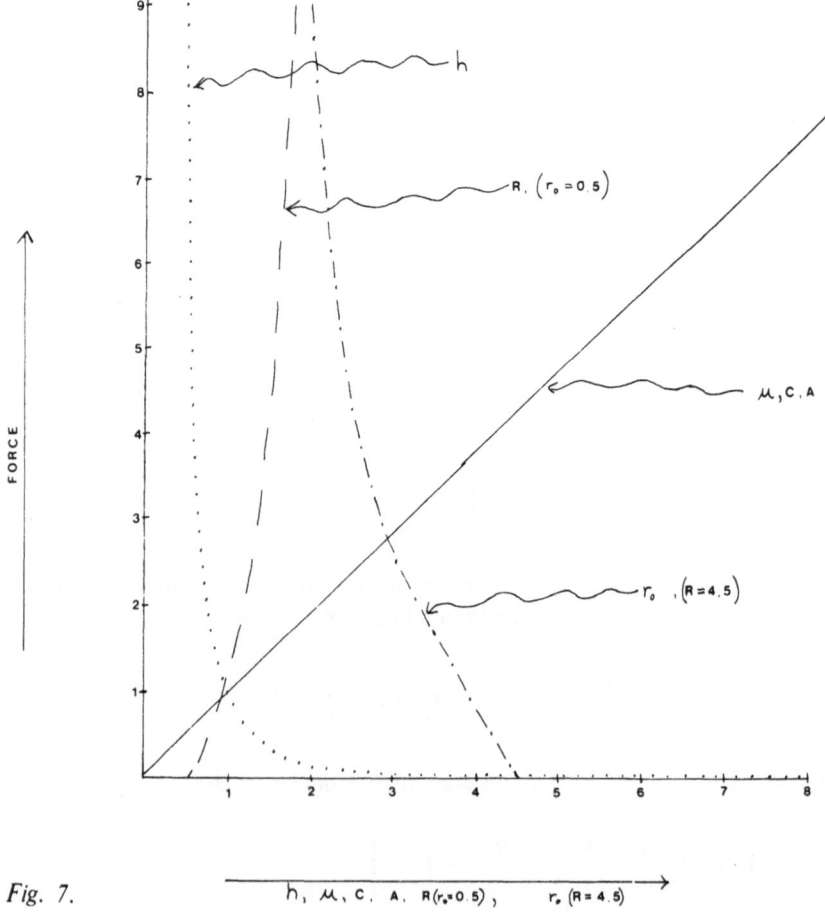

Fig. 7.

These findings correlate well with clinical experience. Since the reapproximating force falls off as the inverse square of the height of the break above the buckle, a relatively sharp cut-off may be expected in the height at which reapproximating force will regularly exceed residual detaching forces. O'Connor found this distance to be about 3 mm clinically. The prediction that reduced viscosity will reduce the reapproximating force correlated with Rosengren's experimental findings and his observation that reduced viscosity in myopes and aphakes may make them more vulnerable to detachment.

A reduced rate of RPE fluid absorption would give a decreased value of C. This would also reduce the reapproximating force proportionally. Escoffery and O'Connor have noted delayed absorption of SRF in senile choroidopathy.

AN ORDER OF MAGNITUDE CALCULATION OF THE RE-APPROXIMATING LIFT FORCE

The calculation of the lift force from the relationship derived above could only be regarded as an order of magnitude calculation of the re-approximating force because so many approximations have been made.

Let us calculate the reapproximating force (F) at the edge of a buckle with a radius (R) of 4.5 mm where the retinal break has a radius (r_0) of 0.5 mm.

The mean relative viscosity of normal owl monkey vitreous is 11.3 (Swan & Constable 1972). The relative viscosity of the vitreous aspirate in an owl monkey 40–180 days after a saline implant varies from 1.6 to 3.3 The later case is more likely to correspond to the viscosity of the vitreous fluid in the detached and syneretic vitreous of most patients with retinal detachments. The relative viscosity of water is 1 (Diem 1962). The absolute viscosity of water at 37 degrees celsius is 0.6947 centipoise (Hodgman 1945). The absolute viscosity of the owl monkey vitreous 180 days after saline implant would be 2.29 centipoise. For ease of calculation let us take $\mu = 2.0$ centipoise.

To calculate the volume of fluid absorbed per unit time we must use clinical experience. It is not uncommon for a one quadrant bullous detach-

←

Fig. 7

h = ½ height of retina above buckle.
μ = viscosity.
C = choroidal absorption rate per unit area.
A = area of RPE exposed by the detachment.
R = radius of a cylindrical buckle.
r_0 = radius of the retinal break.

71

ment to be completely flat 24 hours after buckling without closure of the retinal break.

To calculate the volume of SRF in such a detachment the following spherical approximation was made:

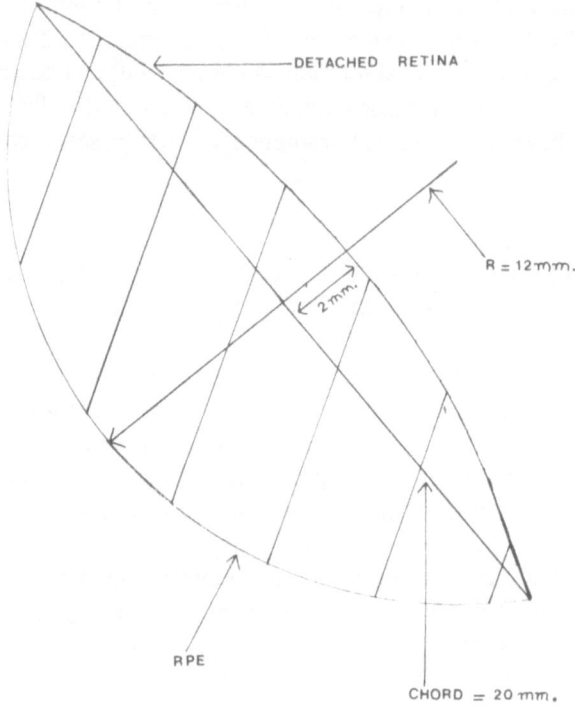

Fig. 8

The volume would then be 1242 mm³. The absorption would then be 52 mm³ hr. The area (A) of the exposed RPE = 405 mm². The rate of absorption by the RPE (C) would be 0.1278 mm³ of SRF absorbed per mm² of RPE per hour. The actual rate could be considerably higher for the healthy choroid since (1) larger volumes of detachment have been noted to flatten in 24 hours and (2) there would be some leakage through the break until it became closed against the RPE on the crest of the buckle.

If the retinal break is 1 mm above the RPE then h = 0.5 (since 2 h is the distance between the RPE and the retina).

The reapproximating force over the crest of the buckle is then:

$$F = \frac{3\,(2.0 \text{ centipoise})}{4\,(0.5 \text{ mm})^3} \left\{ \frac{0.1278 \text{ mm}^3}{\text{mm}^2 \text{ hour}} \right\} (405 \text{ mm}^2)(0.5 \text{ mm})^2 \times$$

$$\times \left\{ \left(\frac{4.5 \text{ mm}}{.5 \text{ mm}} \right)^2 \left\{ \left(\log \frac{4.5 \text{ mm}}{.5 \text{ mm}} \right) - \frac{1}{2} \right\} + \frac{1}{2} \right\}$$

72

$F = 5.95 \times 10^{-4}$ dynes.

If the break is 3 mm above the crest of the buckle, we have h = 1.5 mm and

$F = 2.20 \times 10^{-5}$ dynes.

If the break is 5 mm above the crest of the buckle, we have h = 2.5 mm and

$F = 4.76 \times 10^{-6}$ dynes.

According to O'Connors clinical observations, the detachment forces would frequently exceed the re-approximation force at this elevation of the break above the RPE. A rough estimate of the sum of the residual detachment forces would then be 1×10^{-5} dynes.

THE EFFECT OF CHORIORETINAL INJURY

Chorioretinal injury, e.g., cryopexy, diathermy, photocoagulation, has the major intended effect of making the post-operative chorioretinal adhesion very strong and water tight.

Chorioretinal injury would presumably destroy the capacity of the RPE to absorb SRF. As long as the chorioretinal injury is confined to the crest of the buckle and the total area of the detachment is substantially larger than the treated area the total choroidal reabsorption rate shouldn't be reduced very much. The reapproximating force would remain relatively undiminished.

Successful scleral buckling can be performed without chorioretinal injury (Zauberman & Rosell 1975). Drainage of SRF is usually employed. Although treatment of phakic cases is relatively successful, a high rate of re-detachment is reported in aphakic cases. Decreased viscosity in aphakia may be contributing to both increased detachment forces and decreased attachment forces.

Chorioretinal injury may induce a fibrin clot which would have the net effect of impeding the flow between the RPE and the retina or effectively narrowing the channel available for the SRF to flow through. The re-approximating force could be substantially increased by chorioretinal injury.

Protein exudation through the treated RPE could conceivably alter the viscosity locally. However, Robertson (1979) found no significant alteration in protein concentration of SRF analysed before and immediately after retinocryopexy in 3 patients.

SUMMARY

Retinal breaks up to 3 mm above the crest of a scleral buckle will reliably lead to retinal re-attachment. The RPE is thought to absorb subretinal fluid thereby inducing a 'lift' force which tends to re-approximate the retina to the scleral buckle. A mathematical expression for the re-approximating lift force is derived:

$$F = \frac{3\mu CA\, r_0^2}{4\, h^3} \left\{ \frac{R^2}{r_0^2} \left(\log \frac{R}{r_0} - \frac{1}{2} \right) + \frac{1}{2} \right\}.$$

An order of magnitude calculation of the lift force is made. An estimate of the order of magnitude of residual detachment forces is 10^{-5} dyne.

REFERENCES

Diem, K., Ed. Documenta Geigy Scientific Tables, 6th edition, Ardsley, New York, Geigy Pharmaceuticals, p. 548 (1962).

Escoffery, R. F., E. Okun & I. Boniuk. Vitreoretinal pathology in Retinal Detachment. International Ophthalmology Clinics, Vol. 16, No. 1, Boston, Little Brown and Co., pp. 45-62 (1976).

Fatt, I & K. Shantinath. Flow Conductivity of the Retina and Its Role in adhesions, Exp. Eye Res., 12: 218-226 (1971).

Gass, J. D. M. Stereoscopic Atlas of Macular Diseases. St. Louis, The C. V. Mosby Co., p. 20 (1977).

Goldstein, S. Modern Developments in Fluid Dynamics,. Vol. 1. New York, Dover Publications, Inc., p. 309 (1965).

Hodgman, C. D., Ed. Handbook of Chemistry and Physics, 29th edition. Cleveland, Chemical Rubber Publishing Co., p. 1686 (1945).

Kolker, A. E. & J. Hetherington. Becker and Shaffer's Diagnosis and Therapy of the Glaucomas. St. Louis, The C. V. Mosby Co. p.99 (1970).

Leaver, P. V., G. H. Chester & S. H. Saunders. Factors Influencing Absorption of Subretinal Fluid. Brit. J. Ophthal. 60: 557 (1976).

Lincoff, H. & R. Gieser. Finding the Retinal Hole. Arch. Ophthal. 85: 565 (1971).

Lincoff, H. & I. Kreissig. The Treatment of Retinal Detachment without Drainage of Subretinal Fluid. Tr. Amer. Acad. Ophth. and Otol. 76: 1221 (1972).

Lincoff, H., I. Kreissig & M. Goldbaum. Selection of Patients for Nondrainage Operations, Chapter 30 in: Retina Congress, ed. by R. C. Pruett & C. D. J. Regan. New York, Appleton-Century-Crafts, pp. 397-412 (1972).

Maurice, D. M., J. Salmon & H. Zauberman. Subretinal Pressure and Retinal Adhesion. Exp. Eye Res. 12: 212-217 (1971).

O'Connor, P. R. Absorption of Subretinal Fluid after External Scleral Buckling without Drainage. Amer. J. Ophthal 76: 30 (1973).

O'Connor, P. R. Absorption of Subretinal Fluid with External Buckling without Drainage. Amer J. Ophthal. 76: 30 (1973).

O'Connor, P. R., External Buckling without Drainage in Retinal Detachment. International Ophthalmology Clinics, Vol. 16, No. 1, Boston, Little Brown and Co., pp. 107-126 (1976).

Rachal, W. F. & T. C. Burton. Changing Concepts of Failures after Retinal Detachment Surgery. Arch. Ophthal. 97: 480 (1979).

Robertson, D. M. Delayed Absorption of Subretinal Fluid After Scleral Buckling Procedures. Amer. J. Ophthal. 87: 57-64 (1979).

Rosengren, B., Discussion to Fison: Observations on Retinal Detachments. Trans. Ophthal. Soc. U.K. 75: 43-50 (1950).

Rosengren, B. & S. Osterlin. Hydrodynamic Events in the Vitreous Space Accompanying Eye Movements. Ophthalmologica (Basel) 173: 513-524 (1976).

Swann, D. A. & I. J. Constable. Vitreous Structure II, Role of Hyaluronate. Investig Ophthal. 11: 164 (1972).

Teng, C. C & H. H. Chi. Vitreous Changes and the Mechanism of Retinal Detachment. Amer. J. Ophthal. 44: 335 (1957).

van Heuven, W. A. J & W. K. W. Larn.

Aqueous Humor as the Origin of Subretinal Fluid, ARVO, 1978, 50th Program Abstracts. The Association for Research in Vision and Ophthalmology, Inc., Sarosota, Florida, p.268 (1978).

Zauberman, H. & H. de Guillebron. Retinal Traction *in vivo* and Postmortem. Arch Ophthal. 87: 549 (1972).

Zauberman, H., H. de Guillebron & F. J. Holly. Retinal Traction in Vitro Biophysical Aspects. Investig Ophthal. 11: 46-55 (1972).

Zimmerman, L. E. & A. B. Eastham. Acid Mucopolysaccharide in the Retinal Pigment Epithelium and Visual Cell Layer of the Developing Mouse Eye. Amer. J. Ophthal. 47: 488 (1959).

Zauberman, H. & F. G. Rosell. Treatment of Retinal Detachment without Inducing Chorioretinal Lesions. J. Amer. Acad. Ophth. and Otol. 79: 835 (1975).

Author's address:
University of South Carolina
Department of Surgery
3321 Medical Park Rd., Suite 300
Columbia, South Carolina 29203
U.S.A.

METABOLIC FACTORS IN THE MAINTENANCE
OF RETINAL ADHESION

MICHAEL F. MARMOR, D. SCOTT COHEN &
AZIZ S. ABDUL-RAHIM

(*Stanford and Palo Alto, California, U.S.A.*)

ABSTRACT

The resorption of subretinal fluid was studied by injecting small amounts of fluid under the retina of intact rabbit eyes, and measuring how long the fluid persisted. Retinal adhesion was studied by measuring the force required to peel strips of rabbit retina from the pigment epithelium within a physiologic bathing medium. Both the resorption of subretinal fluid and the peeling force were enhanced by exposure to ouabain, inhibited by exposure to cyanide, and inhibited by the replacement of the physiological medium with normal saline. Thus, dual metabolic systems may hydrate and dehydrate the subretinal space, and normal saline lacks some factor important to the maintenance of adhesion.

INTRODUCTION

As aspect of ocular physiology which has received relatively little attention, beyond the pioneering experiments by Zauberman and colleagues (Zauberman & Berman 1969; Maurice, Salmon & Zauberman 1971; deGuillebon & Zauberman 1972; Zauberman & deGuillebon 1972) is the mechanism of adhesion between the photoreceptors and the retinal pigment epithelium (RPE). These layers are embryonically distinct, and even in the adult when they are apposed, no anatomic junctions have ever been demonstrated between them in mammals. They are not irrevocably glued to one another, however, since separation occurs in a variety of ophthalmic disorders ranging from focal and transient separations (e.g. central serous retinopathy) to more severe and potentially permanent separations (e.g. rhegmatogenous detachment or the detachment after an osmotic load in the vitreous [Marmor 1979]). What forces normally keep the retina in place, and what factors allow it to detach under the stress of disease? What factors allow subretinal fluid to be rapidly resorbed when a retinal hole is sealed? Hydrostatic, osmotic, electrical, and metabolic forces act continually upon the subretinal space, and

Supported in part by National Eye Institute Grant EYO1678 and by the Medical Research Section of the Veterans Administration.

77

we have attempted in a recent series of experiments (Marmor 1979; Marmor, Abdul-Rahim & Cohen 1980), to define some of the mechanisms which normally influence retinal adhesion.

METHODS

Experiments were performed on Dutch rabbits anesthetized with pentobarbital.

Focal *in vivo* detachments were produced by inserting a glass micropipette filled with control or experimental solution through a hole in the pars plana, and advancing it to make contact with the retina so that a small amount of fluid could be injected into the subretinal space (Fig. 1). The minute hole produced by the 15–25 μ tip of the pipette sealed spontaneously, and any blebs in which there was significant tearing of the retina were rejected. Typical blebs had a diameter of 1–3 mm; they were observed with an operating microscope until the subretinal fluid had resorbed, as judged by visibility of the RPE mosaic. Ames' solution (Ames, Tsukada & Nesbett 1967) or Hanks' solution (Grand Island Biological 402S) were used as controls, and compared with the effects of using normal saline or of adding metabolic inhibitors.

The measurement of peeling force was based upon techniques initially developed by deGuillebon & Zauberman (1972), but modified to insure that tissues were maintained and peeled at 37 °C within a control or experimental

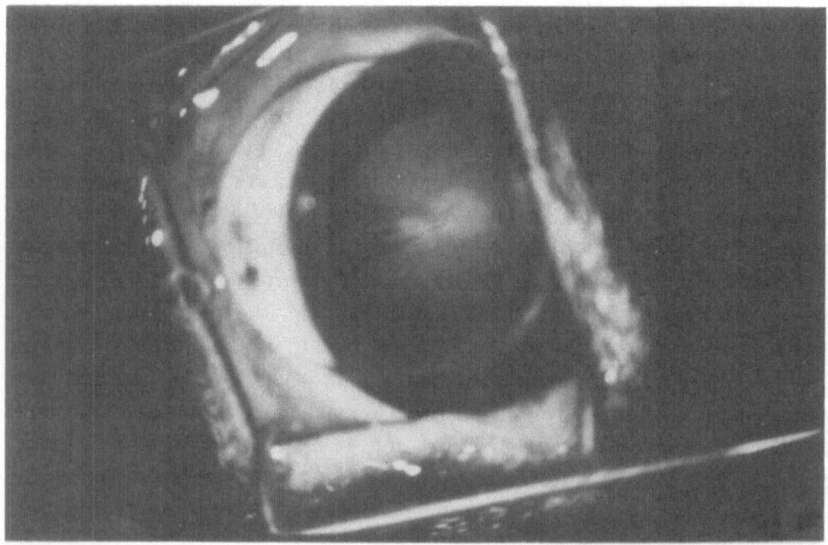

Fig. 1. Rabbit fundus, viewed through a contact lens. A glass micropipette enters near the pars plana and contacts the retina, forming a small bleb.

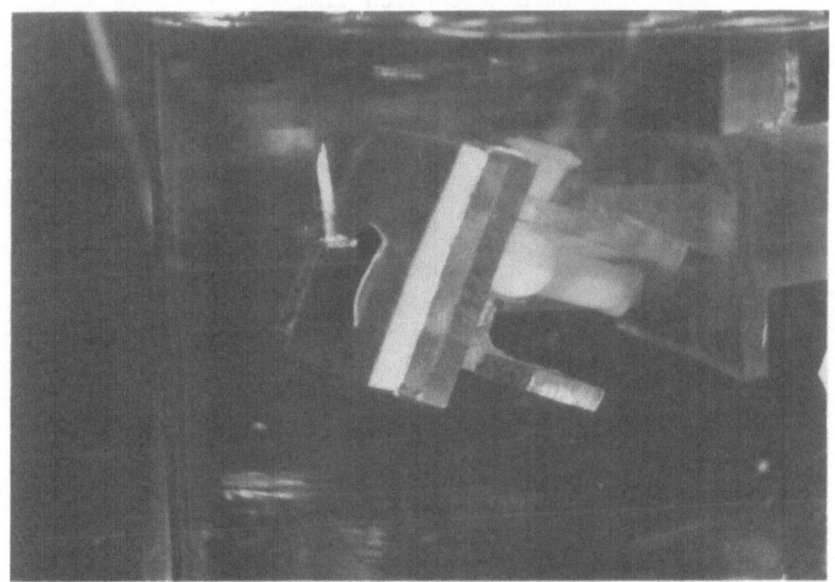

Fig. 2. Retina being peeled from the RPE within a beaker of fluid.

tissue culture medium. Strips of eyecup were mounted to a small plate which could be immersed in a beaker containing the tissue culture medium. A probe from a delicate force transducer (Harvard Instruments model 363) was glued to the retinal surface with cyanoacrylate, and slowly pulled away at an angle of 23° (Fig. 2). Once the retina began to peel, the recordings showed a steady level of force for 15 to 30 sec.

RESULTS

Focal in vivo *detachments*

Blebs made with either Hanks' or Ames' solutions usually persisted for 1–4 hours. Interestingly, the resorption time in a control series of 38 blebs was not related to bleb area. This probably reflects the fact that most blebs had the shape of a flattened dome rather than a spherical segment so that their height did not vary a great deal. Since blebs within each eye tended to resorb in about the same period of time, experimental conditions were only compared with control blebs in the same eye.

Figure 3 shows the effect on bleb resorption time of forming the blebs with various saline media or with fluid containing cyanide or ouabain. The addition of cyanide to Ames' solution slowed down bleb resorption by 29%, but the addition of ouabain to Hanks' solution speeded up resorption. The

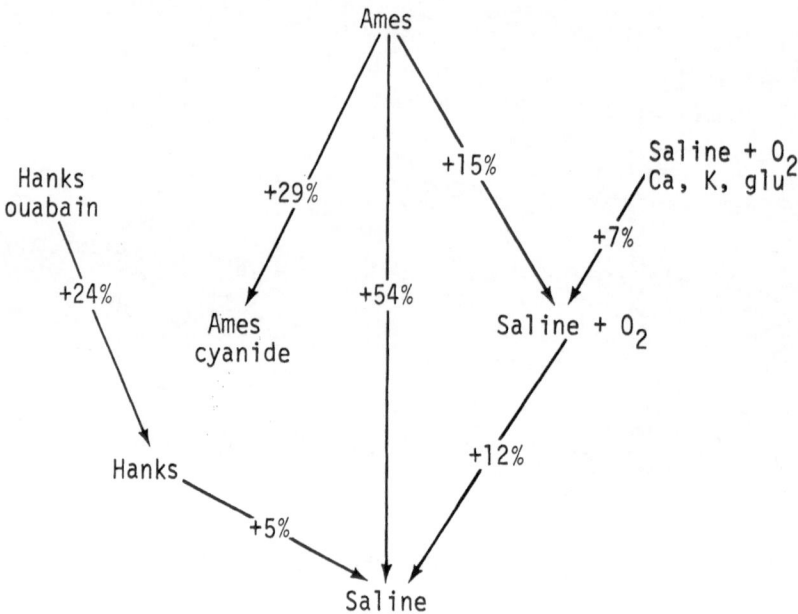

Fig. 3. Relative speed of resorption for blebs filled with different solutions (expressed as the percentage of additional time required by the slower of each pair).

replacement of Ames' solution (which is normally oxygenated to maintain its pH) with normal saline slowed resorption by a remarkable 54%, but the results of various changes in the saline solution were somewhat inconclusive. Oxygenation appears to be a factor, but changes in ionic concentration also have an influence and further experiments will be needed to clarify these relationships.

The fact that filling blebs with ouabain-containing solution speeded up resorption of that fluid was of particular interest, since Zauberman (1972) has reported that retinal adhesion is markedly weakened 12 hours after an intervitreal injection of ouabain. To duplicate his conditions, we injected .05 ml of 10^{-3} ouabain into the vitreous, and waited 12 hours before trying to raise blebs. Unlike the more acute ouabain experiments, we found that fluid from the micropipette now diffused freely under the retina as if the attachment force was nil.

In vitro *peeling experiments*

Peeling forces were first compared between tissues peeled under fluid, or peeled in the air, to evaluate the effects of surface tension. Using 6.5 mm

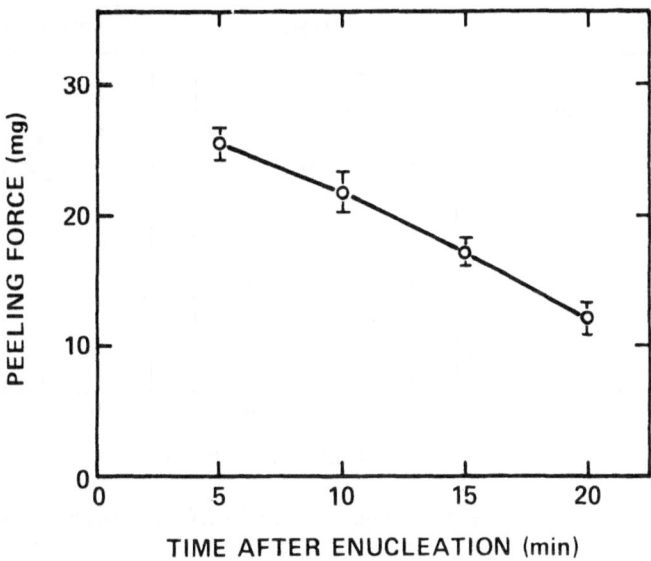

Fig. 4. Force required to peel retina from the RPE in Ames' solution at different times after enucleation.

strips of retina and peeling at 8.7 mm per min, the average force was 125 mg in air and only 25 mg under fluid. However, if the retina peeled in air was allowed to fall back upon the surface of the RPE, the average force upon peeling it a second time was still 59 mm. This can only be accounted for by surface tension. Thus, much of the force recorded in air is probably artifactual, and measurements under fluid mimic more closely the situation inside the eye.

In all subsequent experiments, we used care to keep the tissues within a culture medium, and to take our measurements as soon as possible after enucleation. Nonetheless, the force required to peel 5 mm strips of retina from the RPE at 24 mm/min fell from about 25 mg at 5 min after enucleation, to 12 mg after 20 min (Fig. 4). If this result were dependent on non-specific death of the tissue, one would predict that metabolic inhibitors would accelerate the deterioration. We found appropriately (Fig. 5) that tissues maintained in a cyanide solution required about 5 mg less peeling force than controls throughout the period studied. However, tissue maintained in ouabain solution required slightly *greater* force than the controls, at all times after enucleation. Non-metabolic factors may be even more significant than metabolic ones in controlling the adhesive forces: tissues maintained in normal saline showed much weaker adhesion (10 to 15 mg lower at all times) than tissues maintained in the more complete physiological medium of oxygenated Ames' solution.

The long term effect of inhibitors on the peeling force was somewhat different. In several animals, .05 cc of 10^{-3} M ouabain, 6×10^{-3} M cyanide

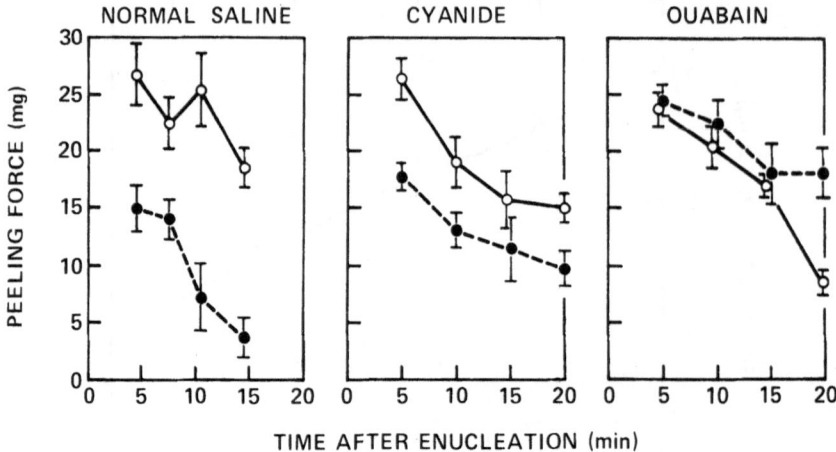

Fig. 5. Force required to peel retina from the RPE in different media (closed circles) relative to Ames' solution (open circles). Cyanide: $3 \times 10^{-3\,M}$; ouabain: $5 \times 10^{-4\,M}$.

or 10^{-3} M dinitrophenol was injected into the midvitreous 12 hours before removing the eyes for measurement of the peeling force. The peeling force for eyes injected with cyanide and dinitrophenol was equal to that of the controls, but the peeling force for eyes injected with ouabain was virtually zero (in contrast to the short term effect of ouabain, which was an increase in adhesive force). Electron micrographs of the peeled retina from a ouabain

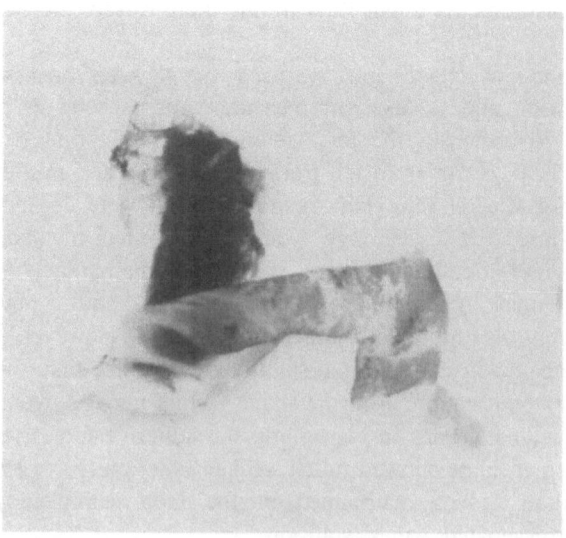

Fig. 6. Fragment of retina peeled from the RPE after 1 hour in Ames' solution plus 5×10^{-4} M ouabain. Firmness of adhesion is shown by the retained RPE pigment.

82

eye showed that separation of the retina had occurred primarily *through* these outer segments, which were severely swollen and fragmented.

To corroborate these observations, we placed freshly enucleated fragments of eyecup into petri dishes containing 37° Ames' solution with and without ouabain. Within 10 min, the retinas maintained in Ames' solution could be peeled cleanly from the RPE, and by 60 min they almost floated off. However, the retinas maintained in ouabain showed a gradual opacification of the retina between 30 and 60 min and were difficult to separate even after 1 hour (Fig. 6). Scanning electron micrographs showed that control retinas separated at the subretinal space, while ouabain-treated retinas had severe receptor damage but were sufficiently adherent that separation took place mostly by rupture of the RPE cells or the outer segments.

DISCUSSION

We have described two new techniques for study of retinal apposition and adhesion. One measures the time required for the resorption of fluid under a small detachment, and depends upon systems which remove fluid from the subretinal space. The second measures the force required to peel retina from the RPE within a fluid medium, and depends upon the firmness of attachment. Subretinal fluid resorption and retinal adhesion are not identical phenomena and do not *a priori* require the same physiological conditions, but it is interesting that they were altered by similar factors in these experiments. We may postulate that the active resorption of subretinal fluid tightens the subretinal space and thus enhances the force of adhesion.

Why does ouabain, which blocks the important metabolic function of sodium-potassium exchange across the cell membrane, speed up the resorption of retinal fluid? This initially puzzling observation is not so surprising in terms of the normal ionic movements across the pigment epithelium. The sodium pump produces a net movement of sodium out of the cell interior, and water is obligatorily carried along. Since the pump is active in the apical membrane of the RPE (Miller & Steinberg 1977), inhibition of the pump will reduce a normal movement of fluid towards the retina, and thereby enhance the resorption of fluid out of the subretinal space by other mechanisms. The possibility that dual metabolic systems are moving fluid in and out of the subretinal space may explain why cyanide acts to slow down subretinal fluid resorption rather than speed it up. Cyanide is a non-specific respiratory inhibitor, and would block not only the sodium pump but also the metabolic systems which normally move fluid *out* of the subretinal space and which normally must be dominant. Bicarbonate transport systems may also be expected to affect the resorption of fluid from subretinal blebs, and experiments are in progress to determine the effects of acetazolamide on our two models.

We were surprised to find that normal saline had greater effect in slowing the resorption of subretinal fluid than any of the toxins used. Oxygenation of the fluid injected into a bleb seems a significant factor, although judging by the data in Fig. 1, it does not account for all of the effect. Other possible factors such as pH, or the presence of a critical anion or cation, are being investigated.

The fact that a peeling force can be measured in excised tissues shows that structures or processes at the RPE-photoreceptor level contribute significantly to retinal adhesion, and that retinal apposition cannot be attributed solely to hydrostatic or osmotic pressure. The peeling force that we measured in fluid was small, typically only 25 mg for the earliest recordings after enucleation. This value is less than others (Zauberman & Berman 1969; deGuillebon & Zauberman 1972; Zauberman 1972; Lincoff & Kreissig 1979) have obtained in peeling experiments, but differences in technique prevent a close comparison. Furthermore, although this force may seem small, it actually represents a considerable adhesiveness since peeling only measures the force along a thin line of separation, whereas retina is normally adherent over a two-dimensional area.

The purpose of maintaining tissue in a physiologic medium was not only to simulate the fluid environment of the eye, but to eliminate or minimize the effects of tissue death. Investigators who work with isolated retina know how quickly the retinal adhesion weakens after death. Our tissue culture medium clearly slowed the deterioration, relative to maintenance of the tissues in a less suitable medium such as normal saline. However, even in Ames' solution the peeling force dropped steadily over 20 minutes. These results caution that *in vitro* data on retinal adhesion are of questionable validity unless the effects of death, and the time after death, are carefully noted and accounted for.

Zauberman (1972) reported that retinal adhesion was greatly reduced 12 hours after an intravitreal injection of ouabain. Thus, we were surprised initially to find tht ouabain enhanced the force required to peel retina *in vitro*. Our longer term experiments explain the discrepancy. Ouabain is especially toxic to the photoreceptors, which have a very active sodium pump, and gross degeneration is visible after about 30 min of exposure. Thus, although the adherence of the RPE microvilli to the outer segments seems to be enhanced, presumably because subretinal fluid resorption is enhanced, the retina can separate easily by fragmentation of the photoreceptors themselves.

These experiments show clearly that an interaction of metabolic, physiologic, and probably physical factors are required to maintain retinal adhesion and to insure the resorption of fluid from the subretinal space. If we can define these specific factors more precisely, we may ultimately be able to modify retinal adhesion – or retinal detachment – by medical means.

REFERENCES

Ames, A., III, Y. Tsukada & F.B. Nesbett. Intracellular Cl^-, Na^+, K^+, Ca^{2+}, Mg^{2+} and P in nervous tissue; response to glutamate and to changes in extracellular calcium. J. Neurochem. 14: 145-159 (1967).

deGuillebon, H. & H. Zauberman. Experimental retinal detachment. Arch. Ophthalmol. 87: 545-548 (1972).

Lincoff, H. & I. Kreissig. Cryogenic and thermal effect on the retinal pigment epithelium. In: The Retinal Pigment Epithelium, ed. K. Zinn and M.F. Marmor, Cambridge, Harvard University Press, PP. 314-333, 1979.

Marmor, M.F. Mechanisms of retinal adhesion and the function of detached retina. In XXIII concilium Ophthalmologicum, Kyoto 1978, Acta. Ed. K. Shimizu, Amsterdam, Excerpta Medica, PP. 712-714, 1979.

Marmor, M.F. Retinal detachment from hyperosmotic intravitreal injection Invest. Ophthalmol. Vis. Sci. 18: 1237-1244 (1979).

Marmor, MF., A.S. Abdul-Rahim & D.S. Cohen. The effect of metabolic inhibitors on retinal adhesion and subretinal fluid resorption. Invest. Ophthalmol. Vis. Sci. In press (1980).

Maurice, D.M., J. Salmon & H. Zauberman: Subretinal pressure and retinal adhesion. Exp. Eye Res. 12: 212-217 (1971).

Miller, S.S. & R.H. Steinberg. Active transport of ions across frog retinal pigment epithelium. Exp. Eye Res. 25: 235-248 (1977).

Zauberman, H. Measurement of retinal adhesion. Israel J. Med. Sci. 8: 1604-1614 (1972).

Zauberman, H. & E.R. Berman. Measurement of adhesive forces between the sensory retina and the pigment epithelium. Exp. Eye Res. 8: 276-283 (1969).

Zauberman, H. & H. deGuillebon. Retinal traction in vivo and postmortem. Arch. Ophthalmol. 87: 549-554 (1972).

Authors' addresses:

Division of Ophthalmology
Stanford University School of
  Medicine
Stanford, California 94305
U.S.A.

and

Ophthalmology Section
Veterans Administration Medical
  Center
Palo Alto, California 94304
U.S.A.

Requests for reprints:
Ophthalmology Section (112B1)
Veterans Administration Medical Center
Palo Alto, California 94304
U.S.A.

TRACER MOVEMENT ACROSS
THE RABBIT RETINA

H. MOSELEY & W.S. FOULDS
(Glasgow, U.K.)

ABSTRACT

Labeled xenon and water move rapidly from the vitreous across the retina and are removed by the choroidal vessels. Between 80 and 100% of the tracer in the mid-vitreous is removed through this pathway. A diffusional mechanism accounts for the results of this study.

INTRODUCTION

The flow of fluid across the retina has been implicated as a possible mechanism for retinal attachment. (Fatt & Shantinath 1971). Moreover, the existence or otherwise of fluid movement across the retina has obvious implications in the formation and drainage of sub-retinal fluid. However, little is known about water movement *in vivo* across the retina. The present experiments were designed to provide basic information which is fundamental to an understanding of fluid dynamics across the retina.

Studies were performed using two radioactive tracers, viz. xenon-133 dissolved in saline and tritiated water. Xenon was used so that a mathematical model could be formulated and compared with the experimental results for this inert molecule. When it was established that the model and experiment were sufficiently close for xenon, the relevant parameters for tritiated water were put into the model.

The hypothesis was that these substances cross the retina from the vitreous and are subsequently removed by the choroidal circulation. The current experiments were designed to test this hypothesis.

MATERIALS AND METHODS

Six Dutch rabbits weighing between 1.7 kg and 2.3 kg were used in the xenon study. Experiments were performed on living animals under general urethane anaesthesia. Twenty-five microCuries of xenon-133 dissolved in 25 µl of saline were injected into the centre of the vitreous of the eye under

87

study. One of the four vortex veins which drain the choroid was cut and the blood was collected using absorbent paper tissue in small glass vials. The vials were changed every two minutes throughout the duration of the experiment and were heat-sealed. All of the blood leaving the vortex vein was collected by this procedure. The xenon-133 activity present in the tubes was determined using a well counter.

In the tritiated water experiments, six Dutch rabbits weighing between 1.6 kg and 2.2 kg were studied using general urethane anaesthesia. Twenty-five microlitres, containing 25 µCi of tritiated water were injected into a mid-vitreal position through the sclera. Blood was collected from an exposed vortex vein using a capillary pipette. As before, all the blood leaving the vortex vein was collected by this procedure. The blood was emptied into scintillation vials and prepared by a wet oxidation technique for radio-assay by liquid scintillation counting (Mahin & Lofberg 1966).

A mathematical model was developed in which a 25 µl volume representing the tracer was allowed to move from the vitreous into the surrounding tissue by diffusion with removal occurring in the choroid. Mean transit time was computed from the model using published values of the diffusion coefficients of xenon in ocular tissue (Strang 1977) and estimated values for water (Wang 1965).

RESULTS

In each of the xenon-133 experiments, isotope was detected in the blood leaving the vortex vein thus showing that transfer had occurred from the vitreous. It was of interest to quantify this movement and measure the rate at which it occurred. The rate of transfer was determined by calculating the mean transit time which is the average time for tracer movement between the injection point in the vitreous and the tube collecting the blood from the choroid. The experiments lasted between 42 minutes and 80 minutes and each two minute blood sample contained, on average, 0.18 ml (Table 1). Comparing the total counts of xenon in each experiment with known stan-

Table 1. Results: Xenon-133

	Duration of experiment (min)	Amount of Xenon in vortex vein (%)	Mean transit time (min)	Volume of blood in 2 mins. (ml)
Mean	61	20	28	0.18
Standard deviation	15	9	5	0.11
Standard error	6	4	2	0.04

dards, the percentage of the isotope injected into the vitreous which was subsequently collected in the blood leaving the vortex vein was obtained. The mean for the six experiments was 20% and the standard error 4%. At the end of each experiment, the eye was enucleated and the number of vortex veins determined. Each eye was found to possess four vortex veins in accordance with that observed by others (Prince 1964). On the assumption that the total amount of xenon leaving the eye in the choroidal blood was four times that in a single vortex vein (Bill 1962), to an accuracy of 16%, 80% of the xenon in the vitreous left the eye by this route. Further analysis revealed that the average of the mean transit times was 28 ± 2 minutes.

Tritiated water was detected in the blood in the second series of experiments showing that transfer of tracer had taken place between the vitreous and the blood of the choroid. The total amount of isotope collected and the mean transit time were calculated. All the experiments apart from the first lasted 80 minutes and the average volume of blood collected in two minutes was 0.26 ml (Table 2). Comparing the total tritiated water activity in each

Table 2. Results: Tritiated water

	Duration of experiment (min)	Amount of ^3H_2O in vortex vein (%)	Mean transit time (min)	Volume of blood in 2 mins (ml)
Mean	77	25	30	0.26
Standard deviation	8	11	5	0.13
Standard error	3	4	2	0.05

experiment with known standards, it was found that the mean percentage of tracer injected into the vitreous and subsequently collected from the blood leaving the vortex vein was $25 \pm 4\%$. At the termination of the experiments, four vortex veins were counted in the enucleated eyes. On the assumption that the total amount of isotope removed in the blood of the choroid was four times that in a single vortex vein, to an accuracy of 16% all of the tritiated water appeared to leave the eye by this route. The mean transit time was calculated for each experiment and the overall mean was 30 ± 2 minutes. Since it is expected that tritiated water behaves in a similar fashion to the ordinary water molecules in the vitreous, it is reasonable to conclude that the ordinary water molecules of the vitreous are in a similar dynamic state as the tracer molecules.

The mean transit time for xenon according to the mathematical model was 27 minutes and, for tritiated water, was 28 minutes (Table 3).

Table 3. Results: Mathematical model

Isotope	Mean transit time (min)
Xenon-133	27
Tritiated water	28

DISCUSSION

The experimental mean transit time for xenon was 28 ± 2 minutes and according to the model it was 27 minutes. Since the difference is small compared to the uncertainties of experiment and model, the mathematical analogue appears to be valid for the diffusion of xenon. The mean transit time for tritiated water by experiment was 30 ± 2 minutes and according to the model it was 28 minutes. These results also show good agreement between the model and experiment. From this it is concluded that the experimental results are consistent with the movement of water by diffusion.

Two points should be borne in mind in the interpretation of these results. Firstly, the consistency of the present results with a diffusional model does not prove that there were no other processes involved in the transfer of water. Some evidence has been presented for the existence of active transport of certain substances, such as organic anions, across the pigment epithelium (Cunha-Vaz & Maurice 1967; Miller and Steinberg 1977). If the water molecules were actively transported at any stage, this was not the limiting factor under the conditions of the experiments. Secondly, our results have shown the extent of a diffusional-limited movement from the vitreous into the choroid. It is not yet known if the outward diffusion across the retina is matched by an equal inward diffusion along the same route. It may be, for example, that the pigment epithelium exhibits diode-like properties in which an easy passage in one direction is not matched in the opposite direction.

These experiments lead to the following conclusions. There is a rapid movement of dissolved xenon and water from the vitreous across the retina with subsequent removal in the choroidal blood vessels. To an accuracy of 16%, between 80 and 100% of the tracer in the mid-vitreous is removed by this route and, finally the results for both isotopes are consistent with an explanation based on their movement by diffusion.

REFERENCES

Bill, A. Quantitative determination of uveal blood flow in rabbits. Arch. Ophthalmol. 67: 62 (1962).
Cunha-Vaz, J.G. & D.M. Maurice. The active transport of fluorescein by the retinal vessels and the retina. J. Physiol. 191: 467 (1967).

90

Fatt, I.& K. Shantinath. Flow conductivity of retina and its role in retinal adhesion. Exp. Eye Res. 12: 218 (1971).

Mahin, D. T. & R. T. Lofberg. A simplified method of sample preparation for determination of tritum, carbon-14, or sulfur-35 in blood or tissue by liquid scintillation counting. Analyt. Biochem. 16: 500 (1966).

Miller, S. S. & R. H. Steinberg. Active transport of ions across frog retinal pigment epithelium. Exp. Eye Res. 15: 235 (1977).

Prince, J. H. The Rabbit in Eye Research. Illinois: Charles C. Thomas (1964).

Strang, R. The determination of the diffusion coefficient of krypton in rabbit ocular tissue. Invest. Ophthalmol. 16: 83 (1977).

Wang, J. H. Self-diffusion coefficients of water. J. Phys. Chem. 69: 4412 (1965).

Authors' address:
Tennent Institute of Ophthalmology
Western Infirmary
Church Street
Glasgow
United Kingdom

PERFUSION OF THE CHORIOCAPILLARIES THROUGH THE VORTEX VEIN

H. ZAUBERMAN, N. SEGAL, S. PHOTIOU & E. BERMAN

(*Jerusalem, Israel*)

ABSTRACT

Perfusion of the choroid through the vortex vein of rabbits using disulphine blue dye and Indian ink showed that the two contrast materials penetrate easily the choriocapillaries. Tritiated retinol administered in the same way was incorporated rapidly into the pigment epithelium. Radioactivity of labeled retinol decreased rapidly in the RPE cytosol and thereafter its concentration increased in the microsomes, where esterification takes place.

The possibility of perfusing in vivo the choriocapillaries in a retrograde way, via the vortex vein, has been explored using the rabbit as an experimental

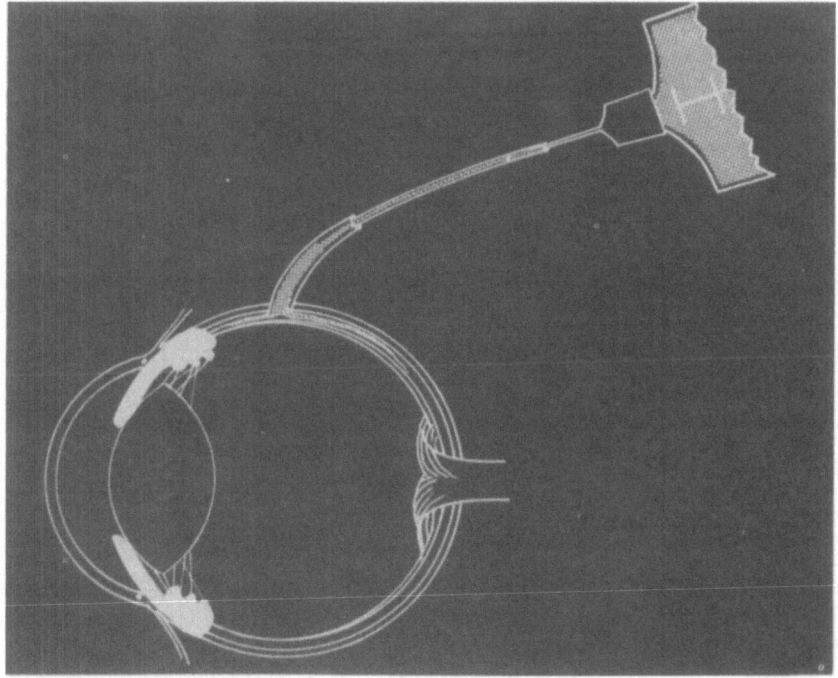

Fig. 1

Docum. Ophthal. Proc. Series, Vol. 25, ed. by H. Zauberman
© *1981, Dr. W. Junk bv Publishers, The Hague*

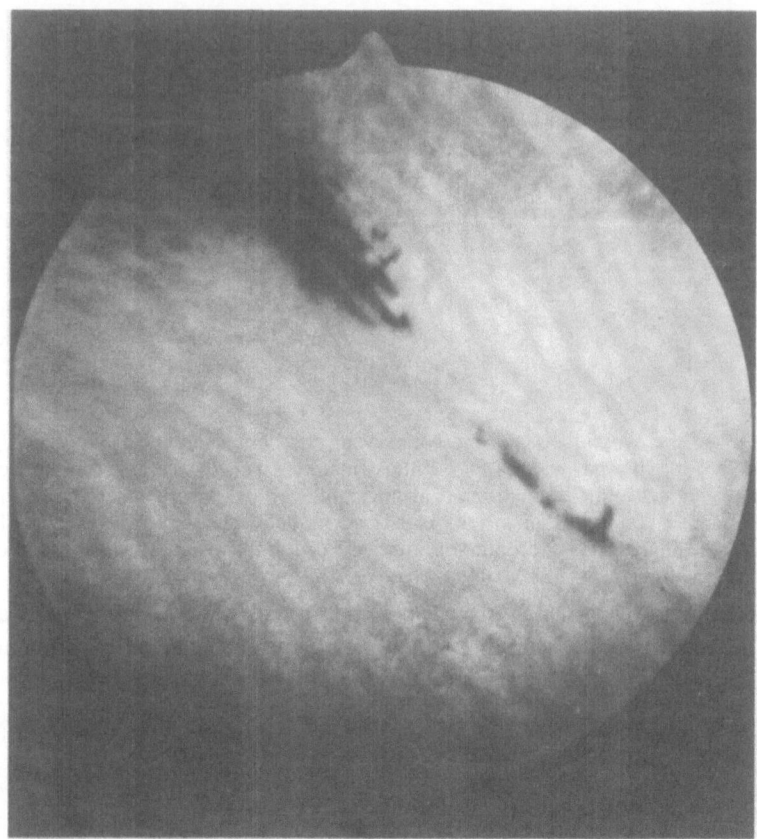

Fig. 2

animal. It is relatively easy to isolate, section and intubate with a fine polyethilene canula one of the nasal vortex veins of the rabbit (Fig. 1). If the hydrostatic pressure of the perfusing, colored fluid is 44 cm H_2O or more, the venous system of the choroid gets easily perfused. The heparinized normal saline stained with disulphine blue dye enters the choroidal veins (Figs. 2 and 3), and then the ball of dye perfuses and stains the optic disc (Fig. 4). Also the iris is stained (Fig. 5), since its circulation is drained in the rabbit by the vortex venous system.

Injection of Indian ink *in vivo* shows a similar perfusion pattern. It can be seen that the choriocapillaries fill well between the larger choroidal vessels (Fig. 6) and also around the optic nerve head (Fig. 7). Histology shows Indian ink filling the large and small choroidal vessels (Fig. 8).

These experiments with Indian ink show that particles injected through the nasal vortex veins of normal rabbits reach the choriocapillaries very

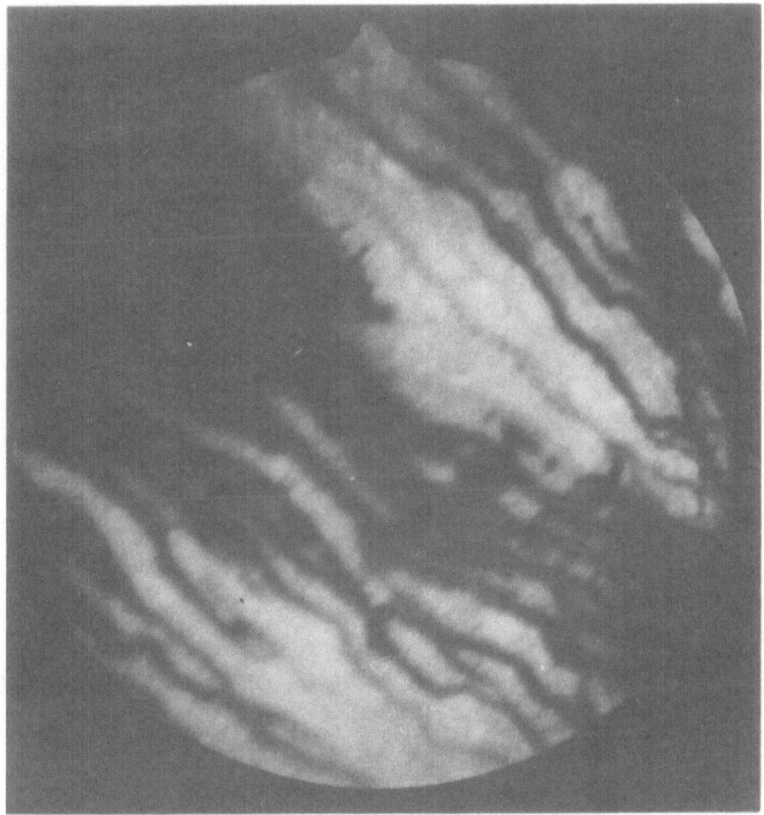

Fig. 3

quickly, but do not pass from the choroid into the pigment epithelium. To answer the question of whether physiological materials, for example blood nutrients, could enter the pigment epithelium when administered through this route, we would need a low molecular weight marker whose fate after injection could be accurately followed. Retinol seemed an ideal choice for this since previous studies in several other laboratories (Young & Bok 1970; Hall & Bok 1974; Hirosawa & Yamada 1976; Robison & Kuwabara 1977) have shown that radioactive retinol injected either intravenously or intraperitoneally finds its way to the pigment epithelium in a matter of minutes or hours, depending on the species used and the design of the experiment. Current theory holds that there are specific receptors on the basal surface of the pigment epithelium which bind the retinol-retinol binding protein that circulates in the blood. This complex does not however pass through the tight junctions of the pigment epithelial cells (Bok & Heller 1976). Rather, the retinol is released and passes into the pigment epithelial cell, while the pre-albumin-retinol binding protein of serum returns to the circulation.

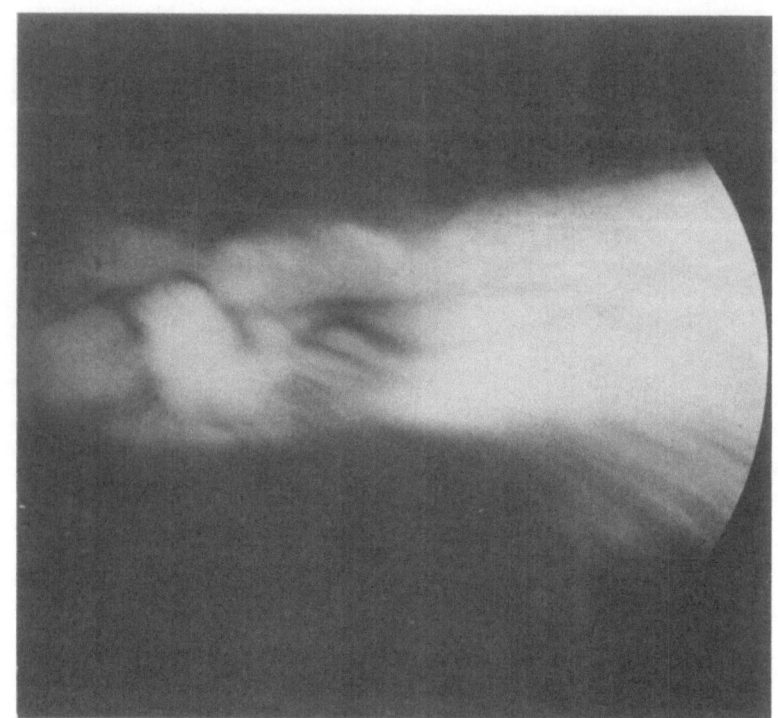

Fig. 4

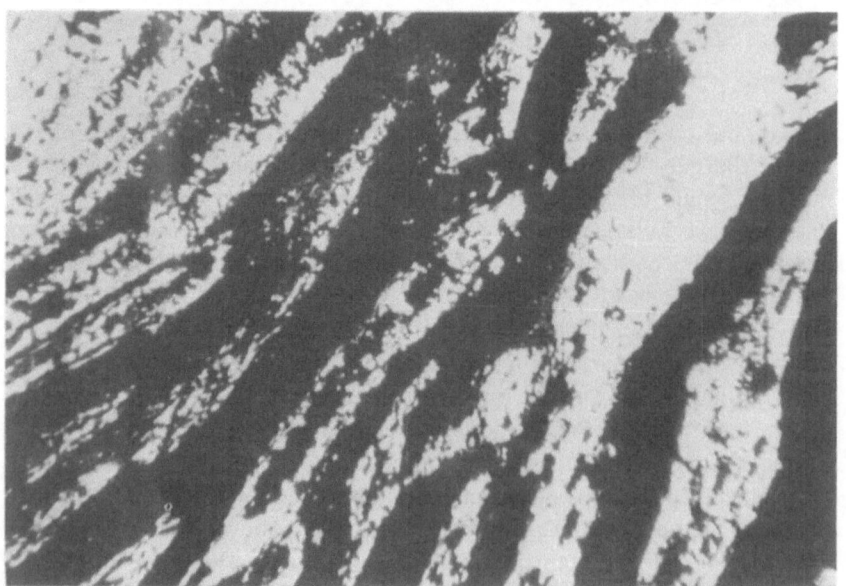

Fig. 5

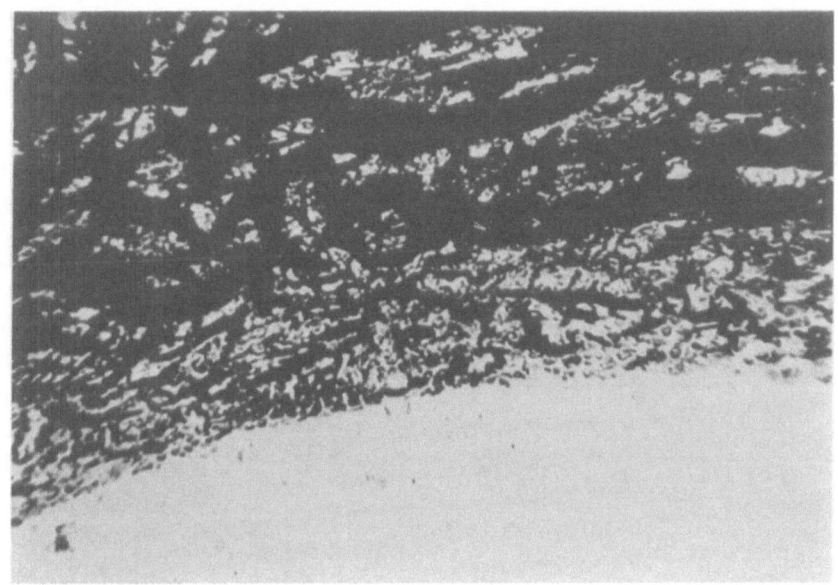

Fig. 6

The fate of retinol administered by perfusion of the vortex vein was studied in the following way: A small amount of tritiated retinol was preincubated with rabbit serum for one hour at room temperature in order to convert the vitamin A to a bound form resembling that present in circulating blood. Approximately 0.5 ml of this solution, containing disulfine blue dye, was perfused through the vortex veins of two rabbits. The eyes were enucleated after 2, 10, 20 and 40 minutes, and the pigment epithelium and rod outer segments dissected out. Vitamin A compounds were extracted and the radioactivity measured in a liquid scintillation counter. The results of these experiments (Fig. 9) show a very rapid uptake of radioactivity into the pigment epithelium after injection. These data are reported as counts/minute of retinyl *ester* (not as retinol) since we know from *in vitro* experiments carried out independently that pigment epithelial microsomes contain one of the most active retinol esterifying enzymes found in any body tissue. Therefore these data corroborate *in vitro* observations, and show that after only two minutes, nearly 30% of the retinol entering the pigment epithelium became esterified and by 40 minutes, close to 90% was in this form. In contrast to this remarkable uptake and esterification of vitamin A by the pigment epithelium, very little radioactive ester was detected in the rod outer segments. It was in fact only barely measurable after 40 minutes.

These findings also support concurrent *in vitro* experiments which showed that, although rod outer segments have esterifying ability, it is far less than

97

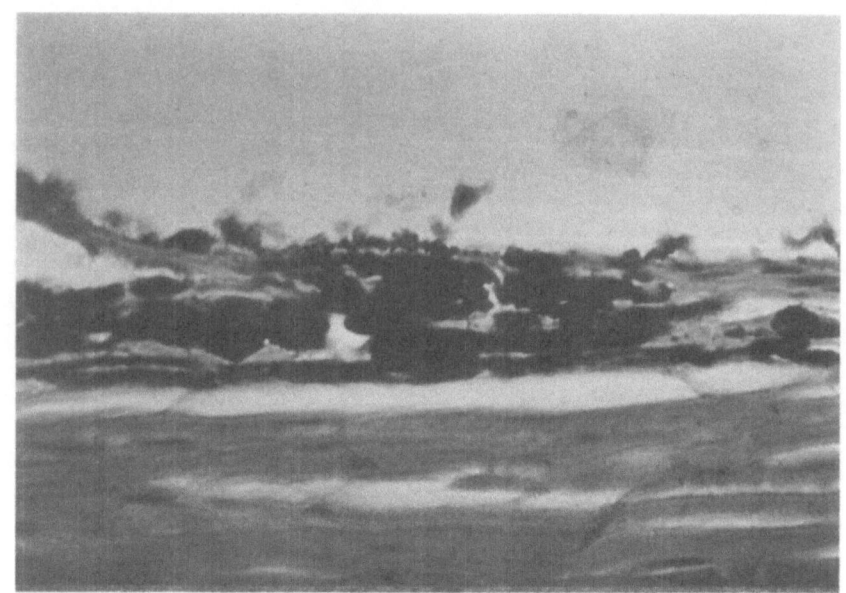

Fig. 7

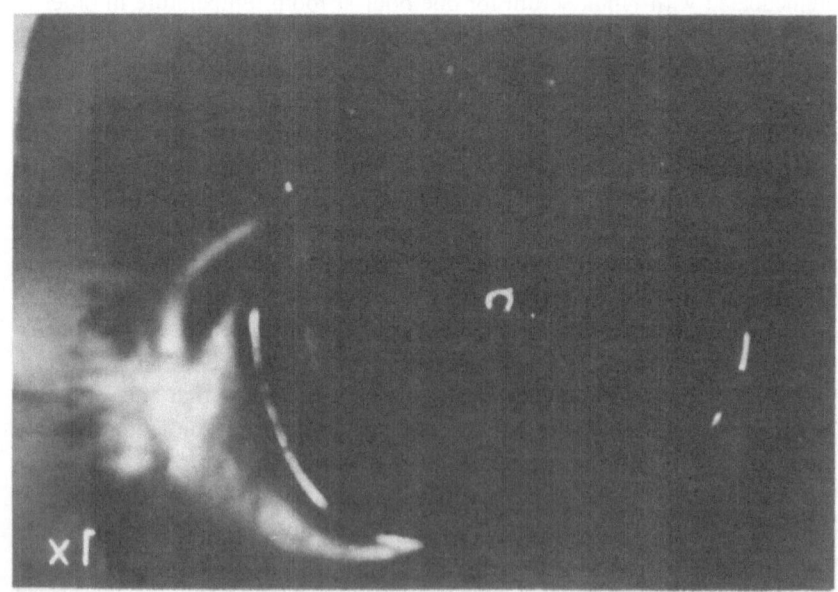

Fig. 8

98

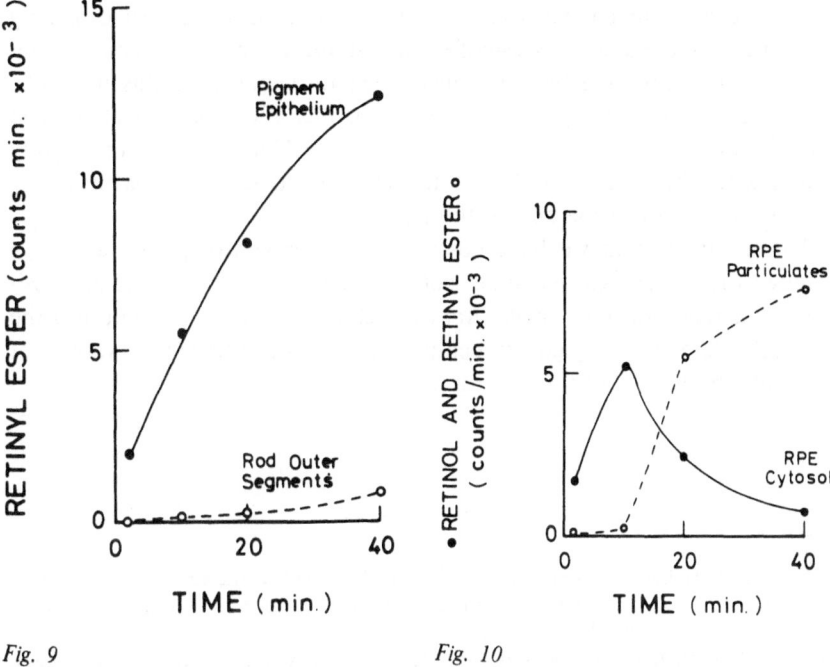

Fig. 9   Fig. 10

that of the pigment epithelium. It seems possible that the radioactive vitamin A ester that we were able to measure in the rod outer segments arose partly by diffusion from the pigment epithelium and partly by esterification *in situ.* These experiments however do not allow us to distinguish between the two possibilities.

We were interested in probing further into the mechanism of vitamin A uptake and metabolism in the pigment epithelial cells because we know that retinol binding protein is localized in the cytosol compartment of the cell, whereas the esterifying enzyme is in the microsomal (or particulate) fraction of the cell. It is also known that retinol bound to cytosol retinol binding protein is an excellent substrate for the esterification. Therefore we not only measured the total radioactivity in the whole pigment epithelial cell, as described above, but we also separated the soluble and the particulate portions of the cell by high speed centrifugation. Fig. 10 shows the results of these experiments. It is an almost classical example of precursor-product relationship. The radioactivity of tritiated retinol is first found in the cytosol, where it is undoubtedly bound to the retinol binding protein. It reaches a peak in about ten minutes, at which time only a small portion is present as the esterified form in the microsomes. Afterward the situation is reversed. The radioactivity representing cytosolic vitamin A drops off and that present as ester rises, both of them in the proportions expected for a precursor-product relationship. These experiments have thus shown in vivo what we could have anticipated from *in vitro* findings, namely that vitamin A is taken up by the pigment epithelial cell, becomes bound to the cytosolic binding protein and subsequently is esterified and stored in the microsomes (endoplasmic reticulum). We had previously tried to demonstrate this metabolic transformation in the pigment epithelium of rats after injection of tritiated retinol, but had failed to get a definitive answer. Not only were they costly experiments, but they also lacked the accuracy that can be achieved by working with an eye the size of the rabbit.

The technique that we have described here for perfusing the rabbit eye through the vortex vein has other potential applications. It should be possible to examine not only uptake from the choroidal circulation, but also the metabolic fate in the pigment epithelium and the retina of a variety of nutrients, hormones and even drugs.

REFERENCES

Bok, D. & J. Heller. Transport of retinol from the blood to the retina: an autoradiographic study of the pigment epithelial cell surface receptor for plasma retinolbinding protein. Exp. Eye Res. 22: 395-402 (1976).

Hall, M.D. & D. Bok. Incorporation of y^{3}HY vitamin A into rhodopsin in light- and dark-adapted frogs. Exp. Eye Res. 18: 105-117 (1974).

Hirosawa, K. & E. Yamada. Localization of vitamin A in the mouse retina as revealed by radioautography, in: The structure of the Eye III, Ed. by E. Yamada and S. Mishima, Jap. J. of Ophthalmology, pp. 165-175 (1976).

Robison, W.G. Jr. & T. Kuwabara. Vitamin A storage and peroxisomes in retinal pigment epithelium and liver. Invest. Ophthal. and Vis. Sci. 16: 1110-1117 (1977).

Young, R.W. & D. Bok. Autoradiographic studies on the metabolism of the retinal pigment epithelium. Invest. Ophthal. 9: 524-536 (1970).

Authors' address:
Hadassah University Hospital
Dept. of Ophthalmology
P.O. Box 12000
Jerusalem
Israel

REGENERATION AND METABOLIC ACTIVITY OF PIGMENT EPITHELIUM IN VITRO

D. BENEZRA, M. TAMAI & A. ZELIKOVICH

(*Jerusalem, Israel*)

ABSTRACT

The regenerating potential and metabolic activity of PE cells *in vitro* is demonstrated by an organ and cell culture. In PE organ cultures derived from the posterior pole of newborn mice, numerous newly-formed microvilli are discovered after 24 hours in culture. These form a confluent densely packed surface after three days in culture. In PE cell cultures derived from the posterior pole of adult guinea pigs, extensive DNA and protein synthesis is observed. These metabolic activities are closely dependent on the serum concentration *in vitro* and are markedly influenced by the addition of epidermal or fibroblast growth factors.

INTRODUCTION

The integrity of the pigment epithelium is essential for the preservation of normal function and metabolism of the photoreceptors. This study was designed to investigate the regenerating capacity of traumatized pigment epithelial cells using an *in vitro* organ culture of PE. Also, an attempt is made to analyze the effect of serum and growth factors on the metabolic activity of PE cell cultures.

MATERIALS AND METHODS

Animals: Normal albino mice 5 and 10 days post natal were used for the preparation of organ PE cells cultures.

Inbred guinea pigs strain 13 were used for the preparation of PE cell cultures.

Cultures: Organ cultures consisting of sheets of PE on Bruch's membrane, choroid and sclera were obtained after dissection of the posterior pole of the albino mice and mechanical gentle separation of the neuro retina. A piece of lens paper 0.5 mm by 0.7 mm inserted below the dissected sheet of PE is used in order to transfer and fix it on tantalum grids bathing in medium 199 supplemented with 15% fetal calf serum (Microbiological Associates) in Falcon plates 3001. The cultures are incubated at 37°C in 100% humid

101

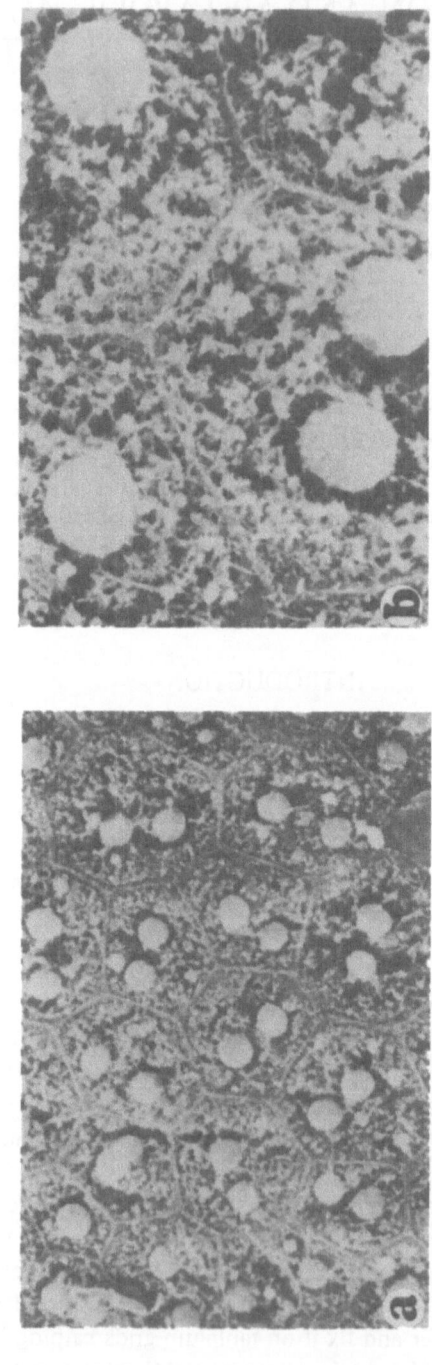

Fig. 1. Pigment epithelium 'organ culture' from the posterior pole of new-born mice after separation from the neuro retina. 1a. magnification ×800; the cell membrane has been disrupted. Many cells harbor two nuclei. 1b. magnification ×3000; bare nuclei.

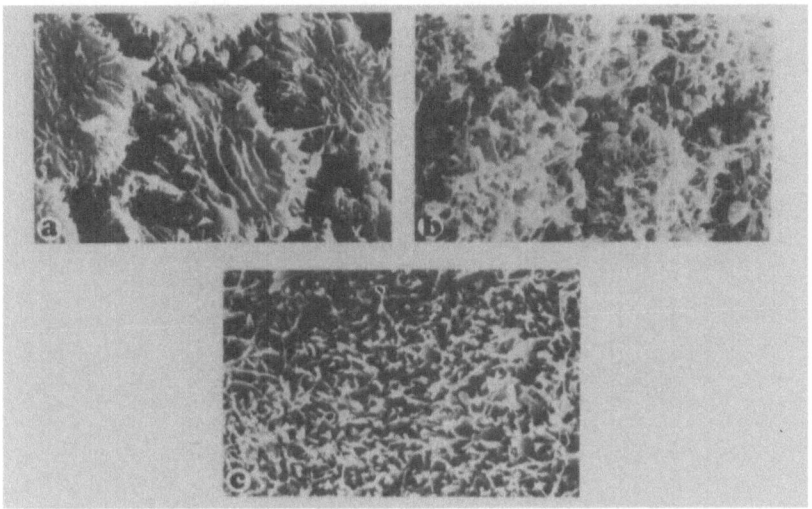

Fig. 2. Regeneration of microvilli after the in vitro culture of PE organ cultures. 2a. one hour after initiation of culture. 2b. 24 hours later; many elongated microvilli are seen. 2c. after three days in culture the PE organ culture is covered with microvilli. 2a and 2b. original magnification ×1200. 2c. original magnification ×1000

atmosphere and a continuous flow of 5% CO_2. Medium was changed every 72 hours. At various intervals after the initiation of culture, samples are processed for scanning electron microscopy.

Cell cultures were initiated with PE cells that adhered to neuro retina of guinea pig eyes after dissection of the sclera and choroid under the operating microscope. The PE cells were stripped of the neuro retina, transferred to petri dishes (Falcon 3001) with RPMI 1640 supplemented with 10% fetal calf serum (Microbiological Associates) and incubated at 37°C in 100% humid atmosphere and a continuous flow of 5% CO_2. Medium is changed every 72 hours. After 10 to 15 days, the PE cells are trypsinized with Dulbecco's PBS medium (without calcium or magnesium) containing 0.25% trypsin and 0.05% EDTA washed, transferred to microculture plates (Falcon 3040) and studied as previously described (BenEzra 1977; BenEzra 1978).

RESULTS

Fig. 1 demonstrates the morphology of the PE cells immediately after the mechanical separation. The cellular membrane of some cells has been torn and the bare nuclei may be seen. As shown, many of the cells have two nuclei and few harbor only one nucleus. After an hour in culture, few fine and elongated microvilli are observed (Fig. 2a). A day later, the microvilli are more numerous and thicker (Fig. 2b). After three days in this particular experiment, microvilli become very densely packed (Fig. 2c).

103

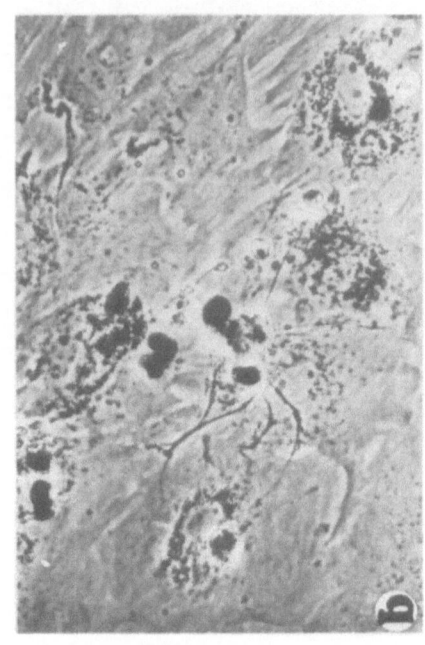

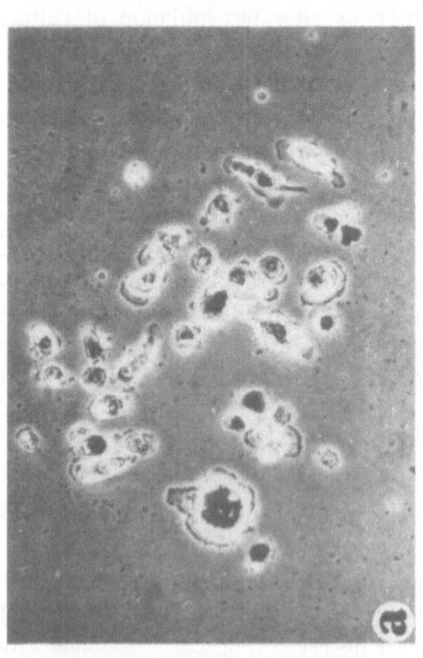

Fig. 3. Pigment epithelium cell culture derived from posterior pole of adult guinea pig. 3a. PE cells after three days in culture; many cells are not firmly attached to the culture plate, others harbor membranous extensions similar to macrophages. At the edges of the culture, mitotic figures are observed. 3b. after 15 days a monolayer of cells is obtained. Original magnifications ×380.

Table 1. Metabolic activity of guinea pig PE cells *in vitro* *

Exp.	Precursor	Day 1	Day 3	Day 5	day 7
1	H^3T	169 ± 5 **	1348 ± 301	4092 ± 358	3576 ± 706
	H^3L	160 ± 11	789 ± 21	2031 ± 152	2938 ± 630
2	H^3T	735 ± 130	2546 ± 179	5320 ± 455	2893 ± 370
	H^3L	234 ± 51	1052 ± 235	2047 ± 236	3125 ± 420
3	H^3T	427 ± 32	947 ± 153	6927 ± 488	2247 ± 537
	H^3L	159 ± 9	526 ± 29	2146 ± 537	2853 ± 439

* Cells were incubated in RPMI 1640 supplemented with 5% FCS and harvested at various intervals after a 24 hr. pulse of 1 μc tritiated thymidine (H^3T) or 0.5 μc of tritiated leucine (H^3L).

** Represent the counts per minute (cpm) of a triplicate set of cultures ± one standard deviation.

Early in cell culture the PE cells harbored the appearance of mobile macrophages (Fig. 3a) and mitotic potential.

After 15 days, a continuous layer of pigment epithelial cells with smaller mitotic potential are obtained (Fig. 3b).

Table 1 illustrates the metabolic activity of the PE cells after trypsinization and transfer to microcultures. In all three representative experiments, marked DNA and protein synthesis is observed. The DNA synthesis activity reached maximal levels after the fifth day in culture, levelling off and even decreasing thereafter. The protein synthesis on the other hand appears to

Table 2. Effect of serum and growth factors on PE metabolic activity *in vitro* *

Serum concentration	Growth factors ***			
	None	EGF	FGF	NGF
None	65 ± 10 **	584 ± 103	929 ± 22	72 ± 20
1%	229 ± 28	1475 ± 85	1864 ± 670	305 ± 37
5%	1241 ± 60	2148 ± 125	4574 ± 464	1098 ± 78
10%	2557 ± 83	2874 ± 317	1914 ± 359	2427 ± 401

* Assessed by the extent of tritiated thymidine uptake on the third day of culture after a 24 hour pulse with 1.0 μc of H^3T.

** cpm ± one standard deviation

*** These factors were added approximately four hours after initiation of the cultures:

EGF : Epidermal growth factor is added at a concentration of 2 ng per microculture.

FGF : Fibroblast growth factor is added at a concentration of 20 ng per microculture.

NGF: Nerve growth factor is added at a concentration of 10 units per microculture.

increase even beyond the fifth day. The concentration of serum is an important factor in the PE cell metabolic activity *in vitro*. The epidermal and fibroblast growth factors could replace the serum promoting growth (at least to some extent) as shown in Table 2. The enhancing capacity of the growth factors is most marked in cultures with low serum concentrations. This effect levels off when higher serum concentrations are used (Table 2).

DISCUSSION

This study demonstrated that PE cells have a rapid regenerating and metabolic activity given the proper conditions in vitro. Periodic scanning electron microscopic observations demonstrated the renewal potential of the PE microvilli and may be interpreted as an indication for the possible healing potential of the PE cells after trauma or infection *in vivo*.

The growth enhancing activity obtained by the addition of epidermal or fibroblast growth factor in PE cell culture is very interesting. Although still preliminary, this activity might be channeled and used for enhancing the potential growth (and activity) of the PE cells in diseases where this capacity is defective. The *in vivo* practical application of these *in vitro* observations is far from becoming a reality at present. However, growth factors induce changes in the cellular membranes and modify their specific receptors affinity. It is not improbable that this potential, if better understood, can be used in order to improve the PE cell – photoreceptor interacton in the early phases of degeneration that occur in retinal dystrophies. The demonstration that epidermal and fibroblast growth factors influence markedly the metabolic potential of the PE cells *in vitro* is a preliminary step in the long journey toward the achievement of this goal.

REFERENCES

BenEzra, D. A microculture technique for the evaluation of corneal cell metabolism in vitro. Invest. Ophthalmol. 16: 893 (1977).
BenEzra, D. & T. Tanishima. Possible regulatory mechanisms of the cornea. I. Epithelial-stromal interaction in vitro. Arch. Ophthalmol. 96: 1891 (1978).

Authors addresses:

D. BenEzra and A. Zelikovich
Department of Ophthalmology
Hadassah Hebrew University Hospital
Jerusalem
Israel

D. BenEzra and M. Tamai
The Clinic Branch
National Eye Institute
Bethesda, Maryland
U.S.A.

THE BIOCHEMISTRY OF PHOTORECEPTOR CELLS
Metabolic effects of light stimulation and light damage

M. J. VOADEN, J. MARSHALL & A. C. I. ORAEDU

(*London, England*)

ABSTRACT

Photoreceptor cells have high rates of metabolism, and enzyme distributions suggest considerable substrate movement. We have used tracer techniques to study the effects of light on photoreceptor metabolism. In vitro, glutamine is metabolized alongside glucose by rat photoreceptors, and is, potentially, a major precursor of the neuroactive amino acids glutamate, aspartate and γ-aminobutyrate (GABA). The utilization of both substrates is decreased by light, as is the turnover of glutamate and aspartate. Tritiated glutamic and aspartic acids are taken up by photoreceptor cells. In the primates all rods but only some cones are labelled, whereas in the guinea pig the picture is reversed. The observations support the premise that glutamate and/or aspartate are photoreceptor neurotransmitters but show that cell and species differences may exist.

We have been unable to find evidence for the involvement of free radical mechanisms in light-induced photoreceptor damage but our initial results suggest a reduced metabolism of glutamine and GABA in damaged cells.

INTRODUCTION

Very high metabolic rates have been observed in isolated mammalian retinas, with respiration reputedly about twice that of brain slices and aerobic glycolysis six times as high (Lolley 1969). Many of the key enzymes of intermediary metabolism have their peak activity in one particular cell type, the photoreceptors, suggesting that much of this 'excess' metabolism may be associated with the functioning of these (Lowry *et al.* 1956, 1961; Lowry 1964; Matchinsky *et al.* 1966; Matchinsky & McDougal 1968). This conclusion is supported by in vitro observations on the metabolic changes occurring in developing and degenerating retinas (Graymore 1969).

Photoreceptor inner limbs are rich in mitochondria. Correlating with this, Lowry and his colleagues (loc. cit.) have found peak activities of the enzymes of the tricarboxylic acid cycle in this region. High levels of pentose phosphate pathway enzymes are also present, needed, no doubt, to supply reducing equivalents for the visual cycle (Futterman 1963, 1974) and for the continual lipid and protein synthesis associated with outer limb growth (Young 1976); and to provide support for the extremely active nucleotide

107

Docum. Ophthal. Proc. Series, Vol. 25, ed. by H. Zauberman
© *1981, Dr. W. Junk bv Publishers, The Hague*

metabolism in both the inner and outer limbs (Ebrey and Honig 1975; Hubbell and Bounds 1979). In contrast, the glycolytic enzymes (phosphohexoisomerase, phosphofructokinase and lactic dehydrogenase) predominate in the inner connecting fibre of the cell.

Clearly, photoreceptors have a complex metabolism involving considerable substrate movement between the outer limb, the inner limb, the nuclear region, the inner connecting fibre and the synapse. Although some progress has been made in the study of the general metabolic effects of light stimulation (see below), we know very little about the overall integration of this metabolism, or the *relative* changes that occur on functional stimulation of the cell. In addition, we need to understand more fully the influence that the extra-cellular microenvironment has on photoreceptor function, and how much individual pathways can substitute to support cell viability in abnormal situations (such as might arise in diabetes or when the blood-retinal barrier is disrupted). The present survey considers some of the metabolic changes that occur on both short term and continuous light exposure of the photoreceptor cells.

LIGHT AND PHOTORECEPTOR METABOLISM

When a dark-adapted photoreceptor cell is exposed to light, oxygen uptake is depressed (Hanawa and Kuge 1961; Sickel 1972a, b), glucose utilization decreases (Basinger *et al.* 1979; Morjaria and Voaden 1979a; Voaden and Morjaria 1980), and, in rats, the turnover of glutamate and aspartate, formed from glutamine, decreases (Voaden & Morjaria 1980; Voaden *et al.* 1980). In contrast, succinoxidase activity (Epstein & O'Connor 1966; *cf.* Enoch 1963, 1967; Marc and Sperling 1976), and turnover of the pentose phosphate pathway (Futterman 1963) may increase. The effect of light stimulation on glycolysis in photoreceptors has not, as far as we are aware, been reported.

Less ATP may be needed in the light-stimulated photoreceptor because of cessation of the sodium current that flows between the inner and outer limbs of the dark-adapted cell, and the consequent decrease in Na^+/K^+ ATPase

$\longrightarrow$

Fig. 1. Light microscope autoradiographs showing the sites of (a) ^{3}H-aspartate and (b) ^{3}H-glutamate uptake in the baboon retina.
Retinas were incubated for 10 mins at 37 °C in Krebs' bicarbonate medium containing 5 µCi/ml ^{3}H-aspartate (178 mCi/mmol) or ^{3}H-glutamate (1.4 Ci/mmol). They were then processed for L.M. autoradiography as described by Voaden et al (1978). Slides were exposed for 3 months at 4 °C.
Uptake has occurred principally into rod photoreceptor cells (black fine arrows), Whereas cone photoreceptors (white fine arrows) are much less labelled. The difference is particularly obvious for ^{3}H-aspartate uptake – cone synaptic pedicles (open arrow) remaining unlabelled whereas grains are present over the rod spherules.
^{3}H-glutamate is also readily accumulated by the glial cells of Müller (arrow heads). The bar marker is 100 µm.

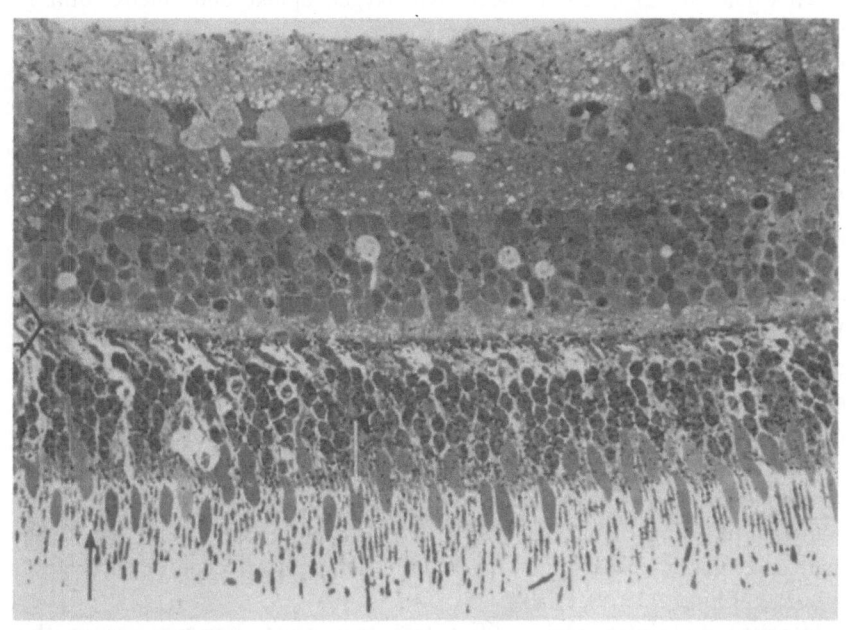

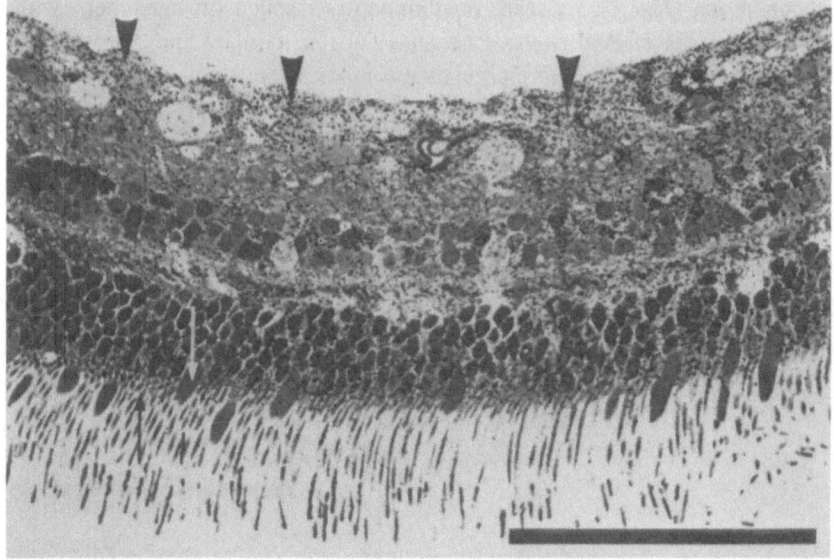

Fig. 1.

activity in the inner limb (Ebrey and Honig 1975). Decreased ATP break-down would, in turn, lead to decreased oxygen uptake and glucose utilisa-tion. It has been suggested that the tricarboxylic acid cycle might also be inhibited by a build up 6-phosphogluconate, occurring because of stimulation of the pentose phosphate pathway (Cohen and Noell 1965). The latter might occur in part because of the reduction of all-trans retinal to retinol (Vitam-in A), in the visual cycle and the consequent reoxidation of NADPH to NADP (Futterman 1974). Increased succinoxidase activity in light-stimulated photoreceptors is, at present, unexplained.

The neuroactive amino acids glutamate and aspartate have, for a long time, been favoured candidates to be photoreceptor neurotransmitters (Neal 1976; Wu & Dowling 1978; Voaden 1979). A decrease in their turnover in photoreceptor cells on light stimulation (Voaden and Morjaria 1980) would be consistent with this as it is now well established that photoreceptor neurotransmitters are released in the dark and that this release is terminated on light stimulation of the cell (Voaden 1979).

In general, released neuroactive amino acids can be taken up again by the neurones releasing them (Neal 1976). It is, therefore, significant that gluta-mate and aspartate can both be taken up by some photoreceptor cells (Fig. 1; Bruun & Ehinger 1974).

Inter-cell and inter-species differences may exist, however, as in the baboon retina (Fig. 1), rods are predominantly labelled (in agreement with the observations of Bruun and Ehinger 1974, on monkey and human reti-nas), whereas in the guinea pig cones are more active (Fig. 2).

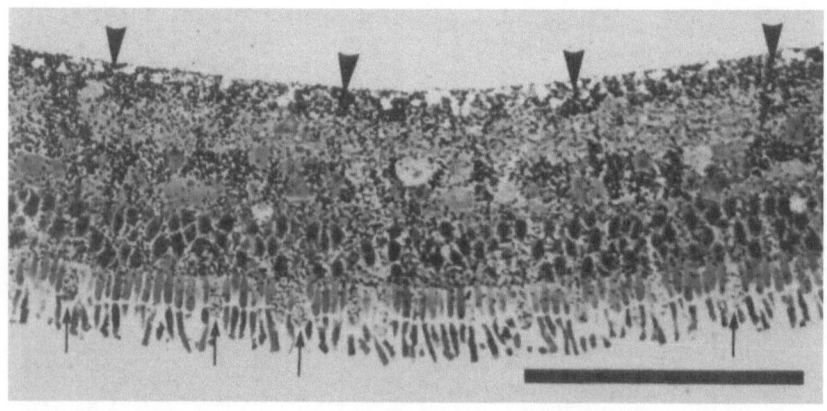

Fig. 2. Sites of ³H-aspartate uptake in the guinea pig retina. Retinas were incubated and processed as described in Fig. 1.
Autoradiographs were exposed for 3 months at 4 °C.
Uptake has occurred principally into Müller cells (arrow heads) and cone photorecep-tors (fine arrows).
A sparse grain distribution is present over rods but their nuclei are, in general, unlabelled.
The bar marker is 100 μm.

METABOLISM IN
THE LIGHT DAMAGED PHOTORECEPTOR CELL

When animals are exposed to continuous illumination their photoreceptor
cells degenerate (Noell *et al.* 1966; Lanum 1978). The molecular mechanisms responsible are unknown but it is established that the action spectrum
of the damaging effect approximates that of visual excitation, suggesting that
the photopigments play a role. This could occur through such side effects as
the generation of free radicals (Daemen 1973; Feeney & Berman 1976;
Delmelle 1978), or via, for example, disturbances resulting from prolonged
alterations in cell activity (Noell & Albrecht 1971). To investigate these
possibilities, we have exposed albino wistar rats to continuous illumination
from a photographic light box containing two 41.5 cm, 15 W Atlas 'tropical
daylight' fluorescent tubes (6,500 K), placed on top of their cage. A sheet of
frosted cinemoid was interposed between the lamps and the cage, and the
maximum illuminance (from the ceiling), was 1544 scotopic lux. Full experimental details and a description of the morphological changes occurring in
the photoreceptor cells on continuous light exposure have been given by

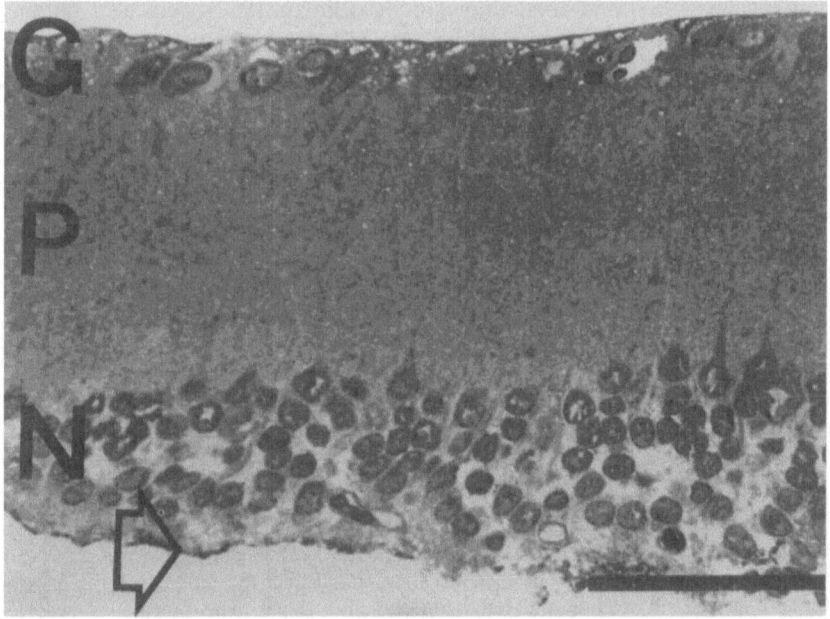

Fig. 3. Section of rat retina, 100 μm depth, obtained by the technique described in
Table 2. Following immersion in glutaraldehyde for 30 mins, the tissue was removed
from the well, postfixed in osmium tetroxide and processed for light microscopy.
G – ganglion cells P – inner plexiform layer. N – inner nuclear layer. The arrow shows
the sectioned surface, and the bar marker is 50 μm.

Oraedu et al. (1980). Typical light damage was observed after 30 hr illumination. However, when animals, exposed for only 18 hr, were returned to their normal environment, extensive outer limb breakdown also ensued. At all the times studied the morphology of the inner retinal layers appeared normal. Photoreceptor outer limbs may be particularly vulnerable to attack by free radicals (Daemen 1973) and it has been postulated that light-damage might result from interaction of the superoxide anion or singlet oxygen with the poly-unsaturated fatty acids there (see e.g. Feeney & Berman 1976). Lipoperoxides would be formed, and, subsequently, the breadkown product of these, malondialdehyde, should be detectable. Malondialdehyde forms a yellow complex with thiobarbituric acid, λ max 532 nm, and increased thiobarbituric acid reactivity has been observed simply on illumination of isolated frog outer limbs (Kagan et al. 1973). However, no evidence for increased reactivity (as compared with normally light or dark-adapted tissue), has been seen in retinas from animals exposed for up to 30 hr to the fluorescent light, or in those left for a further 72 hr under normal laboratory conditions (Oraedu – unpublished observations). In addition there was no change in superoxide dismutase activity. This enzyme is present at high levels in photoreceptor outer limbs (Hall & Hall 1975) and was quantitated in our experiments by its ability to prevent the autoxidation of 6-hydroxydopamine (Heikilla & Cabbat 1976). The concentrations of glutathione (Owens and Belcher 1965) and total thiol groups (Ellman 1959) were also normal. Thus we have so far been unable to obtain evidence for the involvement of free radicals in the photoreceptor damage observed in our studies although,

Table 1. The entry of ^{3}H-2-deoxyglucose into light-exposed rat retinas in vivo

State of Animal	Weight of Retina (mg. wet)	^{3}H-2-Deoxyglucose Uptake (dpm/mg wet wt. retina)
Light-adapted control	13.7 ± 0.5	343 ± 32
* Light exposed 48 hr	12.9 ± 0.5	302 ± 10

* These rats were exposed to the experimental light regime described in the text.
All animals were injected intraperitoneally with 200 nCi/gm body wt 2-deoxy-D-(1-^{3}H)-glucose (17.5 Ci/m.mol) 30 min before sacrifice. After removal of anterior tissue, the back of each eye was dissected out flat, retina uppermost, on a perspex block. A weighed disc of filter paper was then placed over the retina, and the back of the eye peeled off leaving the retina on the filter paper. The preparation was reweighed, the retina solubilized in Triton X-100 and the radioactivity counted by scintillation spectrometry. Results are expressed as the mean $\pm$ SEM (n = 6). Entry of the glucose analogue, 2-deoxyglucose, into the retina provides an index of the rate of glucose utilization (Sokoloff et al. 1977). The results show no significant difference between normal light-adapted retinas and those exhibiting light damage in the photoreceptor outer limbs (cf. Oraedu et al. 1980).

Table 2. ^{14}C-glutamine metabolism in the light-exposed albino rat retina

		DPM $\times 10^{-3}$ / 3 mm dia. disc. retina	
		light-adapted control (n = 4)	light-exposed 48 hr (n = 6)
Photoreceptor cell layer	Aspartate	5.1 ± 0.6	3.5 ± 0.6
	Glutamate	38.4 ± 5.7	26.8 ± 2.8
	Glutamine	79.1 ± 13.3	50.9 ± 5.8
	GABA	12.9 ± 1.8	5.7 ± 0.8 **
	Total radioactivity	146 ± 22	94 ± 10
Inner retinal layers	Aspartate	4.0 ± 1.0	3.4 ± 0.6
	Glutamate	26.8 ± 4.8	24.9 ± 2.6
	Glutamine	53.1 ± 9.7	66.2 ± 6.2
	GABA	26.0 ± 5.4	10.6 ± 1.4 *
	Total radioactivity	121 ± 22	116 ± 10

* $p < 0.5$.   ** $p < .01$.

Retinas were incubated for 30 min under normal room lighting, at $37\,^{\circ}$C, with 600 µM L-[U $-$[14]C] glutamine (15 µCi/ml) in Krebs' bicarbonate medium. They were then sectioned and processed as described by Morjaria and Voaden (1979b). Tissue was floated, photoreceptors downwards onto filter paper. Three mm dia. discs of the preparation were then placed, ganglion cells downwards into 100 µ – depth wells, drilled in blocks of aluminium. These were then frozen ($-80\,^{\circ}$C) and the exposed tissue and filter paper sliced away. This and the section remaining in the well were recovered and separately analysed. Sectioning was approximately at the outer plexiform layer. (cf. Fig. 4). Sections from three retinal discs were combined and processed for the isolation of amino acids (Voaden et al. 1978). Radioactivity was counted by scintillation spectrometry. Results are expressed as the mean ± SEM. There is a significant decrease in the entry of label from ^{14}C-glutamine into GABA, both in the photoreceptor cell and inner retinal layers of the light-exposed as compared with the light-adapted retina.

at the times investigated, vacuolisation and some disorientation of outer limbs was evident. In addition, significant changes were present in the endogenous levels of free amino acids, with taurine reduced, and, in the retinas studied immediately after the illumination, glutamate aspartate, glutamine and glycine increased (Oraedu *et al.* 1980).

As suggested by Noell and Albrecht (1971), it is feasible that cell degeneration could ensue from a prolonged alteration of metabolism induced by continuous light adaption. To investigate this we have looked at the uptake of 2-deoxyglucose in light-exposed as compared with normal, light-adapted animals (Table 1), and have also studied the metabolism of radiolabelled glutamine (Table 2).

The glucose analogue, 2-deoxy D-glucose enters cells on the glucose carrier and is then phosphorylated but not further metabolised. The rate of its intracellular accumulation can, therefore, be used as an index of glucose utilisation in the tissue (Sokoloff *et al.* 1977). There is approximately a 20% reduction in 2-deoxyglucose uptake by the light – as compared with the dark-adapted rat retina. This decrease is localised to the photoreceptor cells and represents a 40% reduction in glucose utilisation in this layer of the tissue (Morjaria and Voaden 1979a). The data in Table 1 show that, on further light exposure, the retina continues to use glucose at the lowered rate. It is probable that the decrease in metabolism in photoreceptors on going from dark to light represents a change from an unusually high rate to a 'resting' more normal situation (*cf.* page 3) and it is unlikely that this would lead to cell death. Damage might result, however, if a further reduction occurred. Although we have found no significant difference between 2-deoxyglucose uptake in light-adapted and light-exposed retinas (Table 1), nevertheless there is a trend in the latter data towards a small decrease. This might prove significant if it were localised to photoreceptors and more studies are needed.

Glucose is the main source of energy and of carbon atoms for the retina. However, potentially, glutamine is also a substrate and, at 500–600 µM, the level present in vitreous (Durham *et al.* 1971; Voaden & Marjaria 1980), it is taken up and metabolised alongside glucose, forming an important precursor of glutamate, aspartate and γ-aminobutyrate (GABA) in both photoreceptor cells and the 'inner' retina (Voaden *et al.* 1978; Morjaria & Voaden 1979b). As discussed earlier, when ^{14}C-glutamine metabolism was investigated in vitro in the normal rat retina, evidence was obtained for a 40–50% reduction in the turnover of glutamate and aspartate in the photoreceptor cell layer of the light-stimulated as compared with the dark-adapted tissue (Voaden & Morjaria 1980). The specific activity of GABA, although greatly reduced in the inner retinal layers on light stimulation, was barely changed in photoreceptor cells. In contrast, when a similar study was done on retinas from rats exposed previously for 48 hr to the experimental light and a comparison made with normal tissue from fully light-adapted animals, the entry of label from ^{14}C-glutamine into the GABA molecule in the photoreceptor cell layer was halved (Table 2). In addition, there was a further 30–40% reduction in the total radioactivity derived from the exogenously-applied ^{14}C-glutamine. There is evidence suggesting the presence of the GABA bypath in rat photoreceptor cells (Hyde & Robinson 1974; Morjaria & Voaden 1979b; Voaden *et al.* 1980). The present results show that its turnover may be significantly reduced in the light damaged photoreceptor. We do not have sufficient information to merit speculation on the significance of these observations but they do raise the possibility that specific aspects of metabolism are curtailed in the light damaged cell.

ACKNOWLEDGEMENTS

We thank Miss Bharti Morjaria and Mr. Peter West for their expert assistance with the metabolic studies and autoradiography respectively, and the Medical Research Council for financial support.

A.C.I.O. is a recipient of an Anambra State, Nigeria, Scholarship.

REFERENCES

Basinger, S., W. C. Gordon & D. M. K. Lam. Differential labelling of retinal neurones by ^{3}H-2-deoxyglucose. Nature 280: 682-684 (1979).

Bruun, A. & B. Ehinger. Uptake of certain possible neurotransmitters into retinal neurons of some mammals. Exp. Eye Res. 19: 435-447 (1974).

Cohen, L. H. & W. K. Noell. Relationships between visual function and metabolism. In: Biochemistry of the Retina. C. N. Graymore (Ed.) pp. 36-49 (1965). Academic Press, London and New York.

Daemen, F. J. M. Vertebrate rod outer segment membranes. Biochim Biophys. Acta 300: 255-288 (1973).

Delmelle, M. Retinal sensitized photodynamic damage to liposomes. Photochem and Photobiol. 28: 357-360 (1978).

Durham, D. G., J. C. Dickinson & P. B. Hamilton. Ion exchange chromatography of free amino acids in human intraocular fluids. Clin. Chem. 17: 285-289 (1971).

Ebrey, T. G. & B. Honig. Molecular aspects of photoreceptor function. Quarterly Reviews of Biophysics. 8: 129-184 (1975).

Ellman, G. Tissue sulfydryl groups. Arch. Biochem. Biophys. 82: 70-77 (1959).

Enoch, J. M. The use of tetrazolium to distinguish between retinal receptors exposed and not exposed to light. Invest. Ophthalmol. 2: 16-23 (1963).

Enoch, J. M. Validation of an indicator of mammalian retinal response: recovery in the dark following exposure to a luminous stimulus. Invest. Ophthalmol. 6: 647-656 (1967).

Epstein, M. H. & J. S. O'Connor, Enzyme changes in isolated retinal layers in light and darkness. J. Neurochem. 13: 907-911 (1966).

Feeney, L. & E. R. Berman. Oxygen toxity: membrane damage by free radicals. Invest. Ophthalmol. 15: 789-792 (1976).

Futterman, S. Metabolism of the retina III. The role of reduced triphosphopyridine nucleotide in the visual cycle. J. Biol. Chem. 238: 1145-1150 (1963).

Futterman, S. Recent studies on a possible mechanism for visual pigment regeneration. Exp. Eye Res. 18: 89-96 (1974).

Graymore, C. N. General aspects of the metabolism of the retina. In: The Eye Vol. 1. Vegetative physiology and biochemistry, 2nd ed. H. Davson (Ed.) pp. 601-645 (1969) Academic Press, London and New York.

Hall, M. O. & D. O. Hall, Superoxide dismutase of bovine and frog rod outer segments. Biochem. Biophys. Res. Commun. 67: 1199-1204 (1975).

Hanawa, I. & K. Kuge. The effect of light intensity upon the oxygen consumption of the isolated outer segments rods. Jap. J. Physiol. 11: 38-43 (1961).

Heikkila, R. E. & F. Cabbat. A sensitive assay for superoxide dismutase based on the autoxidation of 6-hydroxydopamine. Analyt. Biochem. 75: 356-362 (1976).

Hubbell, W. L. & M. D. Bownds. Visual transduction in vertebrate photoreceptors. Ann. Rev. Neurosci. 2: 17-34 (1979).

Hyde, J. C. & N. Robinson. Localisation of sites of GABA catabolism in the rat retina. Nature 248: 432-433 (1974).

Kagan, V. E., A. A. Shvedova, K. N. Novikov & Yu. P. Kozlov. Light induced free radical oxidation of membrane lipids in photoreceptors of frog retina. Biochem. Biophys. Acta 330 : 76-79 (1973).

Lanum, J. The damaging effects of light on the retina. Empirical findings, theoretical and practical implications. Surv. Ophthalmol. 22 : 221-249 (1978).

Lolley, R. N. Metabolic and anatomical specialisation within the retina In : Handbook of Neurochemistry Vol. 2 : structural neurochemistry. A. Lajtha (Ed.) pp. 473-504 (1969) Plenum Press, London and New York.

Lowry, O. H. Biochemical studies on layered structures. In : Morphological and Biochemical Correlates of Neural Activity. M. Cohen and R. S. Snider (Eds) pp. 178-191, (1964) Hoeber, New York.

Lowry, O. H., N. R. Roberts, & C. Lewis. The quantitative histochemistry of the retina. J. Biol. Chem. 220 : 879-892 (1956).

Lowry, O. H., N. R. Roberts, D. W. Schulz, J. E. Clow & J. R. Clark. Quantitative histochemistry of the retina II enzymes of glucose metabolism. J. Biol. Chem. 236 : 2813-2820 (1961).

Marc, R. E. & H. G. Sperling. Color receptor identities of goldfish cones. Science 191 : 487-489 (1976).

Matschinsky, F. M. & D. B. McDougal. Quantitative histochemistry of enzymes and glycolytic intermediates of retina, pancreas and organ of Corti. In : Progress in Clinicochemical Methods (Proceedings of the 6th Int. congress of clin. chem. Munich 1966). 3 : 71-86 (1968) Karger, Basel and New York.

Matschinsky, F.M., J. V. Passonneau & O. H. Lowry. Quantitative histochemistry of metabolites of glycolysis in retina. J. Histochem. Cytochem. 13 : 707-   (1966).

Morjaria, B. & M. J. Voaden. The uptake of (^{3}H)-2-deoxy glucose by light- and dark-adapted rat retinas in vivo. J. Neurochem. 32 : 1881-1883 (1979a).

Morjaria, B. & M. J. Voaden. The formation of glutamate, aspartate and GABA in the rat retina : glucose and glutamine as precursors. J. Neurochem. 33 : 541-551 (1979b).

Neal, M. J. Amino acid transmitter substances in the vertebrate retina. Gen. Pharmac 7 : 321-332 (1976).

Noell, W. K. & R. Albrecht. Irreversible effects of visible light on the retina : role of vitamin A. Science 172 : 76-80 (1971).

Noell, W. K., V. S. Walker, B. S. Kang & S. Berman. Retinal damage by light in rats. Invest. Ophthalmol 5 : 450-473 (1966).

Oraedu, A. C. I., M. J. Voaden & J. Marshall. Photochemical damage in the rat retina : morphological changes and endogenous amino acids. J. Neurochem. In Press (1980).

Owens, C. W. I & R. V. Belcher. A colorometric micro-method for the determination of glutathione. Biochem. J. 94 : 705-711 (1965).

Sickel, W. Retinal metabolism in light and dark. In. Handbook of Sensory Physiology VII/2 : physiology of photoreceptor organs. M.G.F. Fuortes (Ed.) pp. 667-727 (1972a) Springer, Berlin.

Sickel, W. Electrical and metabolic manifestations of receptor and higher order neuron activity in vertebrate retina. Adv. Exp. Med. Biol. 24 : 101-118 (1972b).

Sokoloff, L., M. Reivich, C. Kennedy, M. H. Des Rosiers, C. S. Potlak, K. D. Pettigrew, O. Sakurada & M. Shinohara. The (^{14}C) deoxyglucose method for the measurement of local cerebral glucose utilisation : theory, procedure and normal values in the conscious and anaesthetised albino rat. J. Neurochem. 28 : 897-916 (1977).

Voaden, M. J. The chemical specificity of neurones in the retina. Progress in Brain Res. 51 : 389-402 (1979).

Voaden, M. J. & B. Morjaria, The synthesis of neuroactive amino acids from radioactive glucose and glutamine in the rat retina : effects of light stimulation. J. Neurochem. 35 : 95-99 (1980).

116

Voaden, M. J., N. Lake, J. Marshall, & B. Morjaria. The utilisation of glutamine by the retina: an autoradiographic and metabolic study. J. Neurochem. 31: 1069-1076 (1978).

Voaden, M. J., B. Morjaria & A. C. I. Oraedu. The localisation and metabolism of glutamate, aspartate and GABA in the rat retina. In: Neurochemistry of the Retina. N.G. Bazán and R. N. Lolley (Eds.) Neurochemistry. 1: 151-165 (1980).

Wu, S. M. & J. E. Dowling. L-Aspartate: evidence of a role in cone photoreceptor synaptic transmission in the carp retina. Proc. Nat. Acad. Sci. 75: 5205-5209 (1978).

Young, R. W. Visual cells and the concept of renewal. Invest. Ophthalmol. 15: 700-725 (1976).

Authors' address:
Institute of Ophthalmology
Judd Street
London, U.K.

CHEMICAL FACTORS IN THE INTERTISSUE VASCULAR RELATIONSHIPS IN THE DEVELOPING EYE
A preliminary report

ISAAC C. MICHAELSON & DAVID BENEZRA

(*Jerusalem, Israel*)

In a previous report there were described the intertissue vascular relationships of the fundus of the eye (Michaelson 1965). This report was concerned chiefly with the definitive state. The present report is confined to the developing eye state where attempts will be made to indicate the chemical factors involved under physiological circumstances. The cornea is a suitable workshop for the experimental study of vasculogenesis because of its transparency, avascularity, closeness to the conjunctival vascular system and accessability for an experimental approach. Corneal studies have shown that its experimental neovascularisation is consequent on the formation in the cornea of a diffusable substance which at a critical concentration is capable of stimulating the pre-existing nearby limbal vessels to proliferate towards the maximal concentration of the surmised substance; whose diffusability results in the isoceles triangular distribution of the intra-corneal vascular invasion (Campbell & Michaelson 1948). There have been several efforts to identify the vasogenic substance (Maurice et al. 1966; BenEzra 1978, 1979). The former authors demonstrated that oedema was a necessary although not a sufficient condition for the growth of vessels into the cornea. They suggest that the liberation of some chemical substance from the wounded corneal tissue is necessary to promote the vessel growth. They demonstrated a mathematical treatment of how the vaso-stimulating substance moves through the cornea from a traumatic focus and how the capillaries sense the concentration gradient of the substance. BenEzra has demonstrated in an impressive series of experiments that prostaglandin is capable of inducing vasculogenesis. It is a product of cells that have been traumatised physically, chemically or otherwise or are undergoing rapid growth or multiplication as in development. It is a reasonable assumption that this or allied substances are active in the angiogenic process generally.

A study of the development of the vascular system in the inner eye specially of these stages where foci of cells are undergoing rapid growth and multiplication indicates that the process is understandable on the basis of the formation of the diffusable angionic substance elaborated by these foci of cells whose behaviour in development is controlled enzymatically. It will be

119

Docum. Ophthal. Proc. Series, Vol. 25, ed. by H. Zauberman
© *1981, Dr. W. Junk bv Publishers, The Hague*

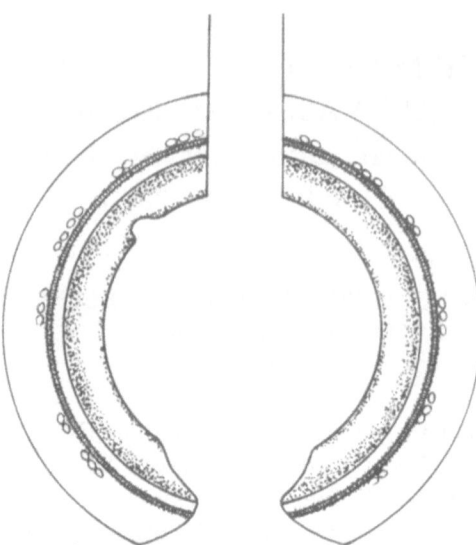

Fig. 1. Diagram indicating the disposition about the 10 mm stage in the human retina of the anlage of the choriocapillaris.

shown that this process is influenced by the local oxygen concentration, which tends to inhibit vasogenesis if at sufficient concentration.

The vascular development of the inner eye is then dependent on three main chemical activities; the onset of the growth of differentiated cells interspersed throughout the growth period at predetermined intervals as dictated by enzymatic activities; the elaboration, as the consequence of such rapid cell multiplication, of a vasogenic substance capable of diffusing through the tissues to the nearest already vascularised zone and of stimulating the accession of new vessels to the cell-multiplying zone; and the controlling influence in this process of the local tissue oxygen concentration as determined by the proximity of blood vessels already present.

The initiating factor is the multiplication of developing cells. Each of these multiplications is now discussed in more detail.

(A) The earliest to take place is in the 5–10 mm stage of the human embryo in the outer zone of the neural layer of the optic cup (Mann 1950). This stimulates the accession of new vessels to the situation of the future choriocapillaris (Fig. 1).

(B) Growth of cells of the posterior lens epithelium which takes place at the 5 mm stage and stimulates the accession through the optic fissure of the hyaloid vessel system. This system begins to recede and regress after the 35 mm stage by which time the posterior lens epithelium has ceased its lens fibre growth which is taken over by the lateral epithelium of the lens (Mann 1950) (Fig. 2).

(C) At the 70 mm stage in the human foetus there is multiplication of retinal cells especially in the inner retina and its temporal half (Mann 1950).

120

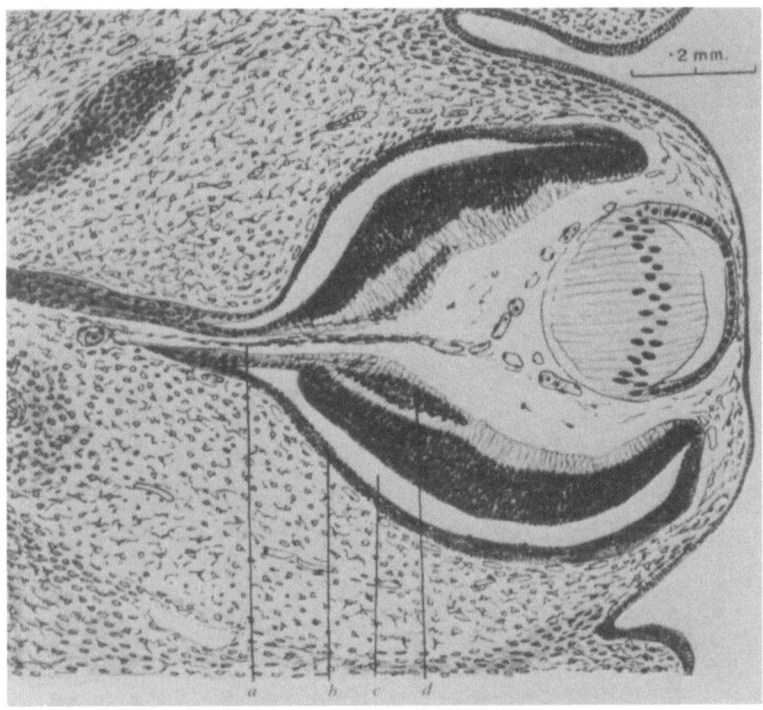

Fig. 2. Section through the optic cup of a 17 non-human embryo showing the hyaloid artery at the upper end of the foetal fissure and its branches behind the developing lens (Mann 1950).

These are mainly ganglion and mural cells. Thickening of the retina results. The cell multiplication increase until the consequently elaborated vasogenic substance stimulates the accession of vessels into the inner retina from the already vascularised optic disc zone, first from its temporal and later from its nasal aspect (Fig. 3). This takes place in the human foetus about the 110 mm stage. It appears to be delayed until this period because of the oxygen concentration which the choriocapillaris manages to supply to the retinal tissue, a function that cannot be maintained in the inner zone of the retina once the retina has achieved the thickness of the 110 mm stage. The restraining influence of a certain oxygen concentration on the vasogenic process is confirmed by the further mode of development of the retinal vessels. This leaves avascular zones around the arterioles, in the outer retina (Fig. 4) and the fovea and retinal periphery because of the thinness of the retina in these localities (Michaelson 1954). With the competing influences of the cell-produced vasogenic substance and the local existing oxygen concentration within the retinal tissue, development has found within the normal body a beautiful way of ordering and monitoring new vessel growth.

121

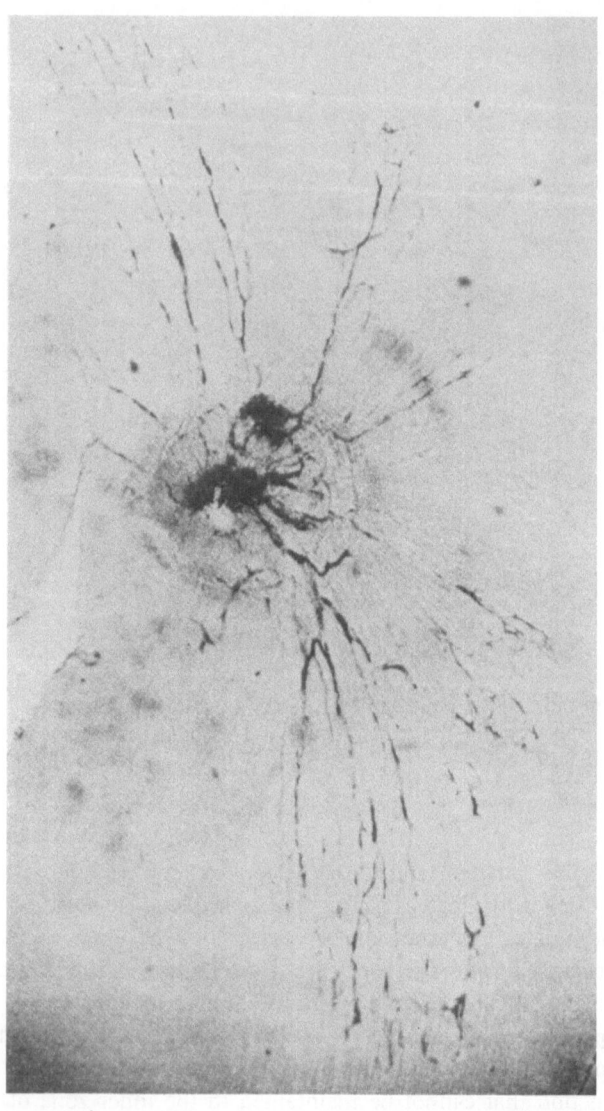

Fig. 3. Injected retina of 110 human foetus. Proceeding from the disc margin these can be distinguished the upper temporal, lower temporal, upper nasal and lower nasal vessels.

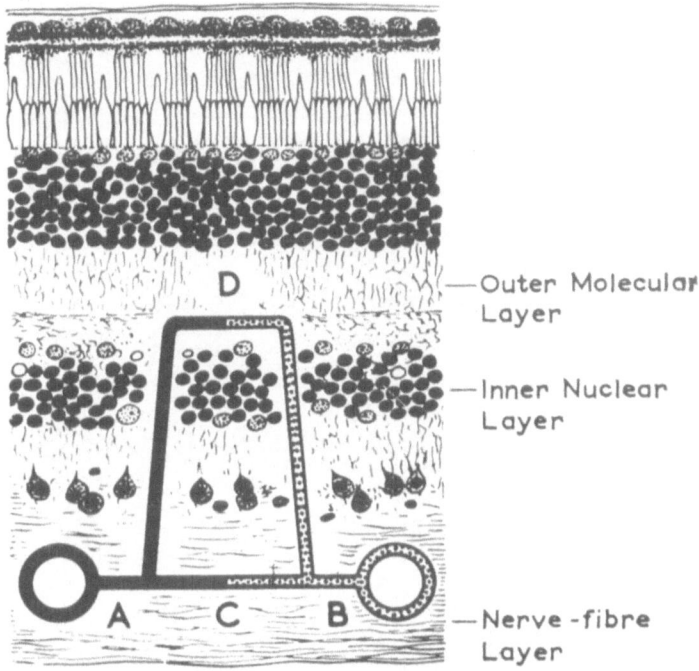

Fig. 4. Diagrammatic presentation of the definitive retinal vascular system showing the inner and outer capillary layers. The zone between the latter and the choriocapillaris is avascular.

REFERENCES

BenEzra, D. Neovasculogenic ability of prostaglandis, growth factors, and synthetic chemoattractants. Vol. 86: 455 (1978).

BenEzra, D. Neovasculogenesis. Triggering factors; possible mechanisms. Survey of Ophthalmology. 24: 167 (1979).

Campbell, F.W. & I.C. Michaelson. Heat injury and new vessel formation in the rabbit's cornea. Proceedings of the Physiological Society. Journal Physiology. Vol. 108: (1948).

Campbell, F.W. & I.C. Michaelson. Blood-vessel formation in the cornea. Brit. Jour. Ophthal. 248: 33 (1949).

Mann, I. The Development of the Human Eye. Grune & Stratton. New York. (1950).

Michaelson, I.C. Retinal Circulation in Mann and Animals. Charles C. Thomas. Springfield. Illinois. U.S.A. (see figs. 34, 35, 45, 48, 49, 62, 64, 74). (1954).

Maurice, D.M., Ch. Zauberman & I.C. Michaelson. The stimulus to neovascularisation of the cornea. Expl. Eye. Res. 5: 168 (1966).

Authors' address:
Straus Health Centre, Hadassah
P.O. Box 499
Jerusalem
Israel

123

NEOVASCULARIZATION,
A UNITARIAN PHENOMENON

DAVID BENEZRA

(*Jerusalem, Israel*)

ABSTRACT

Corneal neovascularization is used as a model for a possible 'heuristic theory' of a unitarian phenomenon of neovascularization in ocular tissues. In this unitarian mechanism, the pivotal role is fulfilled by a local cellular metabolite(s). As prostaglandins are possible and most suitable candidates for this role, the effect of indomethacin on the neovascularization has been studied. It is shown that indomethacin inhibits markedly the extent of neovascularization triggered by different neovasculogenic substances reinforcing the postulation for involvement of the prostaglandins in this phenomenon. However, the role of other factors is still open as the inhibition of neovascularization by indomethacin was not absolute in any of the cases where a strong neovasculogenesis was induced.

INTRODUCTION

In fully developed organisms, blood vessel proliferation is a phenomenon triggered during the healing process of tissues as part of the repair mechanism. In the eye, the neovascularization may be detrimental to vision; therefore, it has attracted the interest of ophthalmologists for decades (Campbell & Michaelson 1949; Cogan 1949; Patz et al. 1952; Imre 1964; Henkind & de Oliveira 1967; Zauberman et al. 1969). Although the possible pivotal role of a chemical substance, coined X-factor, in the induction of new vessel growth has been postulated by Michaelson (1948), little progress has been made in the characterization of such a substance. More recently, a factor released by growing tumor cells – tumor angiogenesis factor (TAF) – has been demonstrated (Folkman et al. 1971). Also, neovasculogenesis has been induced by activated macrophages (Polverini et al. 1977) while the release of a neovascular attracting factor (NAF) has been observed during the process of activation of leukocytes by various mitogens (BenEzra 1977, 1978a). Following these findings, the possibility that the X-factor, TAF, NAF or the factor released by activated macrophages might be a similar substance has been suggested (BenEzra 1978b).

In this study, some of the crucial events in neovascularization are reemphasized and a possible unitarian phenomenon with its possible clinical implications is suggested.

125

Docum. Ophthal. Proc. Series, Vol. 25, ed. by H. Zauberman
© *1981, Dr. W. Junk bv Publishers, The Hague*

MATERIALS AND METHODS

Under various conditions, the extent of neovascularization was assessed by the implantation of the tested substance in the mid-stroma of rabbit corneas.

Animals. Albino rabbits of both sexes weighing 2–3 kg were used.

Implants. These were prepared as previously described (BenEzra 1978b). In brief, neovasculogenic substances were incorporated in a casting solution of 10% ethylene vinyl-acetate copolymer (Elvax-40) in methylene chloride under a laminar flow hood. The methylene chloride is allowed to evaporate and a hardened film of Elvax-40 is obtained within two to three minutes. A one mm^2 piece of this film sequestering a standard concentration of tested material is implanted under the microscope at the mid-stromal level. Two implants are inserted in each cornea, at 6 and 12 o'clock.

Neovascularization of the cornea. Observation of the neovascular attracting ability of the various implants was made under the operating microscope at 24-hour intervals for the first two days and every 48 hours thereafter. The length of the leading vessel from the limbus toward the tested material as well as the active neovasculogenic base at the limbus are recorded on the sixth day after transplantation. Then, the eyes are enucleated, and the corneas subjected to histological studies. ED_{50} of neovascularization was coined when neovascularization was induced in certain conditions in at least 50% of the experiments.

Neovasculogenic agents. Prostaglandin E_1 obtained as a gift from Dr. Pike of Upjohn Company was used in concentrations of 1 to 10 µg/implant and was used as a standard neovasculogenic substance. Lipopolysaccharide W.S. typhimurium (LPS) was purchased from Difco Laboratories. Epidermal growth factor (EGF) and fibroblast growth factor (FGF) were purchased from Collaborative Research Inc. Indomethacin was obtained from Sigma.

RESULTS

Using the corneal implant system the evidence for a specific neovasculogenesis was made based on the following observations:

1. Neovascular budding from pre-existing limbal vessels is initiated and progresses in a triangular shape with its apex toward the implant.

2. The extent of neovascularization is closely dependent on the concentration of the neovasculogenic substance.

3. The distance from implant to limbus determines the size of the active base at the limbus.

4. The more distant the implant from limbal vessels, the more neovasculogenic substance is needed in order to trigger EC_{50} of neovascularization (Table 1).

126

Table 1. Correlation between the distance from limbus to implant and the concentration of stimulating substance inducing EC_{50} of neovascularization

Distance limbus-implant (mm)	Minimal effective concentration *		
	EGF μg/implant	FGF μg/implant	PGE μg/implant
2	5	5	< 1
3.5	20	25	5
4.5	50	> 50	10

* Designating the minimal concentration that induces neovascularization in at least 50% of the tested implants (EC_{50}).

5. The budding of neovascularization is from one side of the initiating vessel(s) and is directed toward the implant.

6. There is a regression of the new vessels on 'emptying' of the implants from the neovascular factor (Fig. 1). Reimplantation of the original implant during the active stage of neovascularization, attracts vessels to the new site. Reimplantation during the regression stage fails to induce neovasculogenesis.

The possibility that the induction of new vessel growth is mediated via the release of prostaglandins and the strong potential of prostaglandins of the E series to induce neovascularization has been reported (BenEzra 1978b). Table 2 illustrates the inhibitory potential of indomethacin on the neovascularization induced by different stimuli. In all cases, indomethacin affected the size of the neovascular tuft. The neovasculogenic ability of the fibroblast growth factor and to some extent that of the epidermal growth factor were markedly inhibited. The LPS capacity tò induce new vessel growth was also affected (Fig. 2). Unexpectedly, the extent of neovascularization induced by PGE implants was also inhibited (Table 2 ad Fig. 2).

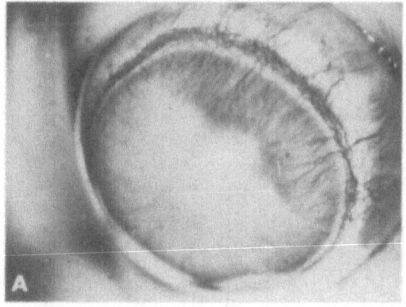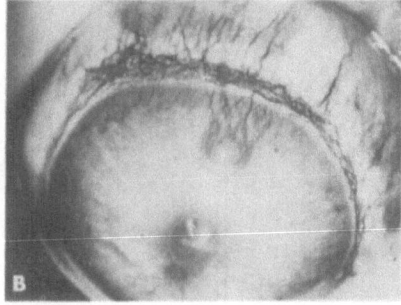

Fig. 1. Strong neovascularization is induced with implant sequestering 5 μg of LPS. A. Six days after implantation; B. After 20 days.

Table 2. Effect of indomethacin on neovascularization

Tested material	µg/implant	Without indomethacin +			With 40 µg indomethacin **		
		No. implants	Active	Surface *	No. implants	Active	Surface
PGE$_1$	5	6	6	16.2±5.4	7	7	6.9±5.1
	10	8	8	20.8±3.1	7	7	13.8±3.8
EGF	10	8	6	3.2±2.8	10	6	1.6±2.0
	20	8	8	6.8±1.7	6	6	3.0±2.2
FGF	10	4	2	1.5±1.8	4	0	0
	20	6	5	2.9±2.2	6	3	1.2±0.6
LPS	1	4	4	18.6±2.0	4	4	8.1±3.2
	5	4	4	25.2±1.8	4	4	16.8±3.8

* Surface, designates the surface of neovascularization calculated as a triangular tuft:

$$\frac{\text{length of leading vessel} \times \text{active base}}{2}$$

** Indomethacin (40 µg) were sequestered into the implant along with the tested material.

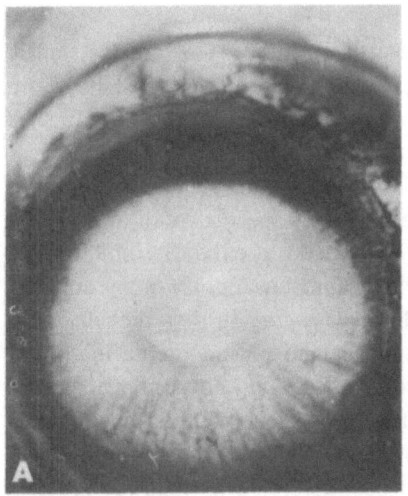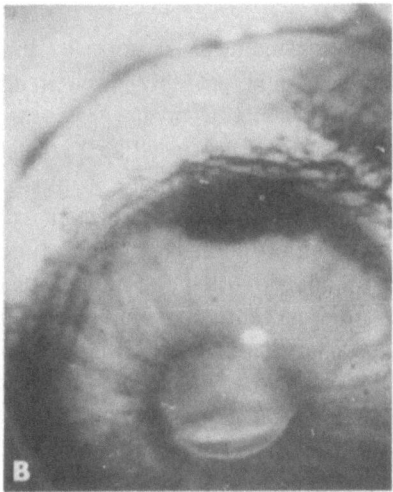

Fig. 2. Neovasculogenesis ability of PGE$_1$ and inhibition by indomethacin. A. 5 µg of PGE$_1$ on day 6 after implantation; B. 5µg PGE$_1$ with 40 µg indomethacin on day 6 after implantation.

DISCUSSION

The data as reported in this study are in line with the observations made by Michaelson (1948, 1954) and reinforce the postulation that neovascularization is triggered by a cell metabolite locally produced. If this is conceivable, then it is logical to assume that this 'metabolite' may be produced or released by cells following various stimuli. Thus, although the triggering phenomenon for corneal vascularization might be different from that of retinal neovascularization, in both cases the chain of events leads to the production and release of the 'neovascularizing metabolite' as the end product. Extensive studies aimed at singling out this metabolite have led to the possible identification with prostaglandins of the E series (BenEzra 1977, 1978a,b, 1979a; 1979b). Due to the strong neovasculogenic ability of PGE and their important role as intercellular messengers and regulators of inflammatory and immune reactions (Goodwin *et al.* 1977; Humes *et al.* 1977) this possibility is very tempting. Growing tumor cells also synthesize and release prostaglandins that may play the role of tumor angiogenic factor (TAF). Activated macrophages as well as activated leukocytes release larger amounts of prostaglandins. Furthermore, platelets from diabetic patients synthesize and release more prostaglandins than platelets from non-diabetic patients (Halushka *et al.* 1976). These findings make it possible to explain the proliferative diabetic retinopathy on the basis of the accumulation of high concentrations of prostaglandins in the retinal blood vessels of diabetics. Hypoxia is also a trigger for prostaglandin release and may explain the retinal neovascularization in hypoxia as an effect of the accumulation of prostaglandins in the tissue.

Prostaglandins used normally as intercellular messengers are constantly produced and probably also circulate; therefore, if these substances are indeed playing a pivotal role in neovascularization it must be further assumed that there need be a crucial concentration for initiating the neovascular events. Furthermore, it must also be assumed that there exists also an inhibitor which becomes inactivated locally in very specific conditions. Thus, inhibition of the neovascularization can be carried out either by inhibition of the production of the stimulating metabolite (prostaglandin?) or by enhancing the concentration of the local inhibitor. Carrying further the idea that prostaglandins may be the crucial initiating metabolite, indomethacin should be a potent inhibitor of neovascularization. Indeed, all neovasculogenic substances that have been tried in this study have been inhibited by indomethacin. However, this inhibition has not been total, when a strong neovasculogenesis is induced. These facts can be interpreted as follows: (a) it is possible that apart from prostaglandins, there exist other factors that stimulate the blood vessel growth. (b) Prostaglandins fulfill only the role of 'helpers' and are not the crucial link of the chain of events. (c) Indomethacin inhibits the activity of the enzyme arachidonic acid cyclo oxygenase and interferes with prostaglandin synthesis. It is possible that in these conditions there might be other pathways of prostaglandin synthesis bypassing the cyclo oxygenase step.

CONCLUSION

It has been assumed that the release of certain metabolite(s) locally induces neovascularization. This metabolite(s) can be produced by many cells given the appropriate conditions that may be specific to the tissue. Therefore a unitarian phenomenon for the ocular neovascularization has been suggested. From extensive studies it appears that prostaglandins may fulfill the role of a pivotal metabolite. Although this possibility is very tempting, it should still remain at the present stage of our knowledge as a 'heuristic theory.' Nevertheless, an attempt to treat early signs of neovascularization with inhibitors of prostaglandins might be warranted even at this early stage of our knowledge.

REFERENCES

BenEzra, D. Mediators of immunological reactions and neovascularization. Presented before the Jerusalem Conference on Impaired Vision in Childhood, Jerusalem, May 12, 1977.
BenEzra, D. Mediators of immunological reactions. Function as inducers of neovascularization. Metabolic Ophthalmol. 2: 339 (1978a).

BenEzra, D. Neovasculogenic ability of prostaglandins, growth factors and synthetic chemoattractants. Am. J. Ophthalmol 86: 455 (1978b).

BenEzra, D. Possible mediation of vasculogenesis by products of immune reaction. The Second International Symposium on Ocular Immunology and Immunopathology. Paris, Masson & Co., p. 315 (1979a).

BenEzra, D. Neovasculogenesis: Triggering factors and possible mechanism(s). Survey Ophthalmol. 24: 167 (1979b).

Campbell, F. W. & I. C. Michaelson. Blood vessel formation in the cornea. Br. J. Ophthalmol. 33: 248 (1949).

Cogan, D. G. Vascularization of the cornea. Arch. Ophthalmol. 41: 406 (1949).

Folkman, J., E. Minder, C. Abernathy & G. Williams. Isolation of a tumor factor responsible for angiogenesis. J. Exp. Med. 133: 275 (1971).

Goodwin, J. S., A. D. Bankhurst & R. P. Messner. Suppression of human T-cell mitogenesis by prostaglandins. Existence of a prostaglandin-producing suppressor cell. J. Exp. Med. 146: 1719 (1977).

Halushka, P. V., C. Weiser, A. Chambers & J. Colwell. Synthesis of prostaglandin 'E like' in diabetic and normal platelets. Adv. Prostagl. Thrombox. Res. 2: 853 (1976).

Henkind, P. & L. N. F. deOliveira. Development of retinal vessels in the rat. Invest. Ophthalmol. 6: 520 (1967).

Humes, J. L., R. J. Bonney, L. Pelus, M. E. Dahlgren, S. J. Sadowski, F. A. Kuehl & P. Davies. Macrophages synthesize and release prostaglandins in response to inflammatory stimuli. Nature 269: 149 (1977).

Imre, G. Studies on the mechanism of retinal neovascularization. Br. J. Ophthalmol. 48: 75 (1964).

Michaelson, I. C. The mode of development of the retinal vessels and some observations of its significance in certain retinal diseases. Trans. Ophthalmol. Soc. U.K. 68: 137 (1948).

Michaelson, I. C. Retinal Circulation in Man and Animals. Springfield, Charles C. Thomas, PP. 118-131 (1954).

Patz, A., L. E. Hoeck & E. DeLaCruz. Studies on the effect of high oxygen administration in retrolental fibroplasia. Am. J. Ophthalmol. 35: 1248 (1952).

Polverini, P. J., R. S. Cotran, M. A. Gimbrone & E. R. Unanue. Activated macrophages induce vascular proliferation. Nature 269: 804 (1977).

Zauberman, H., I. C. Michaelson & F. Bergman. Stimulation of neovascularization of the cornea by biogenic amines. Exp. Eye Res. 8: 77 (1969).

Author's address:
Immuno-Ophthalmology Laboratory and
Pediatric Ophthalmology Unit
Department of Ophthalmology
Hadassah Hebrew University Hospital
Jerusalem
Israel

EXPERIMENTAL SUBRETINAL NEOVASCULARIZATION

STEPHEN J. RYAN

(*Los Angeles, Calif., U.S.A.*)

ABSTRACT

A reproducible model of subretinal neovascularization has been developed. In the opinion of this author, this is an important first step in the study of disciform macular degeneration. The methodology employed in the development of subretinal neovascularization in the primate is detailed in the text.

This reproducible model will be used in subsequent studies of the pathogenesis, and activation of this subretinal neovascularization. Different theories related to ischemia, hemorrhage, inflammatory response, and position in relation to the center of vascular free zone, as factors important in the development and evolution of subretinal neovascularization, will be investigated.

INTRODUCTION

Disciform macular degeneration is the term applied to a characteristic response in the macula occurring in many different diseases. The disciform response is not an etiologic diagnosis, but is a clinical pathologic entity shared by several conditions affecting the retinal pigment epithelium-Bruch's Membrane-choriocapillaris complex with resultant subretinal neovascularization. This terminology has been the subject of many semantic debates, reflecting confusion as to the basic pathogenesis. The author prefers to restrict the term 'disciform' to include those lesions with subretinal neovascularization and its resultant manifestations. This subretinal neovascularization is derived from the choroidal circulation, and many different theories attempt to explain its pathogenesis and activation. In a landmark monograph, Gass (1967) collated the extant knowledge into the hypothesis for the

From the Johns Hopkins University, Wilmer Institute, and the University of Southern California, Department of Ophthalmology and the Estelle Doheny Eye Foundation. This study was supported in part by grant awards from the National Institutes of Health, EY09944 and EY01545.
Dr. Ryan was a recipient of the Louis B. Mayer Scholar Award from Research to Prevent Blindness, Inc., New York, New York.

133

pathogenesis of disciform macular degeneration which is widely accepted at present. His detailed clinical studies as well as histopathologic studies described the wide range of morphology and presenting appearances of this entity.

The number of patients studied clinically with fluorescein angiography whose eyes were subsequently available for histopathologic and ultrastructural correlation is very small. In those few cases with direct clinicopathologic correlation, the eyes can be examined only at the time of the patient's death which is not optimum in terms of clinical interest. Thus, the basic pathogenesis and such considerations as the role of the inflammatory responses, angiogenesis factors, the role of ischemia, etc., cannot be studied in the condition with histopathologic and ultrastructural correlation at desired times in the course of disciform macular degeneration. For these reasons a reproducible experimental model of subretinal neovascularization and the disciform response is particularly desirable.

The subhuman primates involved in this study have an ocular and macular anatomy remarkably similar to that of man. It must be emphasized that this experimental study has no relevance to senile macular degeneration in man. By comparison, this experimental model is acute, and the most relevant clinical comparison in man would probably be subretinal neovascularization after trauma, particularly that after laser photocoagulation. The goal of a reproducible model of subretinal neovascularization has been the subject of long-standing research efforts by the author (Ryan 1979). The methodology and results are outlined in this report.

MATERIALS AND METHODS

Macaca mulatta (Rhesus monkey) and Macaca speciosa (Stumptail monkey) were chosen for this study because of distinct retinal and choroidal circulations and macular anatomy similar to that of man. The voluminous literature documenting utilization of the Rhesus monkey as an experimental animal also made it ideally suited for the multifaceted study reported in this text.

Fundus photography and fluorescein angiography were performed in the standard manner employed clinically.

The series of experiments with enzymatic injections employed either collagenase 25 or 35 units, or hyaluronidase 15 units, or combinations thereof. Physiological saline, the animal's own whole blood, and needle placements alone were utilized as controls. Injections were made in the periphery and compared with results of injections in the macular region (see Tables 1 and 2).

For the laser photocoagulation studies, the coherent radiation system 900 argon laser was used. The laser energy was delivered with the slit lamp and a Goldmann contact lens. The basic approach for this experimental laser pho-

Table 1. Incidence of subretinal neovascularization in transscleral subretinal injections *

Material injected	Site of injection	
	Macula	Periphery
Collagenase	2 of 7	0 of 3
Collagenase-hyaluronidase combination	3 of 36 [1]	0 of 4
Saline	0 of 10 [2]	0 of 5
Blood	0 of 3	0 of 5
Total	5 of 56	0 of 17

[1] Two other monkeys of the remaining 33 developed neovascularization, *but* in a fibrous scar similar to that seen after a perforating injury. This development differs from the desired experimental model in which the subretinal neovascularization leaks fluorescein which can then pool rather than merely stain, as in the case of these two 'scars'.

[2] One monkey in this group has a fibrous scar with neovascularization similar to that described above, i.e., resembling a perforating scar rather than the disciform process sought in the experiments.

* Reprinted with permission. From the *Transactions of the American Ophthalmological Society* (Ryan 1980).

Table 2. Incidence of subretinal neovascularization in transvitreal nicropipette subretinal injections *

Material injected	Site of injection	
	Macula	Periphery
Collagenase	1 of 5	0 of 2
Collagenase and Hyaluronidase	2 of 11	0 of 2
Hyaluronidase	0 of 3	0 of 2
Saline	0 of 5	0 of 2
Total	3 of 24	0 of 8

* Reprinted with permission. From the *Transactions of the American Ophthalmological Society* (Ryan 1980).

tocoagulation was to employ guidelines which are avoided in therapeutic clinical practice, that is:

1. Small spot size – 50 to 100 micron spot
2. Short energy burst – 0.05 seconds
3. High energy density – 500 milliwatts

The goal in this experimental protocol was to produce a disruption of Bruch's membrane; whereas this result should be avoided in clinical practice.

RESULTS

The initial experiments were performed with transscleral subretinal injection. The fundus and site of injection were monitored through the pupil at all times, either with the operating microscope and contact lens or with the indirect ophthalmoscope and Nikon condensing lens. The external approach was monitored with the operating microscope by an assistant surgeon so as to ensure optimal control over the oblique entry of the needle through the sclera.

Although subretinal neovascularization was produced in some animals, the positive cases were low in number and unpredictable in occurrence. Thus, a stereotactic approach was employed, and it was hoped that this more accurate placement of the injected enzymes might improve the results, which it did. By definition, the micropipette traversed not only the vitreous but also penetrated the internal limiting membrane and full thickness of the sensory retina. The discrete puncture of the internal limiting membrane and sensory retina from the introduction of the micropipette usually closed within a few days to a few weeks, as monitored with ophthalmoscopy and stereophotography.

As in the transscleral approach, no subretinal neovascularization occurred after peripheral subretinal injections. Saline and hyaluronidase alone failed to

Table 3. Incidence of subretinal neovascularization produced by laser application *

	Category	Eyes treated	Eyes with srn
Group 1	Laser breaks only in Bruch's membrane (scatter approach)	2	0
Group 2	Branch vein occlusion study	4	0
Group 3	Branch vein occlusion (Both temporal branches)	5	0
Group 4	Laser breaks followed one week later by branch vein occlusion	2	2
Group 5	Branch vein occlusion followed one week later by laser breaks	2	2
Group 6	Laser breaks performed during the same treatment as attempted closure of all macular veins	4	3
Group 7	Laser breaks and brach vein occlusion done at the same laser application	2	2
Group 8	Laser breaks only (grid)	5	4
Group 9	Laser breaks (grid) and branch vein occlusion	11	9

* Reprinted with permission. From the *Transactions of the American Ophthalmological Society* (Ryan 1980).

136

result in subretinal neovascularization, which was noted only when the aforementioned collagenase was a component of the introduced solution.

In contrast to the poor reproducibility and unpredictability in experiments with subretinal injections, 22 out of 26 animals in the nine experimental groups developed subretinal neovascularization after laser photocoagulation (see Table 3). It should be emphasized that in these experiments laser energy was applied in a manner antithetical to clinical criteria with a therapeutic goal. Specifically, short laser bursts of 0.05 seconds, small 50 or 100 micron spot size, and a very high energy density of 500 milliwatts or greater in deeply pigmented animals were employed. A reproducible, predictable experimental model of subretinal neovascularization was thus produced.

DISCUSSION

In the past decade, the author has pursued a number of methodologies attempting to produce subretinal neovascularization. Subhuman primates have been the experimental subjects because they have distinct retinal and choroidal circulations as well as a macular anatomy closely resembling that of man. Initial attempts to produce subretinal neovascularization have included the injection of lytic enzymes, such as collagenase and hyaluronidase, into the choroid, Bruch's membrane, pigment epithelium, and subretinal space. Suitable controls were employed, including the injection of blood and saline as well as needle puncture alone. It is of interest that the only instances of subretinal neovascularization were in the macular region, not in the periphery. It has been noted in some human cases that inadvertent perforation of the globe with a retrobulbar needle can, in fact, lead to disciform processes with frank subretinal neovascularization (Hamilton *et al.* 1975). A more practical reason for discontinuing this experimental approach, however, was the lack of reproducibility and predictability in eliciting subretinal neovascularization when disrupting the RPE-Bruch's membrane-choriocapillaris complex by mechanical and enzymatic means.

Advantages of laser techniques includes production of breaks in Bruch's membrane without associated damage in the sclera or internal limiting membrane, and preferably without through-and-through perforation of the sensory retina. Previous experimental studies by other investigators have demonstrated that photocoagulation can, in fact, disrupt Bruch's membrane, which usually heals as an avascular chorioretinal scar (Campbell *et al.* 1969; Marshall *et al.* 1975; Apple 1977). However, clinical reports by François *et al.* (1975) and Fine *et al.* (1976) indicate that photocoagulation of macular lesions may, in fact, cause proliferation of subretinal neovascularization. Preliminary pilot studies by the author were negative.

The observations of Archer (1976) on the role of branch vein occlusion in the production of retinal ischemia and as a possible causative factor in the development of subretinal neovascularization stimulated an attempt to reproduce this aspect of his experiments using monkeys. The term 'laser break' is used guardedly. Pathologic correlation on each of these injuries at the time of injury is not available since this would, by definition, result in termination of the clinically relevant experiment. Very intense laser burns were applied antithetical to those employed clinically for therapeutic purposes. No practical correlation could be made with clinical associations such as a popping sound or with the appearance of a gas bubble. In approximately one-quarter of these laser injuries there was spontaneous hemorrhage, either choroidal or subpigment epithelial, in rare cases breaking into the sensory retina. In a few cases there was an immediate associated serous detachment. Neither spontaneous hemorrhage nor serous detachment correlated as statistically significant when compared with subretinal neovascularization subsequent to laser without branch vein occlusion. This technique did result in very reproducible subretinal neovascularization.

In the process of establishing suitable controls to investigate the associated variable of branch vein occlusion, it became apparent that the laser lesion in the region of the macula alone resulted in the development of subretinal neovascularization in the absence of branch vein occlusion. Thus, the branch vein occlusion and the resultant retinal ischemia via this mechanism were not essential in the production of the subretinal neovascularization in this experimental model.

At the present time, we are engaged in determining the natural clinical course of this experimental model. Preliminary observations suggest that there is something intrinsic in the macular region causing a very large proportion of these lesions to develop subretinal neovascularization. By contrast, lesions in the periphery, i.e., at the region of the equator as determined by the vortex veins, did not develop subretinal neovascularization. While the goal of identifying a reproducible model of subretinal neovascularization has now been achieved, the fact remains that many variables accompany this model which must be thoroughly studied after the natural course has been carefully delineated. The role of the local break cannot be studied as an isolated phenomenon. The high energy density required to disrupt Bruch's membrane simultaneously elicits an intense inflammatory response, including many macrophages. Analogous to the wound healing process elsewhere, these macrophages might, in fact, release various factors which could stimulate angiogenesis. Hemorrhage itself may play a role in enhancing this inflammatory process. The author clearly recognizes that simple subretinal neovascularization will occur. This has been well documented by Sarks (1973) and other investigators (Green & Key 1977).

One might speculate that local ischemia resulting from destruction of the choriocapillaris by the laser burn may also contribute to eliciting vasoproliferative ischemia and/or resultant vasoproliferative factors. It would seem more appropriate that this ischemia be at the level of the receptor-pigment epithelium-choriocapillaris rather than at the inner retina such as produced by branch vein occlusion. However, this retinal ischemia after branch vein occlusion could, in fact, have a relative ischemic effect on the outer retina and thus contribute to a postulated angiogenesis factor.

Perhaps the most important aspects, however, to be investigated are the factors or conditions that activate subretinal neovascularization. Gass (1967), Sarks (1973) and Green (1977) have pointed out that subretinal neovascularization may, in fact, be present but completely inactive. It would be of critical importance to know what factors are present that activate existent subretinal neovascularization. Thus, the role of 'activated macrophages,' local ischemia, angiogenesis factors, inflammatory response, and other variables might be considered in this experimental model.

The author again emphasizes that this is strictly an experimental model of subretinal neovascularization and that it bears no resemblance whatsoever to senile macular degeneration in man. The experimental subjects are young, otherwise healthy monkeys with an acute injury. The closest approximation to any human lesion is a disciform lesion after trauma, specifically that induced by laser photocoagulation.

The model, however, does provide a relatively uncomplicated, clean methodology for studying subretinal neovascularization and associated variables. This model suggests that there is something peculiar to the macular region. Subsequent morphologic correlation in all stages will provide a pathogenetic basis for understanding many clinical observations and concepts related to disciform macular degeneration.

REFERENCES

Apple, D. J. Histopathology of xenon arc and argon laser photocoagulation. In L'Es-perance, F. A. (ed.): Current Diagnosis and Management of Chorioretinal Diseases. St. Louis, Missouri, C. V. Mosby Co., pp. 25-93 (1977).

Archer, D. B. Neovascularization of the retina. Trans. Ophthalmol. Soc. U.K. 96: 471-493 (1976).

Campbell, C. J., M. C. Rittler, C. H. Swope, et al. The ocular effects produced by experimental lasers. IV. The argon laser. Am. J. Ophthalmol. 67: 671-681 (1969).

Fine, S., A. Patz, D. Orth, et al. Subretinal neovascularization developing after pro-phylactic argon laser photocoagulation of atrophic macular scar. Am. J. Ophthalmol. 82: 352-357 (1976).

François, J., J. J. De Laey, E. Cambie, et al. Neovascularization after argon laser photocoagulation of macular lesions. Am. J. Ophthalmol. 79: 206-210 (1975).

Gass, J. D. M. Pathogenesis of disciform detachment of neuroepithelium. Am. J. Ophthalmol. 63: 573-711 (1967).

Green, W. R. & S. M. Key. Senile macular degeneration: A histopathological study. Trans. Am. Ophthalmol. Soc. 75: 180-254 (1977).

Hamilton A. D., J. Marshall, E. M. Kohner, et al. Retinal new vessel formation following experimental vein occlusion. Exp. Eye Res. 20: 493-497 (1975).

Marshall, J., A. M. Hamilton & A. C. Bird. Histopathology of ruby and argon laser lesions in monkey and human retina. Br. J. Ophthalmol. 59: 610-630 (1975).

Ryan, S.J. The development of an experimental model of subretinal neovascularization in disciform macular degeneration. Trans. Am. Ophthalmol. Soc. 77: 707-745 (1979).

Sarks, S.H. New vessel formation beneath the retinal pigment epithelium in senile eyes. Br. J. Ophthalmol. 57: 951-965 (1973).

Author's address:
Department of Ophthalmology
University of S. California
Estelle Doheny Eye Foundation
Los Angeles, CA.
U.S.A.

140

RANDOMIZED CONTROLLED STUDY
OF PARTIAL LASER RX
OF CHOROIDAL NEOVASCULARIZATION
IN THE HISTOPLASMOSIS OCULAR SYNDROME

L. SINGERMAN, T. SCHLAEGEL, D. ORTH & H. JOONDEPH

ABSTRACT

A program for a randomized controlled study of partial laser photocoagulation of choroidal neovascular membranes in the histoplasmosis is outlined.

Treatment will include the neovascular membrane extrafoveally and if possible the feeder choroidal vessel, and a follow of three years will be implemented.

The clinical examinations will include visual acuity, stereo fluorescein angiography photos, Amsler grid, visual field, ophthalmoscopy and slit lamp examinations.

Available reports give an incidence of legal blindness, from 67% to over 85% for patients with histoplasmosis ocular syndrome and neovascular membranes beneath the fovea. None of the 12 patients who fit these criteria, studied by Drs. Klein, Fine, Knox & Patz (1977) had 20/40 or better vision. To my knowledge, only Dr. Schlaegel has carefully studied and reported the effects of photocoagulation to the extrafoveal portion of such a neovascular membrane involving the fovea (Schlaegel 1974; Schlaegel 1975; Schlaegel et al. 1968, Schlaegel & Weber 1971).

The fundamental principle we have followed in the past has been to photocoagulate only choroidal neovascular membranes which could be safely completely eliminated with dense heavy coagulations. We avoided treating patients with neovascular membranes involving the fovea. This principle has been very helpful and by following it, we have been able to achieve satisfactory results clinically.

Drs. Fine & Klein (1977) reported a 67% incidence and Drs. Gass & Wilkerson (1972), an 86% incidence of legal blindness with choroidal neovascular membranes under the fovea. None of Dr. Klein's patients had 20/40 or better. Of Dr. Schlaegel's 19 cases which had partial treatment of choroidal neovascular membranes, only 40% were legally blind. There was a mean follow-up of 20 months and 9 of 15 patients had the same or better vision. The central scotoma was smaller in 5 out of 6 (Schlaegel 1974, 1975; Schlaegel et al. 1968, Schlaegel & Weber 1971).

As we gain experience with more and more patients with choroidal neovascular membranes involving the fovea left untreated, we see the same

141

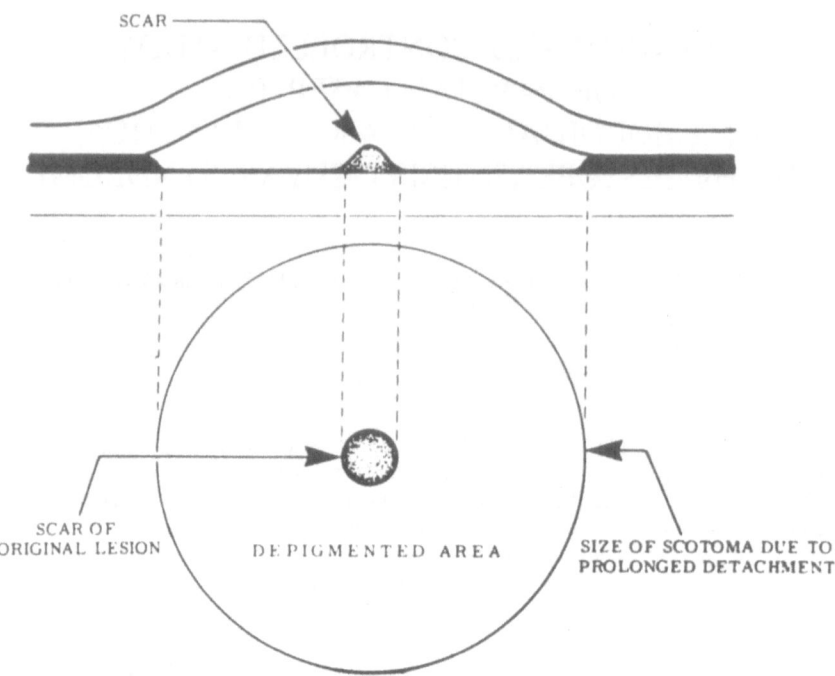

Fig. 1. (Adapted from Dr. T. F. Schlaegel, Jr., *Ocular Histoplasmosis,* Grune & Stratton, 1977).
The diameter of the sensory retinal detachment eventually determines the corresponding size of the permanent partial scotoma.

dismal incidence of blindness reflected in previous reports (Schlaegel 1974, 1975; Schlaegel *et al.* 1968; Schlaegel & Weber 1971; Gass & Wilkinson 1972; Okun 1972).

We are now prepared, after Dr. Schlaegel's lead, to treat selected patients with choroidal neovascular membranes involving the fovea in a randomized control clinical trial.

Histoplasmosis serves as a good model for a partial treatment of choroidal neovascular membranes uncomplicated by superimposed atrophic changes. For example, people with macular choroidal degeneration lose vision on an atrophic basis in the absence of subretinal neovascularization. This complication would be quite rare in histoplasmosis.

Although total photocoagulation is in widespread use, it has not yet been proven to be effective. We look forward to The Macular Photocoagulation Study's elucidation of this issue. The study is chaired by Dr. Stuart Fine, with Drs. Schlaegel, Gass and Burgess on the Organizing Committee and will probably include over ten participating retinal centers.

142

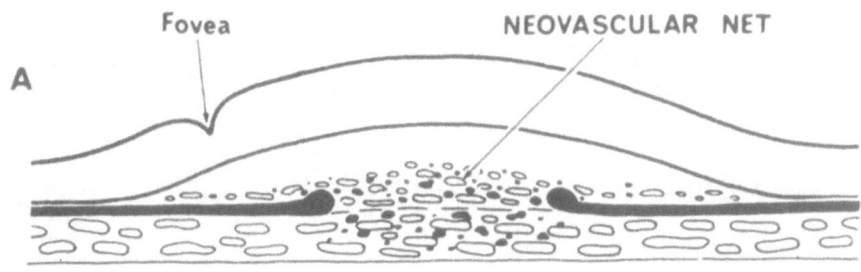

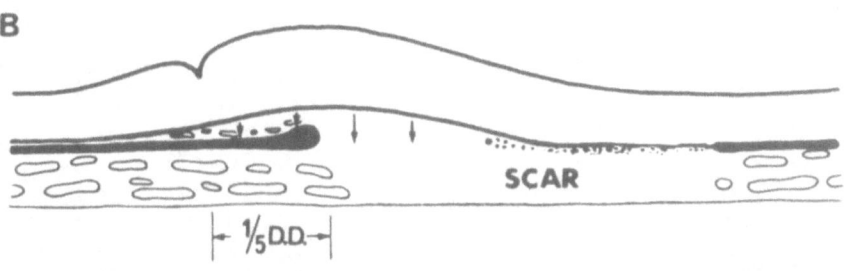

Fig. 2. (Adapted from Dr. T. F. Schlaegel, Jr., Partial Xenon Coagulation of Net in Histoplasmic Choroiditis, *Annals of Ophthalmology*, 7: 476, 1975).
Decrease in elevation, as well as diameter, of sensory retinal detachment over choroidal neovascular membrane after its partial obliteration. (A) Before photocoagulation. (B) after photocoagulation.

The rationale for partial photocoagulation includes: (1) reducing the size of the serous detachment of the sensory retina (Fig. 1); (2) reducing the elevation of the serous detachment to better nourish photoreceptors (Fig. 2); (3) to reduce the spread of choroidal neovascular membranes.

Our criteria for inclusion of cases in this study include an ophthalmoscopic diagnosis of the presumed ocular histoplasmosis syndrome with macular and peripheral punched-out or peripapillary changes. The patient must be between the ages of 18 and 55 and must be able to give fully informed consent. There must be an agreement by the patient and the physician to randomize laser treatment versus no treatment at all. The patient must be available for a five-year study (recruitment two years and follow-up three years) and for all follow-up visits. There should be a symptomatic and worsening course showing increased field defect as documented by Goldmann perimetry. Visual acuity must range from 20/40 to 10/400, utilizing the standard Macular Photocoagulation Study visual acuity chart and lighting criteria (Section 7.11.1, Illumination of the MPS Charts and Room Illumina-

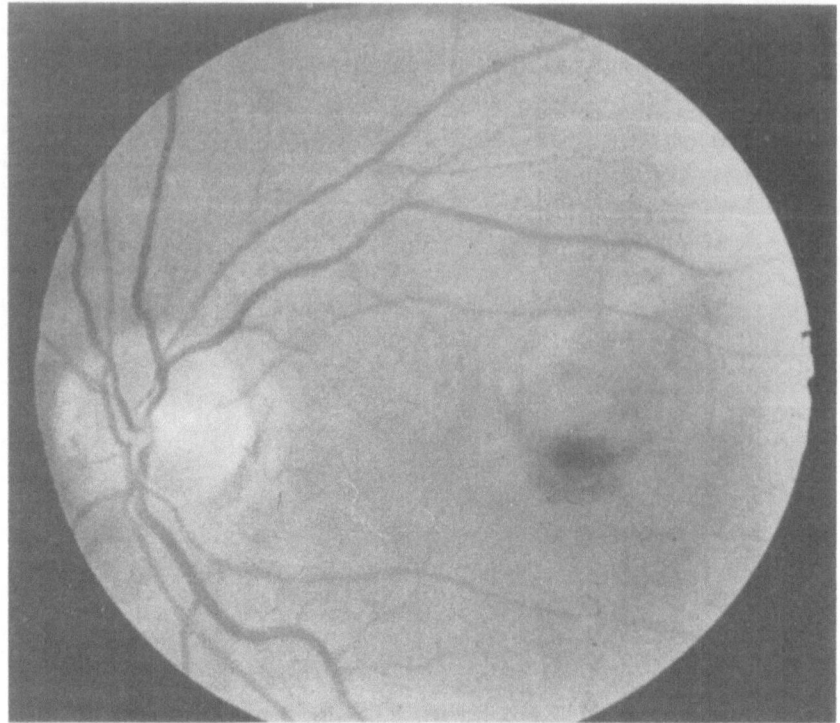

Figs. 3, 4, 5, 6. (Case of Drs. T.F. Schlaegel and L.J. Singerman).
Partial laser photocoagulation of choroidal neovascularization (CNV) resulting in complete obliteration of the neovascular membrane, including the untreated subfoveal portion.
- (3) CNV extending under fovea, with V.A. less than 20/100
- (4) Fluorescein angiogram corresponding to (3)
- (5) Laser treatment to extrafoveal portion of CNV
- (6) Fluorescein angiogram demonstrating post-treatment complete obliteration of CNV, including untreated subfoveal portion, resulting in maintenance of better than 20/30 V.A. to date (more than a year).

tion). The media must be sufficiently clear for adequate photography. There must be fluorescein angiography evidence of a choroidal neovascular membrane extending to less than 200 microns from the center of the retinal avascular zone. The portion of the choroidal neovascular membrane outside that zone should be greater than inside it. The serous detachment of the sensory retina should be greater than two times the choroidal neovascular membrane diameter.

Our criteria for treatment includes: (1) a fluorescein angiogram within 72 hours of the treatment; (2) adequate retrobulbar anesthesia; and (3) treatment 400 microns from the center of the retinal avascular zone, but no closer. We are not intending here to attempt to obliterate the whole mem-

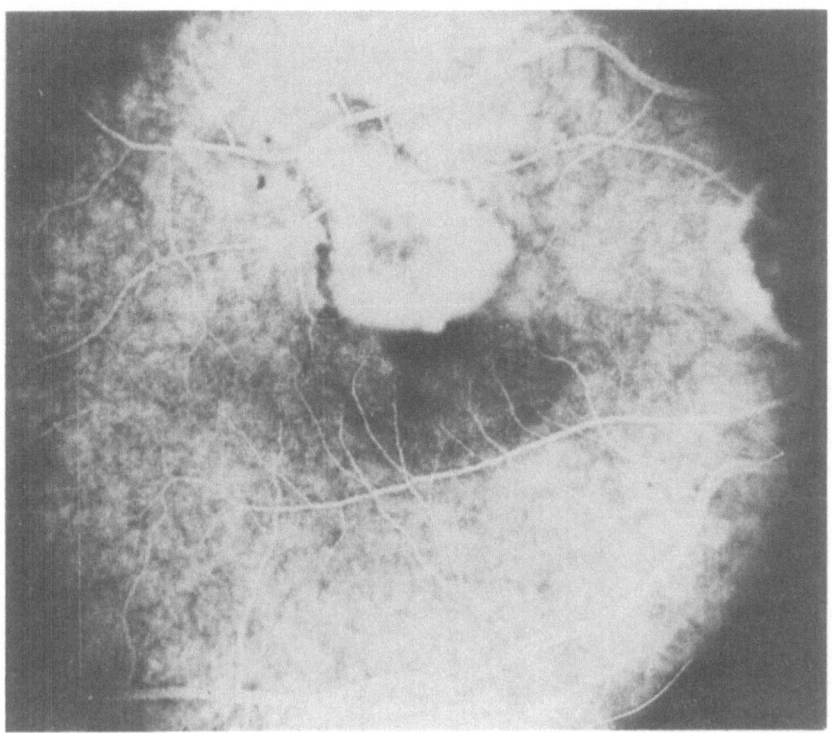

Fig. 4

·brane, so we see no need to take the risk of damaging the rod-free area, (4) end point of treatment is a uniform white lesion which will extend about 100 microns beyond the neovascular membrane along as many borders as possible, (5) intense white burns will be placed (.2–.5 second duration and 200–500 micron spot size). A 50 micron border may be used for visualization purposes, (6) if a choroidal neovascular membrane on follow-up fluorescein angiography shows growth in its extrafoveal portion (the part extending beyond the treatment) it would be treated. We would not treat the foveal portion or extension from that foveal portion.

The minimum follow-up will include a visit at 6 weeks, 3 months, 6 months, 12 months, 18 months and 24 months. At each follow-up, we will study: (1) a subjective questionnaire; (2) best corrected visual acuity; (3) Amsler Grid (completely, using all seven grids and all six questions); (4) visual field with a Goldmann perimeter; (5) direct and indirect ophthalmoscopy; (6) stereo fundus photos and fluorescein angiograms, and (7) slit lamp with fundus contact lens or Hruby lens.

The types of partial photocoagulation will include extrafoveal eccentric choroidal neovascularization, which will be used for the majority of patients

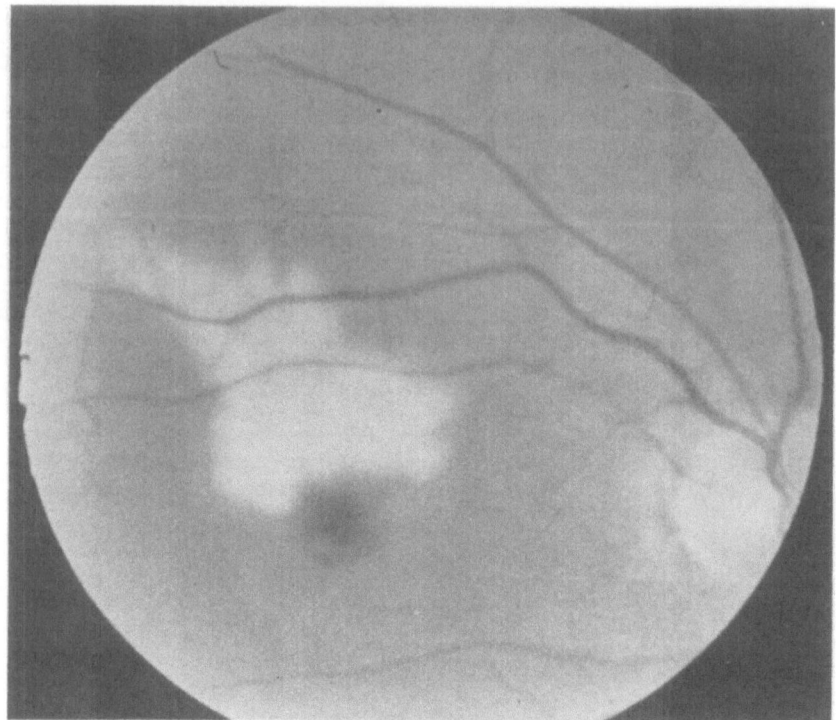

Fig. 5

with membranes extending into the fovea (Figs. 3, 4, 5, 6). If there is blood present around the margins of the extrafoveal choroidal neovascularization, treatment is to extend 100 microns beyond the edge of visible portions of the choroidal neovascularization. Treatment in the papillomacular bundle shall not be performed closer to the optic nerve head than 400 microns. For selected patients with membranes involving the entire fovea and centered around the fovea, a horseshoe-shaped treatment will be placed to surround most of the membrane in its extrafoveal portion. The feeder vessel approach will be used in very select cases where we can demonstrate such a vessel (Fig. 7). We will treat the feeder vessel first if it is identified and then treat the remaining extrafoveal portion of the choroidal neovascular membrane. We feel that it is possible that part of the effectiveness in cases that show marked suppression may be related to the fact that we are inadvertently closing a feeder vessel to the remainder of the net.

The statistics which Dr. Schlaegel listed in the four publications previously related are not statistically significant regarding final scotoma in relation to the size of the net, the proximity of the treatment to the fovea, and the response in the remaining choroidal neovascular membrane. Also, although promising, there is really no statistically significant evidence that the vision

146

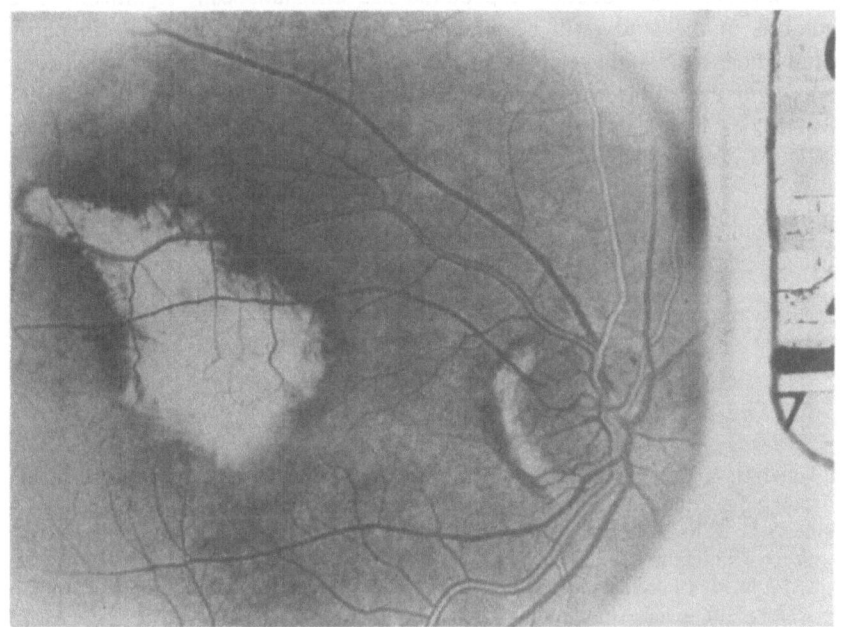

Fig. 6

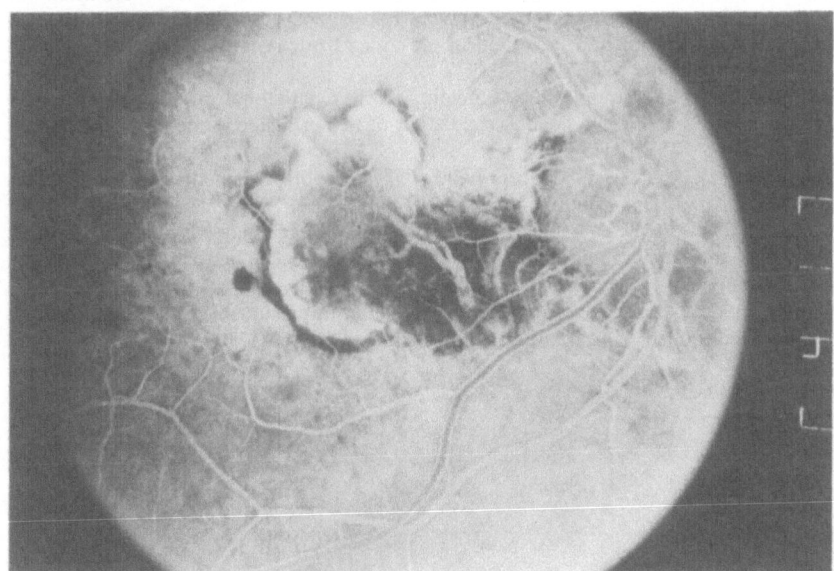

Fig. 7. (Case of Drs. D. Orth and A. Patz). Feeder Vessel to subfoveal choroidal neovascular membrane.

147

will improve. The reduction in scotoma size was statistically significant. The controls in the study will be similar to those in the Diabetic Retinopathy Study and we will have a reading center, coordinating center, statistician, and computer storage of information. Where possible, our criteria and protocol will be identical to those established for the Macular Photocoagulation Study, so as to facilitate comparison of results between these two studies.

In summary, we feel that randomized partial photocoagulation of choroidal neovascular membranes in the presumed histoplasmosis ocular syndrome, is needed because of the poor prognosis in these cases. We feel this is warranted because of the encouraging preliminary results found by Dr. Schlaegel.

REFERENCES

Elliot, J. H. & D. J. Jackson. Presumed histoplasmic maculopathy: clinical course and prognosis in nonphotocoagulated eyes. Int. Ophthalmol. Clin. 15: 29 (1975).

Fine, S. L. & M. L. Klein. Natural history of choroidal neovascular membranes. Perspect. Ophthalmol. 1: 137 (1977).

Gass, J. D. M. Choroidal neovascular membranes – their visualization and treatment. Trans. Am. Acad. Ophthalmol. Otolaryngol. 77: 318 (1973).

Gass, J. D. M. & C. P. Wilkinson. Follow-up study of presumed ocular histoplasmosis. Trans. Am. Acad. Ophthalmol. Otolaryngol. 76: 672 (1972).

Gitter, K. A. & G. Cohen. Photocoagulation of active and inactive lesions of presumed ocular histoplasmosis. Am. J. Ophthalmol. 79: 428 (1975).

Klein, M. L., S. L. Fine, D. L. Knox & A. Patz. Presumed ocular histoplasmosis. Am. J. Ophthalmol. 83: 830 (1977).

Maumenee, A. E. & S. J. Ryan. Phtocoagulation of disciform macular lesions in the ocular histoplasmosis syndrome. Am. J. Ophthalmol. 75: 13 (1973).

Okun, E. Photocoagulation treatment of presumed histoplasmic choroidopathy. Trans. Am. Ophthalmol. Soc. 70: 467 (1972).

Schlaegel, T. F., Jr. Histoplasmic choroiditis. Ann. Ophthalmol. 6: 237 (1974).

Schlaegel, T. F., Jr. Partial xenon coagulation of net in histoplasmic choroiditis. Ann. Ophthalmol. 7: 467 (1975).

Schlaegel, T. F., Jr. & J. C. Weber. Follow-Up study of presumed histoplasmic choroiditis. Am. J. Ophthalmol. 71: 1192 (1971).

Schlaegel, T. F., Jr., D. D. Cofield, G. Clark & j. C. Weber. Photocoagulation and other therapy for histoplasmic choroiditis. Trans. Am. Acad. Ophthalmol. Otolaryngol. 72: 359 (1968).

Watzke, R. C. & P. E. Leaverton. Light coagulation in presumed histoplasmic choroiditis. A controlled clinical study. Arch. Ophthalmol. 86: 127 (1971).

Authors' address:
L.J. Singerman
26900 Cedar Road 323
Beachwood, Ohio 44122
U.S.A.

THE TREATMENT OF EXUDATIVE SENILE MACULOPATHY BY RED CONTINUOUS KRYPTON LASER (647 nm)

Y. YASSUR, N. D. SCHLAEN, R. ȘIEGEL,
B. SILVERSTON & I. BEN-SIRA

(*Tel Aviv, Israel*)

The term Exudative Senile Maculopathy (ESM) has been applied to macular lesions expressed in a serous or hemorrhagic detachment of the RPE, with or without sensory retina elevation, often the result of subretinal neovascularization (SRNV). The etiology of this entity remains obscure, although many causal factors have been advocated. The modern approach to the treatment of this disease is photocoagulation with argon laser of the SRNV. This treatment is often of little benefit to the patient. One limiting factor appears to be the absorption of this type of wave length by blood impregnated nerve fibers and the resulting damage to this important layer.

On the other hand, krypton laser continuous red light of 647 nm is highly transmitted through hemoglobin and xanthophyll and absorbed mainly by the melanin, the RPE, and the choroid, thus theoretically preserving the sensory retinal tissue from being injured in the process of photocoagulation of the subretinal neovascular membrane.

In the present paper, the results of krypton laser treatment of eyes with ESM are compared to the natural history of this disease in untreated eyes. Fifty-one eyes of 35 patients ranging between 46 and 81 years were studied. The follow-up on the patients consisted of visual acuity measurements, stereo color photography and stereo fluorescein angiography before, during and at the end of the follow-up period. The lesions were foveal in two eyes, extrafoveal in nine eyes, and both foveal and extrafoveal in 40 eyes. Thirty-four eyes were treated in a 'horseshoe' pattern around the fovea or directly on the exudative and on the hemorrhagic neovascular lesion, or by a combination of the two modes of treatment. Seventeen eyes were left untreated.

The laser energy was administered with the help of a Lasertek 41 A-K unit and a Haag-Streit 900 Slit Lamp. The power used ranged from 200 to 700 mW, the spot size was between 50 to 500 μ, and the exposure time from 0.05 seconds to a few seconds.

Visual improvement was noted only in the treated eyes: 24% of them had a better VA at the end of the follow-up period than before the treatment. Thirty-two percent (11/34) of the treated eyes and 41% (7/17) of the untreated eyes showed a significant visual loss, while the rest of the eyes in

Docum. Ophthal. Proc. Series, Vol. 25, ed. by H. Zauberman
© *1981, Dr. W. Junk bv Publishers, The Hague*

both groups did not show any significant change in VA. Improvement of vision was always accompanied by reduction of edema and a marked or complete flattening of retina, and decrease or disappearance of the fluorescein active leakage.

Most of the cases which showed improvement had extrafoveal lesions, but three of the improving eyes had also an involvement of the foveal area, and evident SRNV membranes were demonstrated by fluorescein angiography in two of them, and these lesions were treated on the fovea.

The results of this study suggest a beneficial effect of krypton laser treatment of ESM when compared to the course of untreated eyes with a similar type of lesion. Exudative and hemorrhagic lesions in the macular area, which are dangerous to approach by means of argon laser either due to the presence of blood in the nerve fiber layer or due to the proximity of the fovea, should in our opinion be considered for red-krypton laser photocoagulation.

Authors' address:
Department of Ophthalmology
Beilinson Medical Center
The Sackler School of Medicine
Tel Aviv University
Tel Aviv, Israel

PARAFOVEOLAR SUBRETINAL NEOVASCULARIZATION: FEASIBILITY STUDY OF ARGON LASER TREATMENT

GISELE SOUBRANE & GABRIEL COSCAS

(*Creteil, France*)

ABSTRACT

This feasibility study attempts to determine the indication for treatment of macular neovascularization. Photocoagulation offers the only therapeutic possibility of destroying neovascular membranes but the indications are still controversial.

The study shows that laser photocoagulation is possible even very near to the center of the foveola with recuperation or preservation of useful central vision.

A randomized trial needs to be done in order to acquire statistical evidence that this modality of treatment is indeed indicated.

Subretinal new vessels, originating from the choriocapillars, are a dangerous component of disciform macular degeneration.

In most patients, the neovascular tissue underlies the fovea and, sometimes, is located very near the foveola at the initial stage. The early clinical recognition of this membrane is essential. Ophthalmoscopic examination is often sufficient for a proper diagnosis. However, the fluorescein angiogram provides the clinician with a more exact location of the subretinal membrane. This is essential to determine if argon laser photocoagulation can be of potential benefit. The aim of this feasibility study is to determine if it is possible to achieve new vessel obliteration, even in the avascular area, and preserve useful central vision.

A rationale exists for the use of photocoagulation in the treatment of the exudative manifestation that develops following subretinal noevascularization. Recent studies suggest that photocoagulation is justifiable, but its indications are still controversial. Since intense photocoagulation is desired, it is necessary to have a sufficient distance between the edge of the choroidal neovascular membrane and the center of the fovea, to prevent significant damage to the central foveal cones. Usually, 150 microns (150μ = the width

Department of Ophthalmology, University of Paris XII, School of Medicine, Hopital Intercommunal de Creteil; 40 Avenue de Verdun, 94010 Creteil, France.

This study was supported by a grant from I.N.S.E.R.M. and Caisse Nationale d'Assurance Maladie des Travailleurs Salariés, no 900-650-007.

151

of one large vein) beyond the border of the perifoveal capillary ring is considerated as a safe distance for treatment.

In this study, we treated subretinal new vessels extending into the avascular area yet not underlying the foveola centralis. Precise and extensive explanations are given to the patients made them realize that an absolute paracentral scotoma may develop after this treatment.

Criteria for selection of patients: We have included only patients with clearly defined subretinal neovascularization on fluorescein angiogram. Patients with a large amount of blood or exsudate in the subretinal or subpigment epithelial spaces were excluded.

Patients with visual acuity of at least 0.1 and with a neovascular membrane located between 100 to 400 microns from the center of the foveola were considered.

Visual acuity, central visual field (Friedman analyzer) and stereoscopic fluorescein angiograms (KOWA R C W2) were recorded before the first treatment and during the follow-up period which extended from 6 to 24 months.

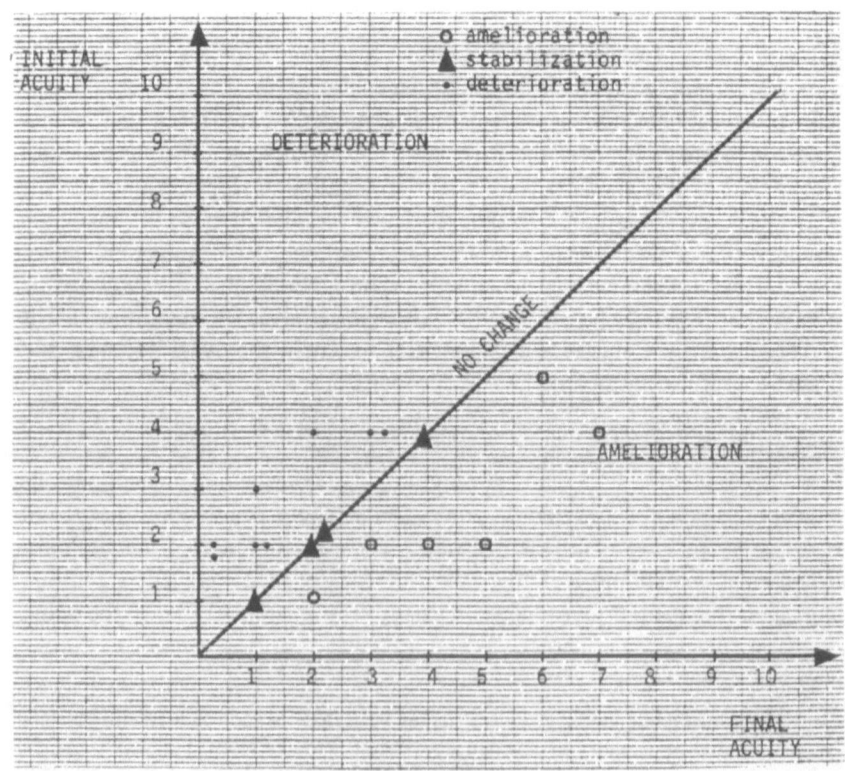

Fig. 1.

We applied photocoagulation with the help of a Coherent Radiation 800 argon laser. The photocoagulation treatment extended 100 microns past the edge of neovascular membrane in all directions. The placement of small spots on the foveal edge of the membrane provided a good visual mark to prevent photocoagulation of the foveola centralis. We applied burns of 100 or 200 μ and a timing of 0.1", with sufficient energy to obtain an intense white burn. The remainder of the peripheral border of the membrane was then treated. After completely surrounding the neovascular membrane, the central portion of the lesion was treated with 200 to 500 μ spots, using 0.2" exposure. Treatment was performed when possible the same day as the clinical examination and fluorescein angiography.

A regular follow-up, that included visual acuity, visual field and fluorescein angiography, was done twice weekly, and once weekly during the first months. Generally, there is sufficient edema to produce marked early hypofluorescence of the treated area. The main problem is residual neovascularization at the edge of the treated area, which needs repeated applications of photocoagulation as soon as possible.

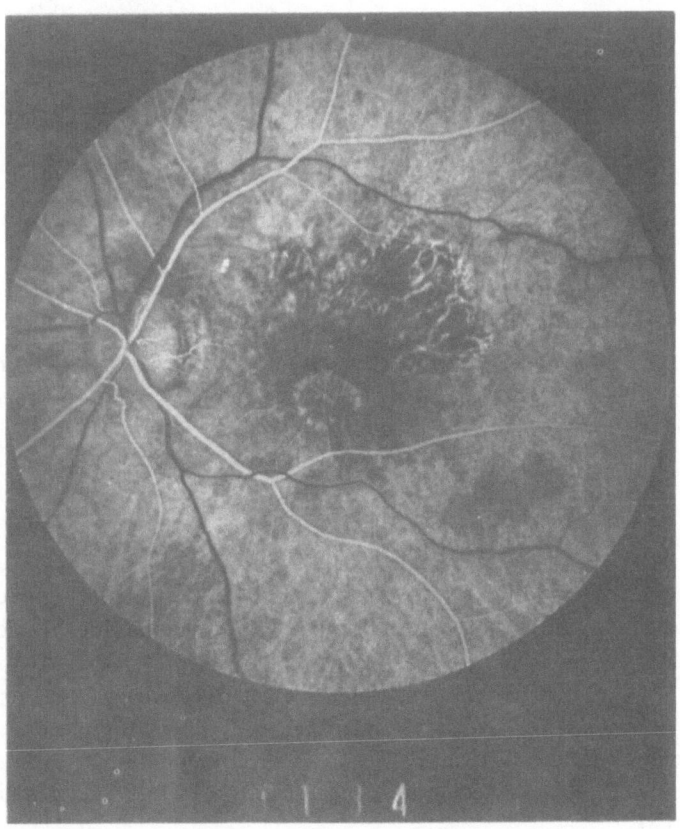

Fig. 2.

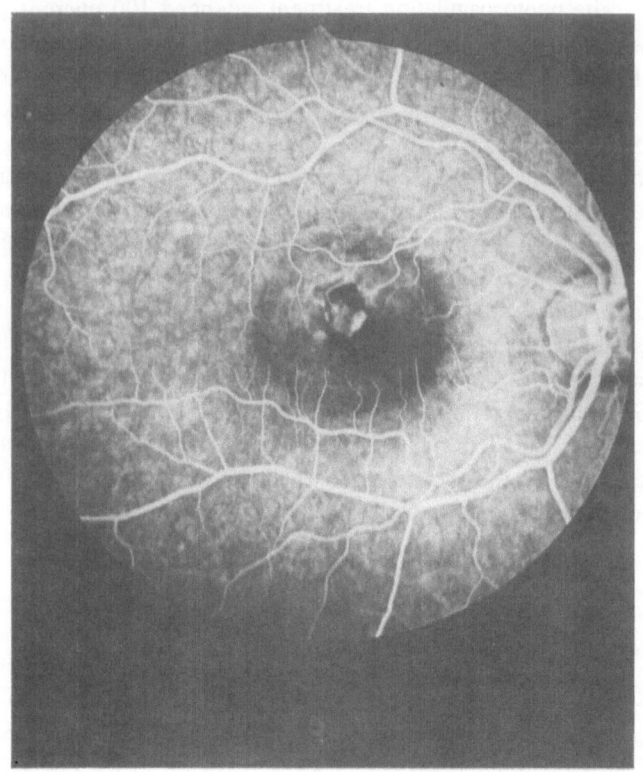

Fig. 3.

Once the lesion was treated, recurrences or a new neovascular lesion may appear, which must be detected as soon as possible using Amsler grid examinations and periodical angiography.

RESULTS

We have considered the results of treatment of 19 patients with clearly defined membranes, located between 100 and 400 microns from the foveola centralis.

The duration of subjective symptoms ranged between 3 to 70 days (mean: 28 days).

The fellow eye had lost central vision in seven patients.

Initial visual acuity varied from 0.1/Parinaud n° 14 to 0.5/Parinaud n° 3 (mean: 0.3).

The age ranged between 20 to 70 years old (mean: 47.9 years).

154

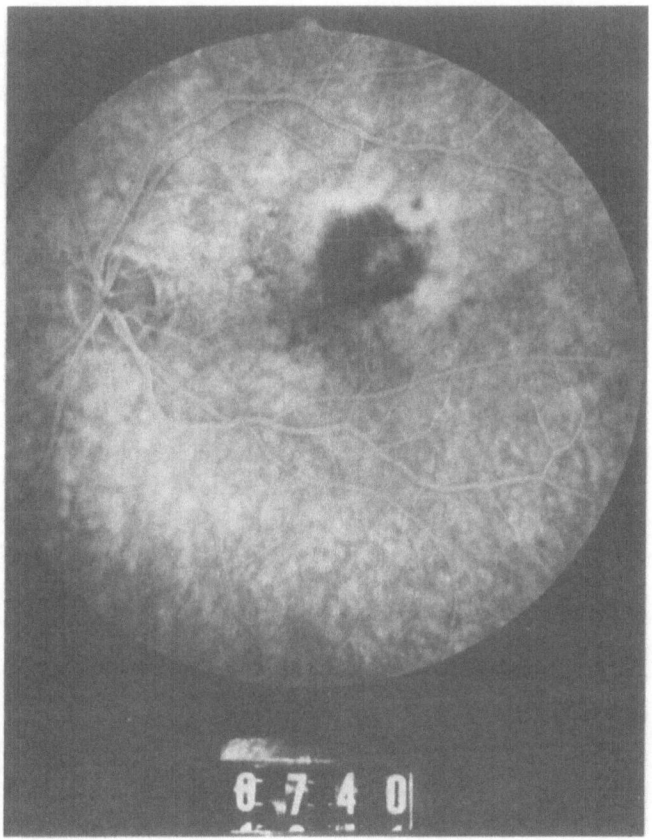

Fig. 4.

Visual acuity improved in four patients, did not change in nine patients, and became worse in six patients (Fig. 1).

Follow-up of these patients ranged from 11 to 26 months (average: 19 months).

Two sessions of treatment were required for three patients and four sessions for one patient with recurrences. Repeated treatment was impossible for two other patients.

COMMENTS

In most papers, improvement or stabilization of the visual acuity after photocoagulation of macular neovascular membrane is said to be obtained in approximately 10%. But nearly all cases of failure are late cases and nearly all good results were obtained in the earliest cases.

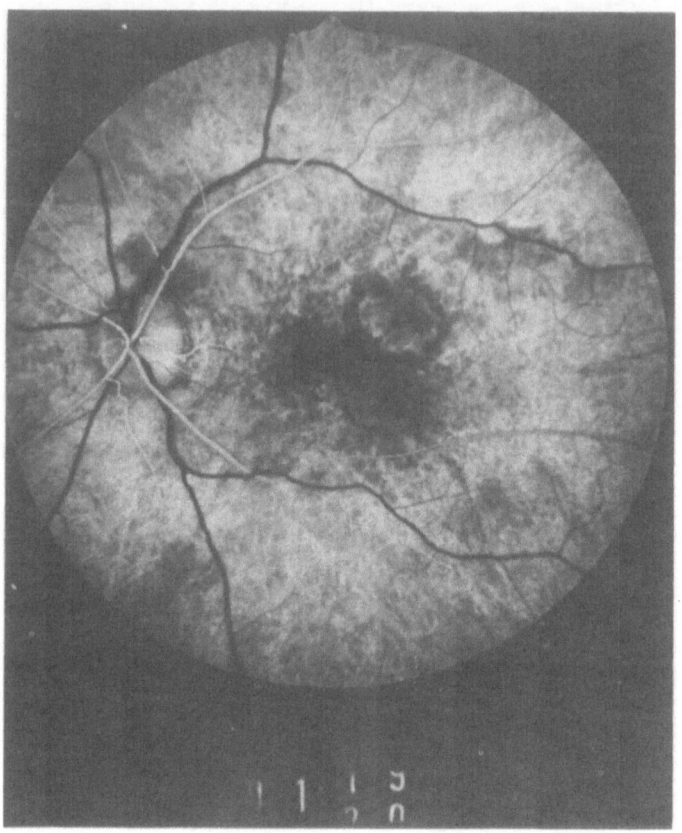

Fig. 5.

The smallest distance to keep free of photocoagulation between the edge of the neovascular tissue and the center of the foveola is still not known.

The level of light energy necessary to achieve obliteration of the new vessels is still difficult to define. There is a poor penetration for a deep thermal effect beneath the pigment epithelium but the light energy is absorbed by luteal pigment and could provoke extensive destruction.

In younger patients, the problem is to know if the end point after laser treatment will show a smaller scar and a better sparing of the foveola, than does natural course.

In older patients, the main difficulty is the management of recurrences at the same location: they may be induced secondarily to laser by rupture of Bruch's membrane.

The natural course of the disease shows a tendency for other areas of the macula to develop new vessels. They may occur soon after treatment, and post-operative follow-up must be intensive with the help of angiography; but photocoagulation does not modify the basic disease process.

156

Our preliminary study shows that positive results may be obtained in cases referred early, treated without delay and regularly followed. This feasibility study shows that destruction by argon laser of macular subretinal neovascularization is possible. Argon laser burns very near to the foveola centralis $(100\,\mu)$ inside the avascular area may be considered and can allow preservation of useful central visual acuity.

Before advising this mode of treatment, we need more statistical evidence, but this data justifies a randomized prospective controlled clinical trial to document the role of photocoagulation in the management of the macular neovascular membranes.

Authors' address:
Department of Ophthalmology
Hopital de Creteil
40 Avenue de Verdun
F-94010 Creteil
France

SUBRETINAL FLUID: ORIGIN, COMPOSITION AND STUDIES ON RETINOL-BINDING PROTEIN

E. R. BERMAN, H. ZAUBERMAN & R. MICHAELI

(*Jerusalem, Israel*)

ABSTRACT

Retinol binding protein of the pigment epithelium is normally present in the cellular cytosol, but can leak out almost quantitatively if pigment epithelial cell membranes are damaged. Subretinal fluid contains fluorescent substances characteristic of vitamin A. They originate entirely from the serum. No evidence could be found for retinol binding protein in subretinal fluid originating from the pigment epithelium. These findings suggest that there is no damage to pigment epithelial cell membranes during retinal detachment in humans.

BIOCHEMICAL AND MORPHOLOGICAL STUDIES OF SUBRETINAL FLUID

The study of subretinal fluid (SRF) has challenged the imagination of clinicians and biochemists alike for nearly forty years. Most investigations have attempted to relate specific chemical markers to the sequence of events associated with retinal detachment.

For example, a direct relationship (in most cases) between protein concentration and duration of the detachment is now well established (Magitot 1934; Smith & Doughty 1960; Heath, Beck & Foulds 1962; Weber & Wilson 1963; Kranias, Kranias & Dobbie 1979). More refined immunological techniques (Cooper, Halbert & Manski 1963; Chignell, Caruthers & Rahi 1971) have brought to light the dynamic process of subretinal fluid formation since not only have serum proteins been identified, but – as the detachment progresses – the protein composition of SRF increasingly resembles that of serum. In terms of reconstructing the sequence of events in its formation, it is not however proteins that enter first but – in cases of rhegmatogenous detachment associated with retinal tears – it is liquid vitreous. The marker in this case is hyaluronic acid which has been identified in many samples (Sweeney, Karlin & Balazs 1965; Berman 1969). Low molecular weight vitreous components such as ascorbic acid (Heath et al. 1962; Weber &

Supported in part by National Institutes of Health Grant EYO1131.

159

Wilson 1964) and lactic acid (Gloor 1970) are present at high concentrations in SRF and may originate from the vitreous as well. On the other hand, their high concentration in retina suggests multicompartmental origin for these – and other – low molecular weight components. Lipids (Lam, Van Heuven, Ray & Feman 1975), probably components of serum lipoproteins (Kaufman 1976), have also been identified in SRF.

Hydrolytic enzymes are a recent addition to the list of SRF components. One of them, butyrylcholinesterase, is an excellent marker (Kaufman & Podos 1973, 1974) since, although present in measurable concentrations in plasma, it is virtually absent in normal ocular tissues and fluids (Leopold & Furman 1970). This enzyme was elevated in about 90% of cases of primary rhegmatogenous detachment where values reached close to 18% of those present in serum. Another hydrolytic enzyme, carboxyl esterase, shows a somewhat more complex pattern (Lam, Constable & Schepens 1972; Lam *et al.* 1974, 1977). Of the three isoenzymic forms present, one is identical to that found in serum while the other two are found in circulating blood monocytes. The presence of the latter isoenzymes in SRF suggests that – characteristic of their behavior in other tissues – monocytes infiltrate the tissue in response to injury and are subsequently transformed into macrophages.

That indeed this is the case has been shown in studies on the sediment obtained after centrifugation of SRF samples (Feeney, Burns & Mixon 1975; Lam *et al.* 1977). Two cellular components have been identified. One consists of free-floating pigment epithelial cells and the other of pigment-laden macrophages. It is the latter that probably secrete the two carboxyl esterases characteristic of blood monocytes (Feman & Lam 1978). These enzymes are not present in the other cell type found in SRF sediments, i.e. pigment epithelial cells.

Considering both the biochemical and morphological findings on the one hand, and the many excellent clinical and experimental investigations of retinal detachment on the other, we are able to formulate a reasonable picture of the sequence of events occurring in primary rhegmatogenous retinal detachment. The tear resulting from traction by the vitreous on the retina allows the immediate entry of fluid into the subretinal space, carrying hyaluronic acid as the most reliable biochemical marker. Increased permeability of the ocular vessels, principally those of the choroid (but also perhaps the retinal vessels), allows the entrance of plasma proteins. Photoreceptor degeneration ensues, one contributing factor possibly being the protein kinases recently reported to be present in SRF (Kranais *et al.* 1979). At this stage, although not proven directly – there is evidence (Foulds 1975, 1979) suggesting that the amount of debris that accumulates may exceed the phagocytic capabilities of the pigment epithelium. In response to this, macrophages – representing transformed circulating monocytes – enter the subretinal space. They not only phagocytize tissue debris, but also secrete certain enzymes into the subretinal fluid. Foulds (1979) believes that the macrophages may represent transformed pigment epithelial cells, but the finding of carboxyl esterase in SRF as well as in circulating monocytes, and the absence of this enzyme in pigment epithelium, would tend to support the extra-ocular origin of the macrophages. Other hydrolytic enzymes should however be examined in order to resolve this point.

VITAMIN A ALCOHOL (RETINOL) IN SUBRETINAL FLUID

The phrase 'transudate from the choriocapillaris' is often used in connection with the entrance of serum proteins into the subretinal space. This frequent- ly invoked mechanism presupposes changes in the permeability of choroidal vessels and Bruch's membrane that would allow the passage of proteins of molecular weight up to perhaps 100,000 to reach and pass through the pigment epithelium. However, to the best of our knowledge, the zonulae occludentes that join the pigment epithelial cells remain intact during retinal detachment. Therefore the proteins would somehow have to pass *through* the cells in order to reach the subretinal space. This raises the question of whether there are any changes in permeability, or damage to plasma mem- branes, of the pigment epithelium during retinal detachment and if so, how can they be detected?

Table 1. Detection of retinol binding protein in pigment epithelial cytosol

---

Incubation (1 hr, room temperature)

    1 ml of tissue cytosol
    ^{3}H-retinol (2.2×10^6 dpm; 1 µCi)

Gel filtration

    Transfer incubation mixture to a column of Sephadex G-100
Elute components in 0.2 M NaCl-50 µM phosphate buffer, pH 7.2
    Measure radioactivity in effluents

A chance observation gave us a clue as to how to approach this question. We have known from recent studies on the transport and metabolism of vitamin A in bovine pigment epithelium (Berman, Segal & Feeney 1979; Berman *et al.* 1980a, b) that as we remove the retinas in order to isolate the pigment cell layer – as gently as we try – there is inevitably enough mechan- ical damage to the apical surface of the cells to cause the almost quantitative loss of cytosol (Saari *et al.* 1977). We also know that pigment epithelial cytosol is one of the richest sources known of a specific tissue retinol binding protein of molecular weight 17,000. If it were present in SRF, we would be able to distinguish it from *serum* retinol binding protein which, in the form of its complex to pre-albumin, has a molecular weight of approximately 85,000 daltons.

Before approaching this problem, we first had to determine whether the cytosol retinol binding protein of human pigment epithelium had similar characteristics to those in other species. The method used for detecting tissue retinol binding protein is fairly simple and straightforward. As shown in Table 1, the cytosol is incubated with tritiated retinol for one hour, and then passed through a column of Sephadex G-100. Examination of the effluents for radioactivity reveals the presence (or absence – as we shall see) of binding protein. Fig. 1 shows an elution profile of cytosol from human pigment epithelium. The first peak, in the void volume of the column, represents the micellar form of ^{3}H-retinol; specific binding proteins are not present in this fraction. The last peak, eluting in the total volume of the column, represents the low molecular weight monomeric form of retinol, also not bound to any specific protein. It is the middle peak, which is measured as the Ve/Vo (the

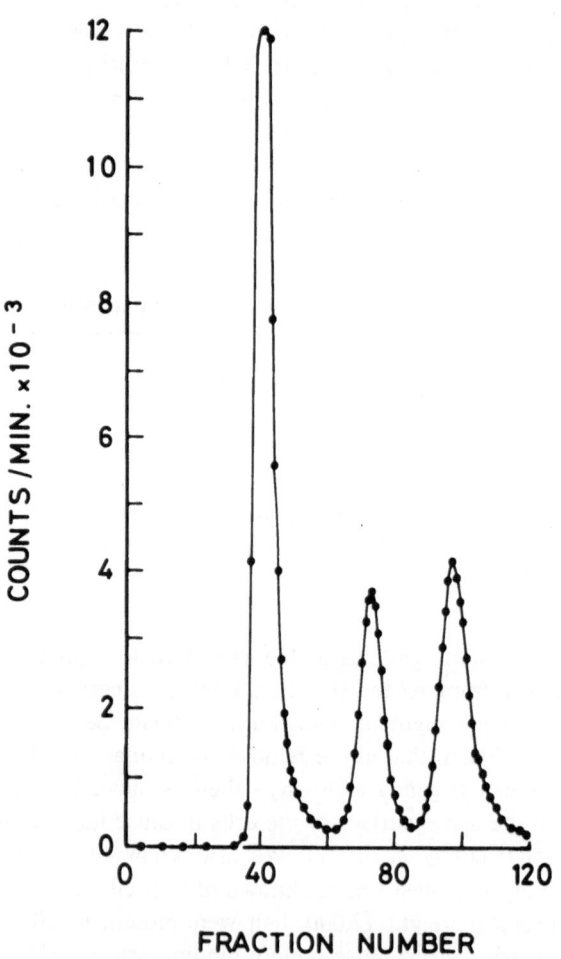

Fig. 1. Elution profile on Sephadex G-100 of retinol binding protein from human pigment epithelial cytosol. See text for explanation of the three peaks.

162

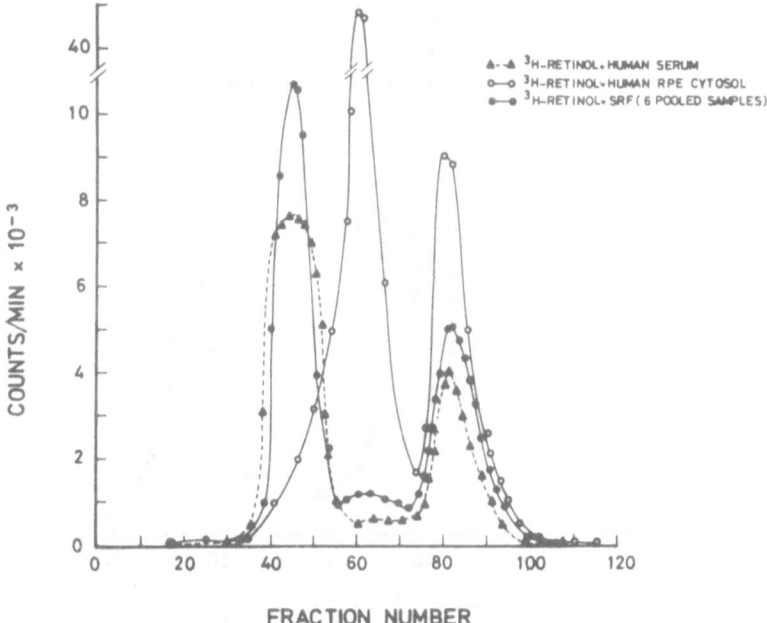

Fig. 2. Comparative elution profiles on Sephadex G-100 after incubating 1 μCi of
³h-retinol with human serum (▲ - - - ▲), human pigment epithelial cytosol (o——o)
and pooled samples of subretinal fluid from 6 patients (●——●). For the sake of clarity,
radioactivity appearing in the void volume (fraction 35) of the column has been
omitted.

ratio of elution volume to void volume), that gives us both the position and
the approximate molecular weight of the specific cytosol retinol binding
protein of the pigment epithelium. Previous calibration of these columns
with proteins of known molecular weight have shown this to be approximately 17,000 daltons. Also from our previous experience with the binding
assay, this elution pattern tells us that human pigment epithelial cytosol
contains a large amount of retinol binding protein. If any of it had escaped
into the subretinal fluid, we would be able to detect it by this technique.

But is there any vitamin A at all in subretinal fluid? This has never been
examined before, as far as we are aware. Using sensitive fluorometric techniques, we did indeed find considerable fluorescence characteristic of vitamin
A (excitation, 325 nm; emission, 470 nm). This would not however tell us
whether it derived from serum, from pigment epithelial cytosol, or both. A
clear picture of specific elution patterns of serum, pigment epithelial cytosol
and SRF provided this information, as shown in Fig. 2. The void volume
effluents have been omitted for the sake of clarity, but this peak emerged at
fraction 35. Looking first at human serum, the first peak elutes at a Ve/Vo
ratio of 1.4, which corresponds to a high molecular weight component,

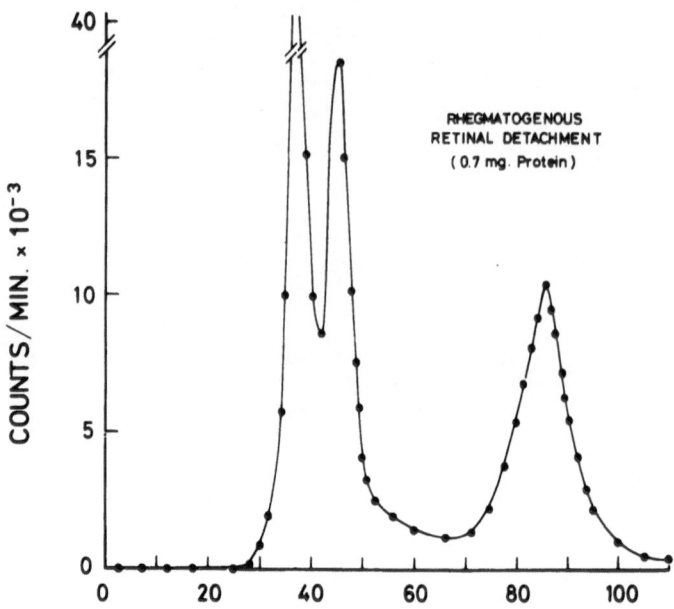

Fig. 3. Gel filtration on Sephadex G-100 of subretinal fluid from a patient with rhegmatogenous retinal detachment after incubation with 1 μCi of ³H-retinol. Fractions of 0.2 ml each were collected at a flow rate of 16 ml/hr.

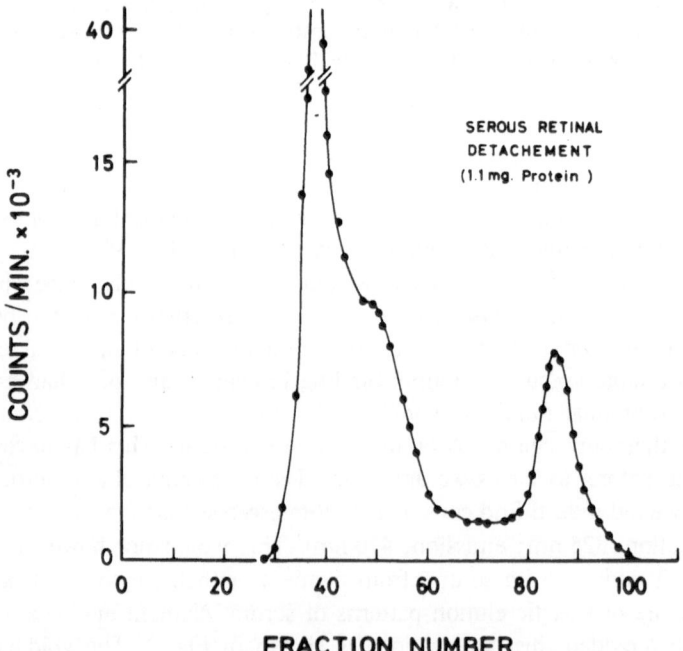

Fig. 4. Gel filtration on Sephadex G-100 of subretinal fluid from a case of vasculitis retinae and exudative retinal detachment after incubation with 1 μCi of ³H-retinol Conditions were the same as in Fig. 3.

probably albumin. As expected, there is no binding in the position where tissue cytosol would appear, namely at about fractions 55–70. As in all gel filtration patterns, the large peak at the end is an unbound monomeric form of retinol. We examined another sample of human pigment epithelial cytosol, which had no binding at the Ve/Vo of 1.4 characteristic of serum, but instead a very large peak at Ve/Vo of 1.8, characteristic of cytosol binding protein. Finally, we pooled 6 samples of SRF, since we did not want to be below the limit of detection in case only a small amount of pigment epithelial cytosol should be present. Not unexpectedly, a very large peak appears at precisely the position of serum. At the position of cytosol (fractions 55–72) there is an indication of a very small amount of pigment epithelial cytosol retinol binding protein present in this SRF sample. Considering that this represents six pooled samples, it is indeed very little.

To summarize, native SRF has fluorescence characteristic of vitamin A. Incubation with tritiated retinol and gel filtration on Sephadex G-100 enables us to determine whether the vitamin A derives from serum or from pigment epithelial cytosol. An analysis of six samples of SRF indicated that virtually all of it represents serum; only a trace can be attributed to pigment epithelial cell cytosol.

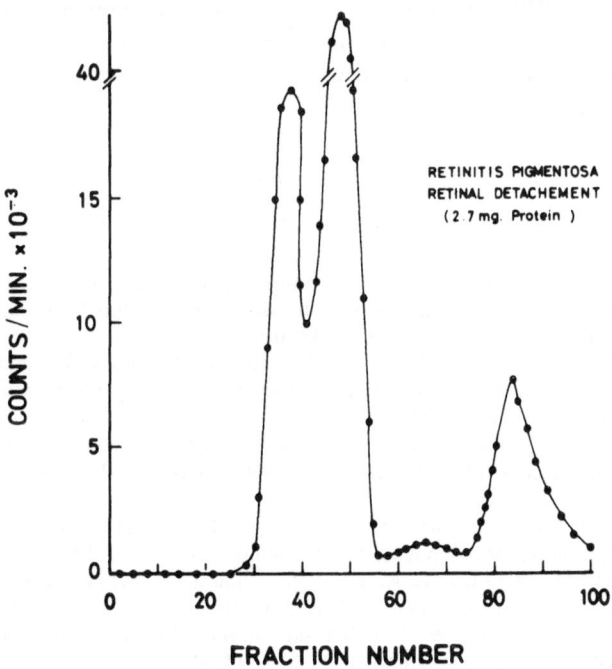

Fig. 5. Gel filtration on Sephadex G-100 of subretinal fluid from an aphakic patient with retinitis pigmentosa after incubation with 1 μCi of ^{3}H-retinol. Conditions were the same as in Fig. 3.

165

That indeed there appears to be little or no damage to pigment epithelial cell membranes during retinal detachment was shown in further analyses of individual SRF samples. In this case, we modified the procedure to increase the sensitivity by carrying out the gel filtration on specially designed microcolumns. SRF samples obtained from three different clinical cases were incubated with tritiated retinol and examined by gel filtration. In the first case of rhegmatogenous detachment (Fig. 3), containing relatively little protein (0.7 mg), all of the retinol present could be accounted for as serum. If any pigment epithelial cytosol had been present, a peak would have occurred at about fractions 55–65. Fig. 4 shows the pattern of a patient with vasculitis retinae and exudative retinal detachment. Again there was no evidence for cytosol leakage from the pigment epithelium. There was a very large serum component, and incomplete separation from the void volume peak. Finally, Fig. 5 shows the elution pattern of a very rare sample of SRF from an aphakic patient with retinitis pigmentosa, traction retinal detachment and congenital deafness. The protein content was fairly high (2.7 mg), and most of the retinol could be accounted for as the form originating from serum. Interestingly enough, a small amount of pigment epithelial cytosol binding protein (fractions 62–70) was also detectable. We do not believe however that it is large enough to conclude that there had been extensive pigment epithelial damage in this particular case, or any other, of retinal detachment studied by this technique. This leaves us with the question still unanswered of the origin of serum components in subretinal fluid. If not as a transudate from the choriocapillaris, then can we consider retinal vessels as an important site of leakage?

REFERENCES

Berman, E. R. Mucopolysaccharides (glycosaminoglycans) of the retina: Identification, distribution and possible biological role, in Mod. Probl. Ophthal. vol. 8, ed. by R. Dufour, L. Fison and G. Meyer-Schwickerath, pp. 5-31 (1969).

Berman, E. R., N. Segal & L. Feeney. Subcellular distribution of free and esterified forms of vitamin A in the pigment epithelium of the retina and in liver. Biochim. Biophys. Acta 572: 167 (1979).

Berman, E. R., J. Horowitz, N. Segal, L. Feeney & S. Fisher. Enzymatic esterification of vitamin A in the pigment epithelium of cattle retina. Biochim. Biophys. Acta, 630: 36 (1980).

Berman, E. R., N. Segal, A. Schneider & L. Feeney. An hypothesis for a vitamin A cycle in the pigment epithelium of bovine retina. Neurochemistry 1, 113 (1980).

Chignell, A. H., M. Carruthers & A. H. S. Rahi. Clinical, biochemical, and Immunoelectrophoretic study of subretinal fluid. Brit. J. Ophthal. 55: 525 (1971).

Cooper, W. C., S. P. Halbert & W. J. Manski. Immunochemical analysis of vitreous and subretinal fluid. Invest. Ophthal. 2: 369 (1963).

Feeney, L., R. P. Burns & R. M. Mixon. Human subretinal fluid. Arch. Ophthalmol. 93: 62 (1975).

Feman, S. S. & K. W. Lam. An enzyme histochemical analusis of human subretinal fluid. Arch. Ophthalmol. 96: 129 (1978).

Foulds, W. S. Clinical significance of trans-scleral fluid transfer. Doyne Memorial Lecture, 1976. Trans. Ophthal. Soc. U.K. 96: 290 (1976).

Foulds, W. S. The retinal-pigment epithelial interface. Brit. J. Ophthal. 63: 71 (1979).

Gloor, B. P. Physiology of the vitreous. In: Adler's Physiology of the Eye, Ed. By R. A. Moses, 5th ed., P. 311, C. V. Mosby, St. Louis (1970).

Heath, H., T. C. Beck & W. S. Foulds. Chemical composition of subretinal fluid. Brit. J. Ophthal. 46: 385 (1962).

Kaufman, P. L. Letter to Editor, Invest. Ophthal. 15: 237 (1976).

Kaufman, P. L. & S. M. Podos. Subretinal fluid butyrylcholinesterase. 1. Source of the enzyme and factors affecting its concentration in subretinal fluid from primary rhegmatogenous retinal detachment. Amer, J. Ophthal. 75: 627 (1973).

Kaufman, P. L & S. M. Podos. Subretinal fluid butyrylcholinesterase. 2. Reoperated rhegmatogenous detachment and diabetic traction detachments. Amer. J. Ophthal. 77: 19 (1974).

Kranias, G., E. Kranias & J. G. Dobbie. Protein kinases in the subretinal fluid. Exp. Eye Res. 29: 1 (1979).

Lam, K. W., I. J. Constable, C. Y. Li & C. L. Schepens. Studies on the cellular constituents and hydrolytic enzymes in human subretinal fluid, in Retina Congress, Ed. by R. C. Pruett and C. D. J. Regan, pp. 281-288, Appleton-Century-Crofts, New York (1974).

Lam, K. W., I. J. Constable & C. L. Schepens. Subretinal fluid: Isoenzymes and cytologic studies. Invest. Ophthal. 11: 1037 (1972).

Lam, K. W., S. S. Feman, G. S. Ray & W. A. J. Van Heuven. A biochemical characterization of the carboxyl esterase in human subretinal fluid: A study comparing the enzymes in serum, in leukocytes and in subretinal fluid. Exp. Eye Res. 24: 467 (1977).

Lam. K. W., W. A. J. Van heuven, G. S. Ray & S. Feman. Subretinal fluids: Lipid analyses. Invest. Ophthal. 14: 406 (1975).

Leopold, I. H. & M. Furman. Cholinesterase isoenzymes in human ocular tissue homogenates. Amer. J. Ophthal. 72: 460 (1971).

Magitot, A. The subretinal fluid in idiopàthic detachment of the retina. Arch. Ophthal. 11: 159 (1934).

Saari, J. C., A. H. Bunt, S. Fu.:erman & E. R. Berman. Localization of cellular retinol-binding protein in bovine ᵣᵢ:ᵢₐ and retinal pigment epithelium, with a consideration of the pigment epithelium isolation technique. Invest. Ophthalmol. and Vis. Sci. 16: 797 (1977).

Smith, J. L. & E. Doughty. Electrophoresis of subretinal fluid. Arch. Ophthal. 64: 144 (1960).

Sweeney, D. B., D. B. Karlin & E. A. Balazs. Biochemistry of subretinal fluid, Ed. by C. L. Schepens and C. D. J. Regan, Controversial Aspects of the management of Retinal Detachment, p. 316, Little, Brown and Co., Boston (1965).

Weber, J. C. & F. M. Wilson. Biochemical studies of subretinal fluid. II. Total protein and albumin of subretinal fluid and blood serum in patients with retinal detachment. Arch. Ophthal. 69: 119 (1963).

Weber, J. C. & F. M. Wilson Biochemical studies of subretinal fluid. III. Ascorbic acid of subretinal fluid in patients with retinal detachments. Arch. Ophthal. 71: 556 (1964).

Authors' address:
Hadassah Hospital
Eye Biochemistry Lab.
Jerusalem
Israel

167

IMMUNOGLOBULINS OF THE SUBRETINAL FLUID
Their significance for the prognosis of the surgical treatment of the retinal detachment

A. ZAVARO, Z. SAMRA, J. KAM,
D. SOMPOLINSKY & R. BARISHAK

(*Zerifin and Ramat Gan, Israel*)

INTRODUCTION

The formation of subretinal fluid (SRF) in rhegmatogenous retinal detachment is a complex process involving the vitreous (Cooper, Halbert & Manski 1963), the sensory retina and retinal pigment epithelium (Leopold & Furman 1971; Feeney, Burns & Nixon 1975) and the choriocapillaris (Kaufman & Podos 1973). It is generally agreed that the greatest part of the protein content of the SRF derives from the choroid (Liotet & Rouchy 1972; Chignell, Carrhuters & Rahi 1971) and that the choriocapillaris-retinal pigment epithelium barrier is an effective barrier, the permeability of which increases with the duration of the retinal detachment (Chignell, Carrhuters & Rahi 1971). It has been stated that, not the total protein content of the SRF but rather the differential protein study is a good indicator of the damage of this barrier (Chignell, Carrhuters & Rahi 1971; Rahi & Chignell 1975).

Rahi & Chignell (1975) took into consideration the studies on the differential protein clearance in the urine and suggested that a similar mechanism might control the composition of the SRF and its protein concentration. They studied the crossing of the immunoglobulins G, A and M and of the low molecular weight protein, transferrin which are all characteristic for the blood serum. They calculated the clearance C of each protein by evaluating their level in the SRF and in the serum. In addition, they determined the Selectivity Index (SI) of each of them by comparing their clearance values to that of transferrin.

They recognized three types of Barrier Damage Pattern (BDP):

In Type I, the SRF contains the serum proteins except Ig A and IgM.

In Type II, it contains the serum proteins except IgM,

In Type III, it contains also IgM.

They presumed that the presence of Ig M in the SRF is associated with a severe damage in the choriocapillaris-retinal pigment epithelium barrier. That the examination of the SRF can give a clue as to the prognosis of the retinal detachment has been negated by some authors (Liotet & Rouchy

169

1972). Rahi & Chignell (1975) proposed using the immunoglobulin analysis of the SRF as a means of differentiating rhegmatogenous retinal detachment from that due to a neoplastic invasion. Robertson (1978) showed a positive relationship between protein concentration in the SRF and duration of detachment but no relationship to other factors which included also delayed resorption of the SRF.

In this study, we applied the notions of Barrier Damage Pattern, of Clearance and Selectivity Index of the Immunoglobulins G, A and M in a trial to determine the prognosis of retinal detachment operations which required drainage of the SRF. In the evaluation of the clinical results we considered only the anatomical one, that is the reattachment of the retina. We postulated that the persistence of SRF in cases where all tears have been well closed, no technical error committed and no periretinal vitreous retraction occurred, could be attributed to the damage of the choriocapillaris-retinal pigment epithelium barrier. Functional results have not been considered as they depend on other parameters which have no connection with the condition of the choriocapillaris-retinal pigment epithelium barrier.

MATERIAL AND METHODS

The SRF of 23 patients who underwent retinal detachment operation with drainage and without any complication has been examined. The radial

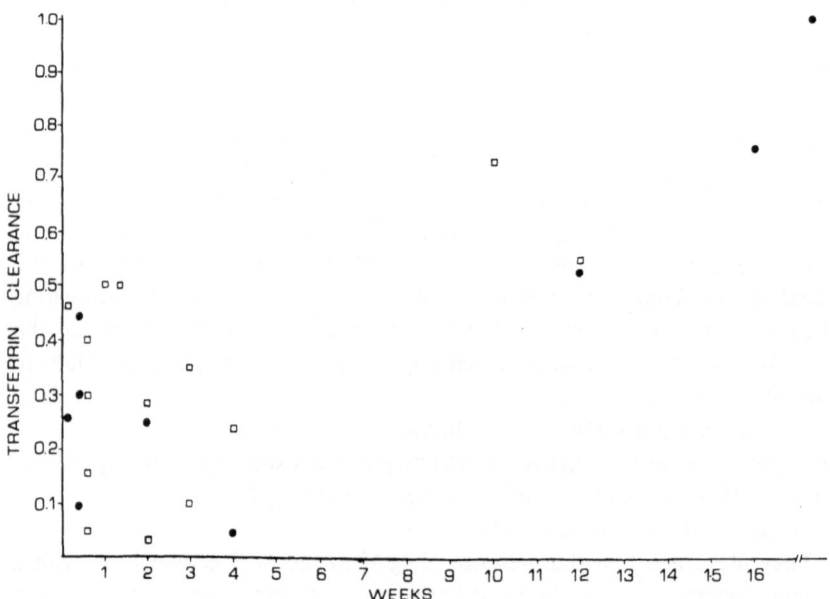

Fig. 1. Distribution of transferrin clearance in relation to barrier damage pattern (BDP) and duration of detachment: ☐ BDP I+II (14 cases). ● BDP III (9 cases).

immunodiffusion technic (Davis 1976) was used in the quantitation of immunoglobulins and transferrin in the SRF and in the serum. Details of the technic have been reported (Zavaro *et al.*, 1980). We determined the clearance of Ig G, Ig A and Ig M and deduced the type of Barrier Damage Pattern for each case. Furthermore, we evaluated the Selectivity Index of each of the immunoglobulins G, A and M and determined whether there was a selective leakage (SI value less than 0,3) or a non selective one (SI value more than 0,3). The limit value of 0,3 has been chosen by Rahi and Chignell (1975) arbitrarily. We used the same limit value for convenience and in order to be able to compare our results with those of Rahi and Chignell. As the molecular weight of IgA is quite near to that of IgG we grouped the BDP types I and II into one, the Type I–II.

The biochemical and clinical results were evaluated independently by different research workers.

RESULTS

We divided the 23 cases into 2 groups: the 1st group includes the 13 cases who had their retina reattached. The 2nd group includes the 10 cases in which the operation failed. We evaluated the distribution of the BDP types in both groups (Table 1). In the 1st group, 11 cases presented the type I–II

Table 1. Distribution of BDP types according to clinical result (anatomical)

Anatomical result	Number of cases	BDP Type	
		I – II	III
Success	13	11	2
Failure	10	3	7

BDP: Barrier Damage Pattern.
I – II: Subretinal fluid contains Ig G or Ig G + Ig A.
III   : Subretinal fluid contains Ig G + Ig A + Ig M.

and 2 cases the type III. In the 2nd group, 3 cases presented the type I–II and 7 cases the type III.

We compared the type of BDP with the SI values for Ig G, IgA and Ig M in both groups. In the 1st group (Table 2), 7 cases showed a type II of BDP and low SI for Ig G and Ig A. Of the remaining 4 cases with a type II, 2 showed a high SI for Ig G and Ig A and 2 showed a high SI for one of them. The 2 cases with a type III of BDP showed a low SI for all the 3 immunoglobulins.

171

Table 2. Distribution of BDP types and SI values in group I (successful cases)

Case No.	Anatomical result	BDP Type	SI Ig G	SI Ig A	SI Ig M
18	+	II	Low	Low	—
15	+	II	Low	Low	—
22	+	II	Low	Low	—
25	+	II	Low	Low	—
20	+	II	Low	Low	—
26	+	II	Low	Low	—
27	+	II	Low	Low	—
21	+	II	High	High	—
6	+	II	High	High	—
28	+	II	Low	High	—
10	+	II	High	Low	—
8	+	III	Low	Low	Low
16	+	III	Low	Low	Low

Anatomical result (+): Success.
BDP   : Barrier Damage Pattern.
SI   : Selectivity Index.
Low SI : Less than 0,3.
High SI: More than 0,3.

Table 3. Distribution of BDP types and SI values in group II (Non-successful cases)

Case No.	Anatomical result	BDP Type	SI Ig G	SI Ig A	SI Ig M
5	—	III	Low	—	Low
13	—	III	Low	Low	Low
19	MVR	III	Low	Low	Low
11	—	III	High	Low	Low
12	MVR	III	High	Low	Low
17	—	III	Low	Low	High
29	—	III	High	High	High
14	—	II	High	Low	—
23	—	II	High	High	—
9	—	I	Low	—	—

Anatomical result (—): Failure.
Low SI value: Less than 0,3
High SI value: More than 0,3.
BDP: Barrier Damage Pattern.
SI: Selectivity Index.
Anatomical result MVR: Massive vitreous retraction.

172

In the 2nd group (Table 3) 7 out of 10 cases had a type III BDP. Only 1 case presented a type III of BDP and a high SI for Ig G, Ig A and Ig M. Of the other 6 cases, 3 showed a low SI for all the 3 immunoglobulins, 2 presented a high SI for Ig G and a low SI for Ig A and Ig M and 1, a low SI for Ig G and Ig A and a high SI for Ig M. The 2 cases with a type II of BDP showed a high SI for one or both of the immunoglobulins G and A. The case No. 9 presented a type I of BDP and a low SI for Ig G.

DISCUSSION

The immunoglobulin pattern of the SRF reflects the functional condition of the choriocapillaris-retinal pigment epithelium barrier. The types of Barrier Damage Pattern as described by Rahi & Chignell (1975) correspond to different degrees of damage of this barrier. When the damage is mild only low molecular weight proteins such as transférrin and albumin cross the barrier. When the damage is moderate the immunoglobulins G and A cross the barrier and this condition corresponds to the types I and II of BDP. If the damage is severe Ig M, a high molecular weight protein crosses the barrier and the composition of the SRF corresponds to that of Type III of BDP.

We noted a correlation between the BDP type and the clinical result (Table 1). In the 1st group, 11 cases showed a type II of BDP. That means that in 11 out of 23 cases, that is in 48% of cases the type II correlated the clinical success. In the 2nd group, 7 cases showed the type III. So in 7 out of 23 cases, that is in 30% of cases the type III correlated the clinical failure. So, to determine the presence or absence of Ig M in the SRF helped in 78% of cases to evaluate the prognosis of the retinal detachment operation. Rachal et al. (1979) mentioned the 'inadequate chorioretinal reaction' as one of the factors of failure of the retinal detachment operation. We presume that in cases of failure due to such a reaction, the composition of the SRF would present a type III of BDP if the SRF had been examined biochemically. Incidentally we have to emphasize that the type III of BDP was noted in cases of failure due to massive periretinal vitreous retraction. Taking into consideration the fact that the permeability of the choriocapillaris-retinal pigment epithelium barrier increases with the duration of the retinal detachment, we tried to determine whether there is a greater percentage of cases with a type III of BDP among the cases of long duration of retinal detachment. We observed (Table 4) that in the group of cases with a duration of less than 1 month, the proportion was 6/17 and in the group of cases with a duration of more than 2 months the proportion was 2/4. With the limited number of cases available, we could not show a direct relationship between the number of cases with type III and the duration of the detachment.

We tried to correlate the BDP types to the SI values. One could presume that a type II of BDP should be associated to low SI values and that a type

Table 4. Distribution of BDP types according to duration of detachment

Duration of detachment	BDP Types	
	I – II	III
Less than 4 weeks	11	6
4–8 Weeks	1	1
More than 4 weeks	2	2

BDP: Barrier Damage Pattern.
I – II: Subretinal fluid contains Ig G or Ig G + Ig A.
III   : Subretinal fluid contains Ig G + Ig A + Ig M.

III of BDP should be associated to high SI values. However, we observed a marked discrepancy between the BDP types and the SI values, discrepancy more marked in the group II including the unsuccessful cases (Tables 2 & 3). It is possible that the BDP type expresses another facet of the damage of the choriocapillaris-retinal pigment epithelium barrier. Than the SI values of the immunoglobulins. It should be considered that the SI value depends not only on the leakage of the immunoglobulin but also on the leakage of transferrin. For instance, the SI might be high not because of a severe leakage of the immunoglobulin but because of a very low clearance of transferrin.

The transferrin, a low molecular weight protein crosses readily the choriocapillaris-retinal pigment epithelium barrier and one could presume that its Clearance C value must show a relation to the degree of damage of this barrier. But we observed a great variability in the C values of transferrin, not always in accordance with the type of BDP. 14 of our cases presented a type I + II of BDP and 9 cases a type III (Fig. 1). The mean C value in the group of cases with type II was 0,333 and in the group of cases with type III was 0,415. But in the group of type I + II the C value varied between 0,033 and 0,736 and in the group of type III between 0,05 and 1,056. So the variability of the C value of transferrin remained high in both groups and as a result, the variability in the SI values is expected also to be high. Such a great variability is also noted in the C values of the immunoglobulins G, A and M.

Our conclusion is that a very specific permeability is present at the choriocapillaris-retinal pigment epithelium barrier and that the molecular weight is not the only factor which regulates the crossing of proteins in cases of damage of this barrier.

Does the immunoglobulin analysis of the SRF give us a clue regarding the prognosis of the retinal detachment operation? In 78% of cases we noted a positive correlation between the BDP type and the clinical result. But the discrepancy between the BDP types and the SI values demands a critical appraisal of these values.

REFERENCES

Chignell, A. M., M. Carrhuters & M. S. Rahi. Clinical, biochemical and immunoelec-trophoretic study of the subretinal fluid. Brit. J. Ophthalmol. 55: 525-531 (1971).

Cooper, W. C., S. P. Halbert & W. J. Manski. Immunochemical analysis of vitreous and subretinal fluid. Invest. Ophthalmol. 2: 369-377 (1963).

Davis, N. & M. O. Monto. Manual of clinical immunology, American Society for Microbiology, Washington D. C. p. 4-16 (1976).

Feeney, L., R. P. Burns & R. M. Nixon. Human subretinal fluid. Its cellular and subcellular components. Arch. Ophthalmol. 93: 62-69 (1975).

Kaufman, P. L. & S. M. Podos. The subretinal fluid in primary rhegmatogenous retinal detachment. Survey of Ophthalmology, 18: 100-116 (1973).

Leopold, I. M. & M. Furman. Cholinesterase isoenzymes in human ocular tissue homogenates. Amer. J. Ophthalmol. 72: 460-463 (1971).

Liotet, S. & J. P. Rouchy. Etude des proteines de liquides de decollement retinien. Arch. Opht. (Paris). 32: 323-332 (1972).

Rachal, W. F. & T. C. Burton. Changing concepts of failure after retinal detachment surgery. Arch. Ophthalmol. 97: 480-483 (1979).

Rahi, A. M. S. & A. M. Chignell. Immunoelectrophoretic analysis of subretinal fluid and its diagnostic significance. Trans. Ophthal. Soc. U.K. 95: 180-183 (1975).

Robertson, D. M. Delayed absorption of subretinal fluid after scleral buckling proce-dures: the significance of subretinal precipitates. Trans. Am. Ophthal. Soc. 76: 557-583 (1978).

Zavaro, A. Z. Samra, R. Barishak & D. Sompolinsky. Proteins in tears from healthy and diseased eyes. Docum. Ophthal. 50: 185-199 (1980).

Authors' address:
Assaf Harofe Hospital
Zerifin and Bar Ilan University
Ramat Gan
Israel

SEASONAL VARIATIONS ON THE CORTISOL CONCENTRATION OF THE SUBRETINAL FLUID IN RHEGMATOGENOUS RETINAL DETACHMENT

J. GÄRTNER, K. SINTERHAUF, K. H. SCHICKETANZ & G. BÖHM

(*Mainz, F.R.G.*)

ABSTRACT

Probes of the subretinal fluid were obtained from 115 nonselected retinal detachments, operated on during the period from November 19, 1973 to December 20, 1974. All patients had no known endocrine abnormalities and had not ever received topical or systemic corticosteroid therapy. Subretinal fluid cortisol was determined by competitive protein binding analysis. A statistically significant increase in mean subretinal fluid cortisol concentration was found for the winter season ($3.3\,\mu g/100$ ml), as compared with the summer months ($1.5\,\mu g/100$ ml). This finding sharply contrasts with the seasonal incidence of the idiopathic retinal detachments which reaches its maximum in the months June to August, whereas during the winter months it is at its lowest.

INTRODUCTION

The level of various constituents of the subretinal fluid (SRF) in rhegmatogenous retinal detachments has been studied by several authors (Kaufman & Podos 1973; Akhmeteli *et al.* 1975). However, to the best of our knowledge, the cortisol content of SRF has so far not been investigated.

It may be adopted as a working hypothesis that, as in other extracellular matrices, for instance the trabecular meshwork of the chamber angle (Spaeth *et al.* 1977), the corticosteroids contribute in some way to the maintenance of the extracellular matrix of the subretinal space. Therefore an investigation was undertaken in which the level of this hormone in the SRF was determined. With regard to the seasonal rhythm in the occurence of idiopathic retinal detachments observed in central Europe (see Gärtner *et al.* 1977), special attention was given to chronobiological aspects.

MATERIAL AND METHODS

The investigation was carried out on 115 specimens of SRF from 49 men and 69 women suffering from bullous retinal detachment, operated on during the period November 19, 1973 to December 20, 1974. The patients

177

ranged in age from 16 to 80 years, with an average age of 57.5. Retinal surgery of 105 patients was performed under general anesthesia. In ten cases local anesthesia was used. All patients had no known endocrine abnormalities, had not recently taken drugs known to alter plasma cortisol levels, and were not given such drugs preoperatively.

SRF was taken during surgery at the highest point of the detachment. The incision of the sclera, suprachoroidea and choroidea was performed step by step under the microscope, using transillumination during the perforation of the choroid (Freeman & Schepens 1975; Gärtner 1975). Thus, the release of SRF was an absolutely controlled microsurgical procedure, avoiding contamination by blood in the operative field. All surgery was performed by one surgeon between 9:00 A.M. and 1:00 P.M. During this period the mean plasma cortisol concentration in men has been found to be relatively constant (Sinterhauf et al. 1975).

The specimens were pipetted off and the fluid was then stored without centrifugation at $-20\,°C$. Specimens of SRF with an admixture of even a minimum amount of blood, visible under the microscope, were not frozen. The randomized cortisol determinations were done in a large series, at the end of the whole study, by means of competitive proteinbinding analysis (Berson, Yalow 1968; Fiorelli et al. 1972). All quantitative hormone assays were performed by the same person, using the cortisol radioassay kit (^3H) from Schwarz/Mann. For quality control we tested the accurancy at 5, 15, and 60 µg/100 ml in 20 single runs by addition of cortisol and the precision by intra- and interassayvariances. Further details concerning the biochemical procedure are published elsewhere (Böhm 1977).

For statistical analysis of the seasonal trends an analysis of variance in an unbalanced design was performed. Because of the distinct skewness of the empirical distributions the analysis of variance was applied to the logarithmically transformed data. In addition linear contrasts by Scheffé's method were calculated.

The different anesthetic techniques (halothane, neurolept, local anesthesia) were compared by means of the chi – square test with respect to the seasonal distributions of the retinal detachments. Further details concerning the statistical methods are published elsewhere (Gärtner et al. 1977).

RESULTS

The data of cortisol concentrations are listed in Table 1.

As antilogarithms of the mean values of the transformed cortisol levels the following data for the meteorological seasons were obtained: Spring (March – May) = 2.3 µg/100 ml, summer (June – August) = 1.5 µg/100 ml, autumn (September – November) = 2.3 µg/100 ml, and winter (December – February) = 3.3 µg/100 ml.

178

Table 1. Cortisol concentration (µg/100 ml) in the subretinal fluid of 115 eyes with retinal detachment

Month	Serial no.	Sex	Age (years)	Cortisol concentration
November 1973	1	male	51	3,5
	2	female	58	2,0
	3	male	51	1,6
	4	male	64	1,6
December 1973	5	male	67	1,4
	6	male	41	1,4
	7	female	66	2,3
January 1974	8	male	55	6,5
	9	male	80	7,5
	10	male	60	1,6
	11	female	59	5,5
February 1974	12	female	63	3,9
	13	male	32	3,7
	14	male	68	7,7
	15	female	52	3,4
	16	female	53	4,4
March 1974	17	male	33	1,4
	18	female	67	2,1
	19	female	65	2,3
	20	female	59	2,6
	21	female	65	1,3
	22	female	64	3,6
	23	female	67	4,0
	24	male	54	3,6
	25	male	67	5,4
April 1974	26	female	51	0,8
	27	female	51	3,4
	28	male	64	2,5
	29	female	51	1,5
	30	female	51	1,3
	31	male	69	4,7
	32	female	63	2,6
	33	male	68	3,3
	34	male	67	7,4
May 1974	35	male	74	1,0
	36	male	46	1,0
	37	female	69	0,8
	38	female	57	1,5
	39	female	66	4,4
	40	female	75	4,5
June 1974	41	female	75	1,3
	42	male	58	0,4
	43	female	68	0,6
	44	female	64	1,5

Table 1. Cortisol concentration (continued)

Month	Serial no.	Sex	Age (years)	Cortisol concentration
	45	female	66	0,4
	46	male	60	1,9
	47	female	53	0,9
	48	male	69	0,6
	49	male	73	1,7
	50	male	80	4,1
	51	female	63	0,9
	52	male	51	1,4
July 1974	53	female	69	0,6
	54	female	61	1,3
	55	male	69	1,6
	56	female	69	2,0
	57	female	29	0,6
	58	female	25	0,7
	59	male	57	0,6
	60	female	74	1,7
	61	female	49	1,0
	62	male	61	0,7
	63	female	62	4,2
	64	female	65	6,5
	65	female	54	1,1
	66	male	24	0,6
	67	male	60	2,7
	68	female	30	4,1
	69	female	77	5,6
	70	female	72	3,8
August 1974	71	female	63	2,3
	72	female	65	2,4
	73	male	52	4,9
	74	female	71	5,9
	75	male	74	1,0
	76	female	26	1,9
	77	male	58	4,4
September 1974	78	female	60	4,4
	79	female	75	3,9
	80	female	75	3,2
	81	female	51	0,9
	82	male	66	3,5
	83	male	67	1,1
	84	female	43	1,1
	85	female	55	1,7
	86	female	69	0,8
	87	male	17	4,8
	88	female	54	2,7
	89	male	19	0,7
	90	female	63	0,7
	91	female	29	3,6

Table 1. Cortisol concentration (continued)

Month	Serial no.	Sex	Age (years)	Cortisol Concentration.
October 1974	92	female	42	5,1
	93	female	73	0,9
	94	female	69	0,8
	95	female	60	2,4
	96	female	62	1,8
	97	female	68	1,4
	98	male	55	2,2
	99	male	55	5,7
	100	female	63	5,5
	101	male	55	4,5
	102	female	52	6,1
November 1974	103	female	47	9,1
	104	male	55	5,4
	105	male	49	2,7
	106	female	38	1,1
	107	male	65	1,8
	108	female	60	2,1
	109	male	60	1,7
	110	male	18	2,0
	111	male	16	1,9
December 1974	112	male	39	7,8
	113	male	60	1,6
	114	male	50	1,5
	115	female	71	3,3

For the F-statistic we obtained the value of F = 4.72, which is compared with the qualities of a F-distribution with degrees of freedom $k_1 = 3$ and $k_2 = 111$. Correspondingly the differences between the transformed cortisol levels can be considered as significant at a level of 1%. The analysis of individual mean differences by Scheffé's method yielded a significance at the same level (1%) for the comparison summer versus winter. All other contrasts were not significant.

The chi-square test for dependence between anesthetic techniques and season was not significant at the 5% level. An influence of the different anesthetic techniques on the circannual rhythm of the cortisol concentration in the subretinal fluid therefore could be excluded.

DISCUSSION

Our results give evidence that cortisol is present in the subretinal fluid of rhegmatogenous retinal detachment. Furthermore, a circannual cycle in subretinal fluid cortisol concentration was found, showing a statistically significant increase in mean concentration of the hormone in the winter season (December to February), as compared with the summer months (June to August). The observation of such a circannual rhythm in subretinal fluid cortisol corresponds with the increase in mean plasma cortisol concentration for the autumn winter seasons, as compared with the spring and summer (Weitzman *et al.* 1975). In winter the general 17-ketosteroid secretion is higher than in summer (Tromp 1963).

A possible influence of contraceptives on the seasonal pattern of the mean cortisol concentrations has to be discussed, because a higher cortisol level induced by contraceptives could be indicated by competitive proteinbinding analysis. However, none of our altogether five female patients under the age of 45 was operated on in winter. If one assumes an influence of a possible intake of contraceptives on the pattern on the cortisol concentration curve, it could only be active as an apparently too high mean cortisol concentration during the other seasons. Thus, an influence of possible intaken contraceptives, causing a too high mean concentration of the subretinal fluid cortisol in winter, does not come into question in our cases.

There exists an inverse correlation (Fig. 1) with the seasonal incidence of the retinal detachments which reaches its maximum in the months of June to August, whereas during the winter months it is at its lowest. This seasonal difference, already observed by other authors, was confirmed in a

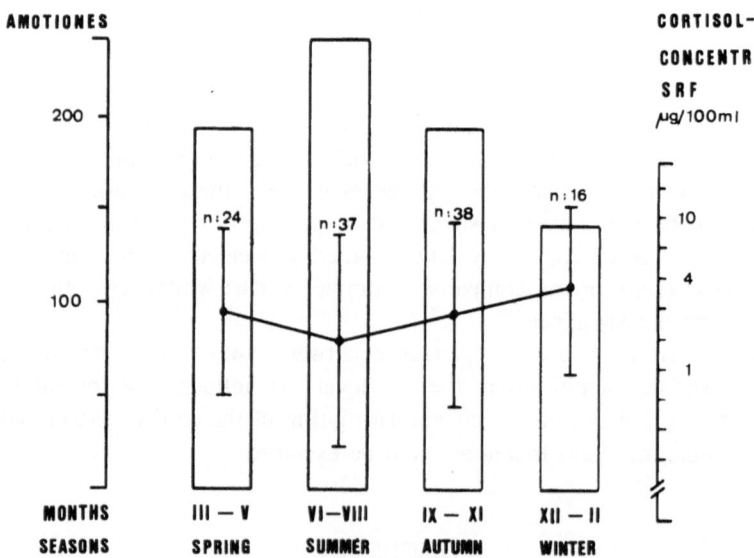

Fig. 1. Subretinal fluid cortisol concentration (mean values) and frequency of idiopathic retinal detachment, correlated with the meteorological seasons. After Gärtner *et al.* (1977).

182

study of 771 patients seen over a period of 26 years with a chronologically well-defined onset of an idiopathic bullous retinal detachment. Of these detachments, 242 occurred in the summer months and only 141 in the winter season. Both in spring and in autumn 194 cases were counted (Gärtner et al. 1977). At the outset of detachment, all patients lived around Mainz under similar climatic conditions.

Since retinal tears or holes do not always lead to detachment, the state of the extracellular matrix located between the photoreceptors and the pigment epithelial layer obviously plays an important role at the outset, in the rapidity of spreading and in the final extent of the separation of the two walls of the primary optic vesicle (Schepens 1976; Gärtner 1977). It is suggested that glycosaminoglycans, forming the predominant component of this matrix, are the 'sticky substances' which serve as an adhesive between these cell layers (Berman 1969; Zauberman et al. 1972). One might speculate on the possibility of a seasonal influence of the free cortisol on these matrix glycosaminoglycans. Such influence could be exerted via the well-known action of the steroid on the lysosomal membranes. As cortisol stabilizes lysosomal membranes, its higher concentration in winter may inhibit the liberation of the catabolic enzymes of glycosaminoglycans from the lysosomes of the pigment epithelial cells, which is essential for the irreversible degradation of the matrix glycosaminoglycans in the subretinal space at the outset of any retinal detachment.

The higher concentration of urine 17-keto-steroids, plasma cortisol, subretinal fluid cortisol and presumably also aqueous humor cortisol in the winter season may be caused by cold stress, creating hypertrophy of the adrenal cortex (Tromp 1963).

REFERENCES

Akhmeteli, L. M., B. S. Kasavina & G. A. Petropavlovskaja. Biochemical investigation of the subretinal fluid. Brit. J. Ophthal. 59: 70-77 (1975).

Berman, E. E. Mucopolysaccharides (Glycosaminoglycans) of the retina: Identification, distribution and possible biological role. Mod. Probl. Ophthal. 8: 5-31 (1969).

Berson, S. A. & R. S. Yalow. General principles of radioimmunoassay. Clin. Chim. Acta 22: 51-69 (1968).

Böhm, G. Jahreszeitliche Schwankungen der Cortisolkonzentration in der subretinalen Flüssigkeit. Dissertation, Mainz 1977, p. 17-22.

Fiorelli, G., P. Piolanti, G. Forti & M. Serio. Determination of plasmacorticosteroids and urinary cortisol by a competitive portein-binding method using dextran-coated charcoal. Clin. Chim. Acta 37: 179-187 (1972).

Freeman, H. M. & C. L. Schepens. Innovations in the technique for drainage of subretinal fluid: Transillumination and choroidal diathermy. Mod. Probl. Ophthal. 15: 119-126 (1975).

Gärtner, J. Release of subretinal fluid with the aid of the microscope. Report on 100 cases. Mod. Probl. Ophthal. 15: 127-133 (1975).

Gärtner, J., K. H. Schicketanz, K. Sinterhauf & G. Böhm. Jahreszeitliche Schwankungen im Vorkommen der idiopathischen Netzhautablosung und der Cortisolkonzentration in der subretinalen Flüssigkeit. Klin. Mbl. Augenheilk. 171: 506-519 (1977).

Kaufman, P. L. & S. M. Podos. The subretinal fluid in primary rhegmatogenous retinal detachment. Survey Ophthalmol. 18: 100-116 (1973).

Schepens, C. L. Retinal detachment. Jap. J. Ophthal. 20: 291-329 (1976).

Sinterhauf, K., P. Herzog & D. Lommer. Beurteilung des circadianen Cortisolrhythmus an Hand von Dreipunkt-Tagesprofilen des Plasmacortisols. Verh. dtsch. Ges. Inn. Med. 81: 1537-1540 (1975).

Spaeth, G. L., M. M. Rodrigues & S. Weinreb. Steroid-induced glaucoma: A. Persistent elevation of intraocular pressure. B. Histopathological aspects. Tr. Am. Ophth. Soc. 75: 353-381 (1977).

Tromp, S. W. Medical biometeorology. Weather, climate and living organism. In cooperation with 26 contributors. Elsevier, Amsterdam 1963, p. 279, 280.

Weitzman, E. D., A. S. Degraaf & J. F. Sassin. Seasonal patterns of sleep stages and secretion of cortisol and growth hormone during 24 hour periods in northern Norway. Acta endocrin. (Kbh.) 78/1: 65-76 (1975).

Zauberman, H., H de Guillebon & F. J. Holly. Retinal traction in vivo. Biophysical aspects. Invest. Ophthal. 11: 46-55 (1972).

Authors' address:

Netzhautabteilung, Univ.-Augenklinik und Poliklinik
der Universität Mainz
6500 Mainz
F.R.G.

DRAINAGE OF SUBRETINAL FLUID
A comparison of external and internal observation techniques

EDWARD OKUN & GLEN PAUL JOHNSTON

(St. Louis, Miss., U.S.A.)

ABSTRACT

Two techniques for drainage of subretinal fluid are described and compared: (1) externally observed drainage through an 'L' shaped sclerotomy with a sharp wire needle; and (2) ophthalmoscopically observed (internal) drainage through a limbus parallel sclerotomy with Wilder picks. Complications encountered are similar and minimal. Drainage under ophthalmoscopic control is utilized in cases with shifting fluid, shallow detachments, choroidal plus retinal detachments, thickened choroids, and following failure to obtain fluid with the external observation technique.

Since drainage of subretinal fluid is a potentially hazardous step in retinal detachment surgery, it should be avoided whenever possible. However, if there is any doubt about whether or not a procedure will be successful without drainage, it has been our policy to drain. Sometimes the hazards of nondrainage are greater than those associated with drainage. These include rupture of the sclera in cases with weakened ocular coats, closure of the central retinal artery, and failure to achieve reattachment with one operative procedure. Since reoperations have a higher incidence of failure, usually because of excessive vitreous reaction, greater tendency toward infection, and choroidal hemorrhages, it is wise to strive for cure with the first procedure.

TECHNIQUE OF EXTERNALLY OBSERVED DRAINAGE

Over the past ten years, we have developed and tested a method of draining subretinal fluid which has had a very low incidence of complications, giving us the confidence to drain when in doubt (Johnston *et al.* 1975). When a lamellar undermining has been performed and adequate subretinal fluid is present in the area of the groove, it has been our preference to drain within the resection bed. However, if there is not enough subretinal fluid in this location, a site is localized where there is sufficient subretinal fluid to avoid perforation of the retina. This is usually posterior to the resection bed. Care

185

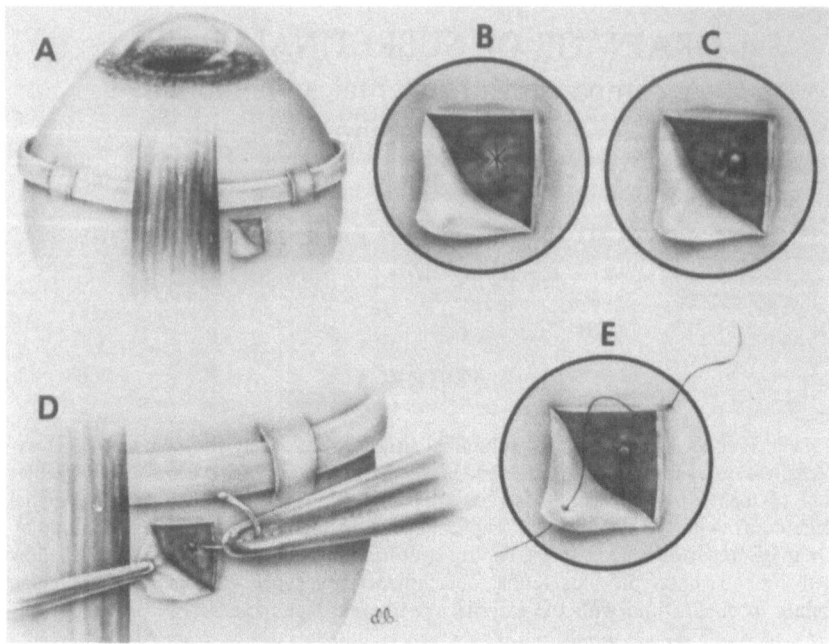

Fig. 1. a. Artist's drawing of band in place and 'L' shaped sclerotomy adjacent to horizontal rectus muscle. b. Bed of 'L' sclerotomy further thinned until, c. tiny bulge of choroid appears. d. Thinned zone (after inspection with magnification fails to reveal any large vessels) is touched with the sharp wire needle of a 6–0 silk suture. e. After drainage the 'L' shaped flap is closed with a suture. © Retina Consultants, Ltd.

is taken to avoid the vortex vein drainage siphon and to stay as far away as possible from large retinal holes. When an episcleral procedure is performed, similar considerations are used in selecting the drainage site, which is usually either just above or below one of the horizontal recti muscles. Localization of this spot is as important as localization of the retinal breaks.

Once the site for the perforation is chosen, an 'L' shaped incision is made in the sclera, and a triangular lamellar undermining is performed (Fig. 1a). This allows the thinly supported choroid to bulge slightly. This thinned bed is examined with intense light and magnification to be certain no large choroidal vessels are in the site intended for perforation. If in doubt, trans-illumination is performed. Once the exact site is determined, the scleral fibers are further thinned until a dark, slightly bulging zone is created (Fig. 1b, c). This spot is then touched with the point of a 6–0 silk wire needle resulting in drainage 90% of the time (Fig. 1d). Note that just prior to perforation with the needle, all tension is removed from the globe by relaxing traction on the extraocular muscles and allowing the eye to sit freely in the orbit. If drainage is not effected with the first try, the site of intended

186

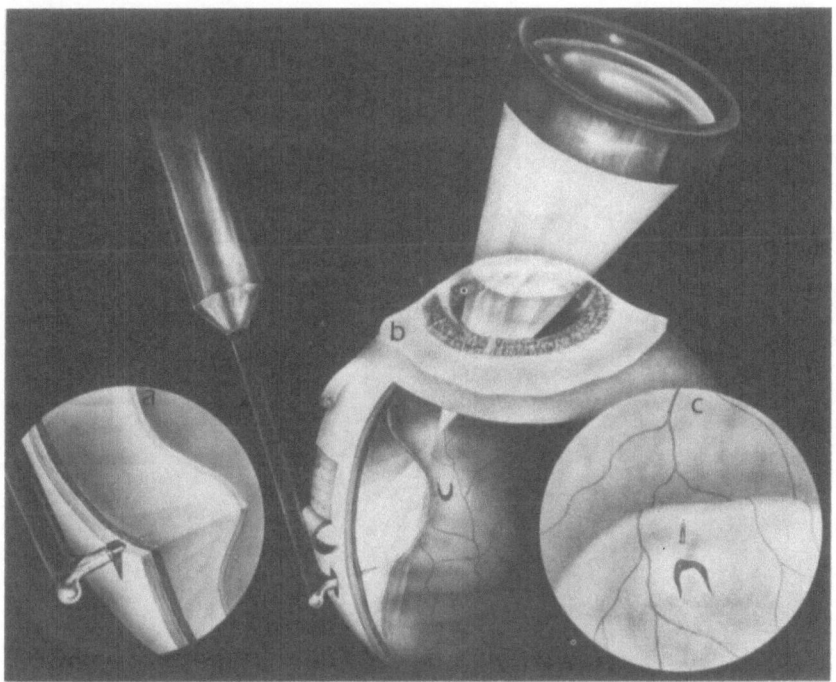

Fig. 2. a. Cibis combination electrode enters subretinal space. b. Conical needle is obscured under the retina by means of the indirect ophthalmoscope, c. Ophthalmoscopic appearance of the electrode under the retina. © Retina Consultants, Ltd.

perforation is reinspected with the indirect ophthalmoscope and another estimate is made regarding the height of retinal elevation. If no hemorrhage is detected, a slightly deeper penetration is made with the drainage needle. Once adequate drainage is secured, the sclerotomy is usually closed with a 5–0 dacron suture (Fig. 1e).

Following the perforation and while drainage is being achieved, the larger breaks are tamponaded by tying the preplaced sutures over the implant material, pulling up on the encircling element, or closing an undermined lamellar bed. Sometimes a cotton-tipped applicator is used to temporarily tamponade the retinal tear thus preventing liquified vitreous from being drained via the open retinal hole.

The eye is always evaluated while in the intended position for perforation to be certain that the subretinal fluid has not shifted away from the area to be drained. Any shift might endanger the retina during the choroidal perforation.

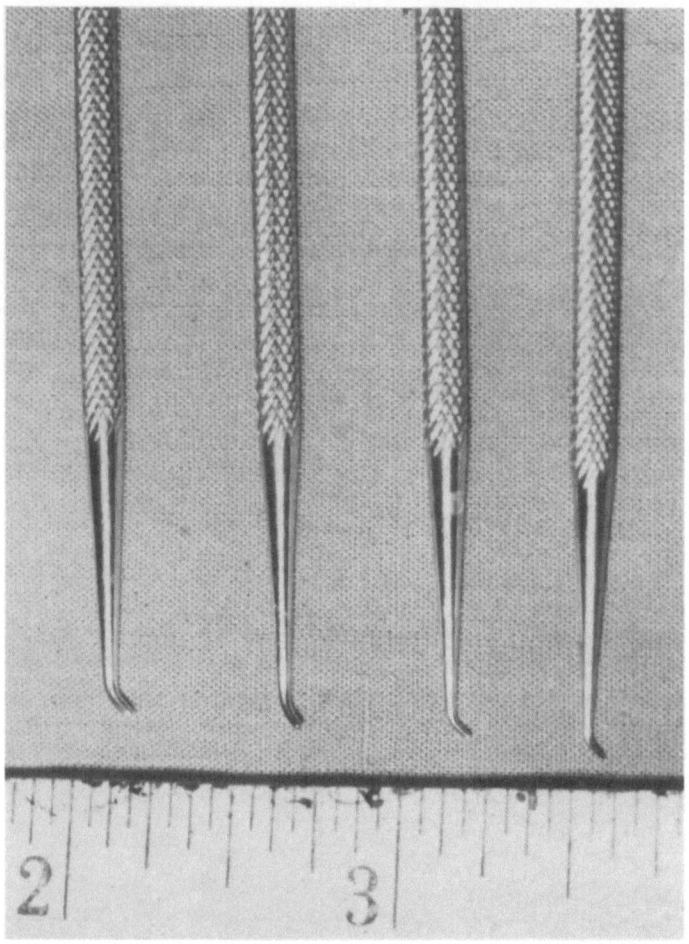

Fig. 3. Photograph of the four Wilder picks, No. 4 to No. 1 left to right. No. 1 is the narrowest and sharpest.

TECHNIQUE OF OPHTHALMOSCOPICALLY OBSERVED DRAINAGE (INTERNAL)

From 1961 to 1965, Paul Cibis drained subretinal fluid under indirect ophthalmoscopic control. For the perforation he utilized the conical tip of a combination ball and cone electrode. The conical needle electrode was quite sharp, but not as sharp as a needle. The conical shape allowed the puncture site to remain sealed until the electrode was withdrawn, thus preventing premature loss of subretinal fluid. The highly reflective needle could be

188

readily seen within the subretinal space, eliminating any doubt about the adequacy of perforation or the possibility of retinal injury (Fig. 2). However, because of its shape, the electrode sometimes twisted during removal and premature loss of subretinal fluid occasionally led to retinal injury. Hemorrhage was very rare. Because of the fear of retinal injury and incarceration this technique was used only occasionally during the period from 1965 to 1978.

In 1977, Howard Wilder reported to the American Retina Society on his technique of evacuating subretinal fluid under ophthalmoscopic control utilizing one of a series of modified lacrimal punctum dilators which he designed (Fig. 3). We have found these dilators to be excellent for perforating and obturating the choroidal opening, and the procedure which we have found to work very well is as follows:

A sclerotomy site is chosen where retinal elevation is the highest, away from vortex veins and large retinal tears, if possible (Okun, 1979). Since drainage can be performed with the eye in its natural position of rest, there is no need to worry about shifting fluid. The sclerotomy is made limbus parallel and shelved posteriorly (Fig. 4a, b). The incision is carried down until the dark blue-black color of thinned sclera is visible. A 5–0 dacron suture is then placed across the sclerotomy (Fig. 4c). The No. 1 or No. 2 Wilder pick is introduced into the sclerotomy until the back recess is felt. With the pick engaged against this posterior recess of the sclerotomy, the eye is next

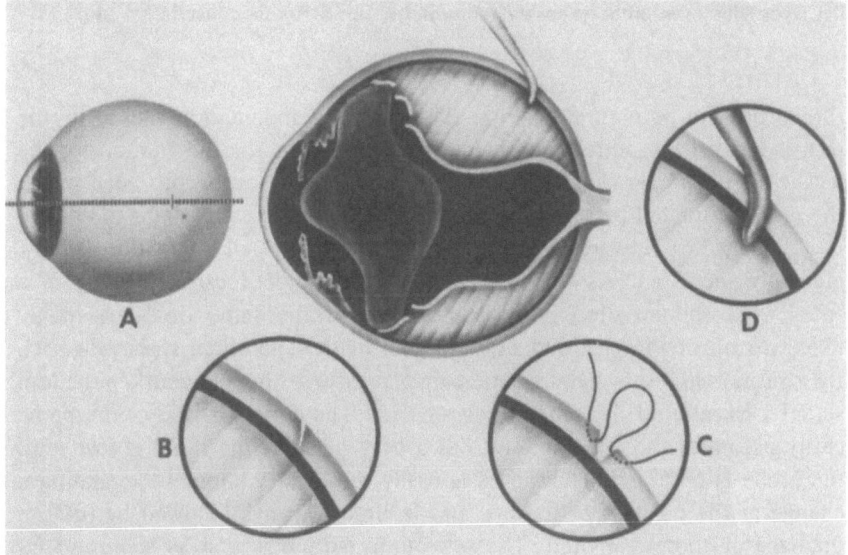

Fig. 4. Techniques for drainage with Wilder pick. a. Limbus parallel sclerotomy, b. sclerotomy slants posteriorly, c. preplaced suture, d. pick obturates the choroidal opening, preventing premature loss of subretinal fluid. © Retina Consultants, Ltd.

189

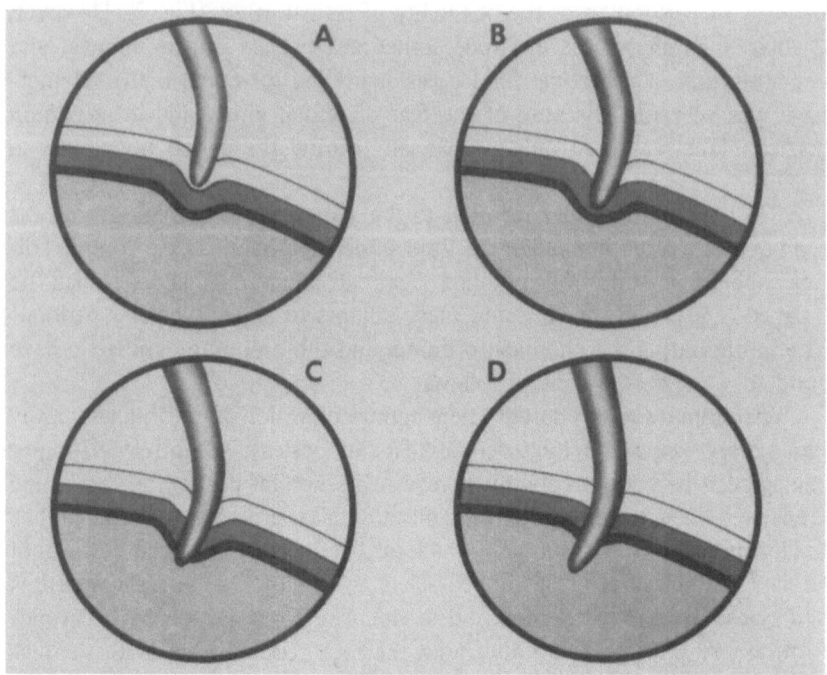

Fig. 5. a. Pick within sclerotomy indenting choroid and Bruch's membrane – pigment epithelial layers. b. Pick working its way through choroid. C. Pick 'pops' through Bruch's membrane – pigment epithelial layer. D. Bruch's membrane – pigment epithelial layer slips over probe exposing more of the tip. © Retina consultants, Ltd.

turned back to its natural position. The choroidal indentation caused by the pick is located by indirect ophthalmoscopy, much as the indentation for the localization of a tear (Fig. 5a). After a positive identification has been made, the probe is rotated between thumb and index finger with a slight to and fro motion (Fig. 6). Inward pressure toward the center of the globe is now gradually increased. As this happens, there is sometimes the feeling of a 'pop' or a sudden drop in resistance, and at the same time the highly reflective tip of the pick suddenly appears in the subretinal space (Fig. 5c). By continuing very slight rotation and pressure, the pigment epithelium settles back around the probe (Figs. 4d, 5d). The conical shape of the probe easily obturates the opening, and not a drop of subretinal fluid is lost until the probe is removed. This probe is easily removed without necessitating a change in the position of the eye and is almost always followed by profuse drainage of subretinal fluid. The sclerotomy suture is tied as soon as adequate drainage has been obtained.

If drainage stops and must be restarted, a duller and wider probe (No. 3) can be safely reintroduced into the previously perforated choroid. As it enters,

190

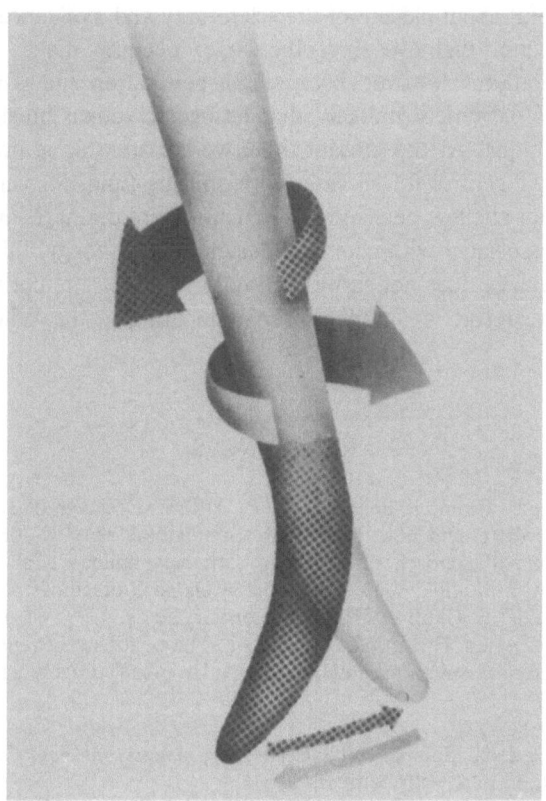

Fig. 6. Drawing illustrates lateral to and fro movements of the tip of the probe that occurs when the shaft is rotated between the thumb and index finger. © Retina Consultants, Ltd.

this will dilate and block the choroidal opening. Greater care is necessary with this large opening to prevent retinal incarceration after completion of drainage.

COMPARISON OF TECHNIQUES

In a review of 795 cases of drainage performed with the 'L' shaped sclerotomy, there was a 5% incidence of significant subretinal hemorrhage, 2% retinal incarceration, and 3% iatrogenic retinal holes (Okun 1972). In the first 50 cases of drainage under ophthalmoscopic control, there was a 4% incidence of organized subretinal hemorrhage, 4% retinal incarceration, and no iatrogenic retinal holes. Both methods have a small acceptable incidence of similar complications, which can perhaps be lowered still further by

191

meticulous attention to technique. With the Wilder picks, one must be extremely careful about closure of the sclerotomy and avoidance of excessive manipulation after drainage since the larger opening makes it easier for retinal incarceration. However, because the perforation site is monitored at all times, it is extremely unlikely that iatrogenic retinal breaks will occur with this technique. At the present time, we are advocating drainage under ophthalmoscopic control for all cases with shifting fluid, for very posteriorly located fluid, for shallow detachments which require drainage, and for retinal detachments associated with choroidal detachment or boggy, thickened choroid. When drainage does not easily occur after the first attempt with external observation, we resort to internal observation utilizing the Wilder picks.

REFERENCES

Johnston, G. P., E. Okun, I. Boniuk & N. P. Arribas. Drainage of subretinal fluid: Why, when, where, and how. Mod. Prob. Ophthalmol. 15: 197-206 (1975).

Okun, E. Simplified approach to a case of extremely bullous total aphakic retinal detachment with multiple holes at multiple levels, in Proceedings of the Paul Cibis Club, 1979, Eds. E. Okun & G. P. Johnston, St. Louis, 1979, pp. 104-113.

Okun, E., in discussion, H. Lincoff & I. Kressig. The treatment of retinal detachment without drainage of subretinal fluid. Trans. Amer. Acad. of Ophthalmol. and Otol. 76: 1221-1232 (1972).

Portions of this presentation are contained in *Proceedings of the Paul Cibis Club, 1979*, and are reproduced here with permission.

Authors' address:
4949 Barnes Hospital Plaza
Suite 17413/East Pavilion
St. Louis, MS 63119
U.S.A.

COMPENSIBILITY IN TRAUMATIC RETINAL DETACHMENT

FRED GOTTLIEB

(*Brooklyn, New York, U.S.A.*)

INTRODUCTION

Ocular trauma is responsible for 10 to 14% of rhegmatogenous retinal detachments in large series of patients (Witmer 1972). Since many patients wish to attribute their retinal disease to an injury in order to be reimbursed by their insurance or Workman's Compensation, it behooves the attending ophthalmologist to know what factors to consider in determining the role of trauma in a given case of detached retina. Large amounts of money may hinge on his evaluation and judgment.

In this paper, the various types of trauma-induced retinal detachments will be outlined and illustrated. Criteria will be presented in judging individual cases as compensible.

CLASSIFICATION OF TRAUMA-RELATED RETINAL DETACHMENTS

Table 1 outlines the types of retinal detachment induced by trauma.

I. *Retinal detachment following perforating ocular injury*

a. Retinal detachment due to direct retinal laceration

Case 1. The spectacles of a 16 year old myope were shattered, and pieces of glass penetrated the interior of the right eye. Three months later, a retinal detachment developed. A linear tear was seen in the 6 o'clock position, surrounded by several pieces of glass. A small wisp of silvery fibrous tissue was seen in the far periphery, presumably the site of perforation (Fig. 1). The retinal detachment was repaired without removal of the glass foreign body. Six months later, the retina appeared to be well attached, both the hole and the glass fragments resting on the buckle. Considerable vitreous fibrous proliferation had occured, bridging the vitreous cavity from inferiorly to the superior periphery (Fig. 2).

193

Table 1. Trauma-related retinal detachment

I. Retinal detachment following perforating ocular injury:
    a. retinal break due to direct laceration of the retina
    b. retinal break due to vitreous contraction on same side as perforation
    c. retinal break due to vitreous contraction on side opposite to perforation

II. Retinal detachment following blunt injury to a healthy eye:
    a. avulsion of vitreous base with a retinal dialysis
    b. equatorial tear due to retinal necrosis
    c. giant tear
    d. macular hole

III. Retinal detachment following blunt injury to an eye predisposed to detachment of the retina

IV. Retinal detachment following indirect injury

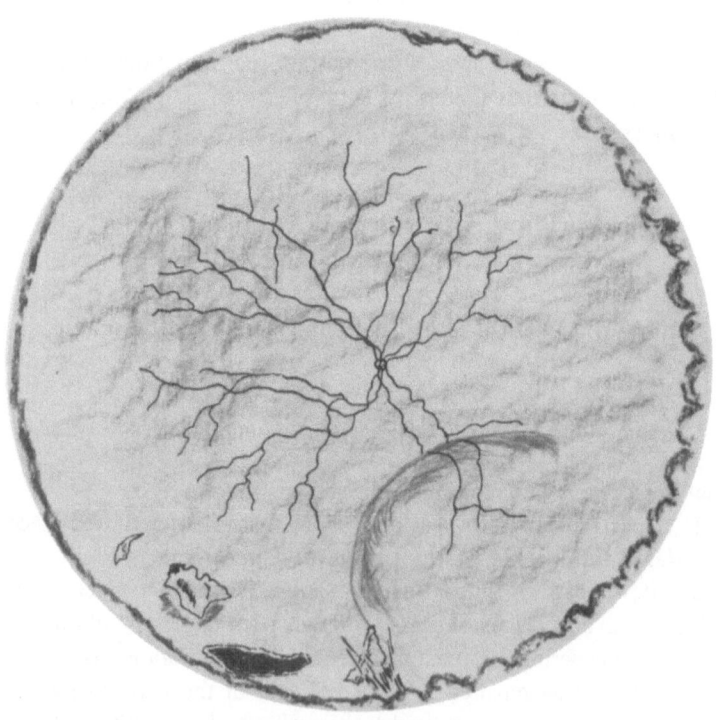

Fig. 1. (Case 1) Subtotal retinal detachment from a linear tear caused by penetrating glass. Small wisp of vitreous fibrous tissue is growing in 5: 30 periphery.

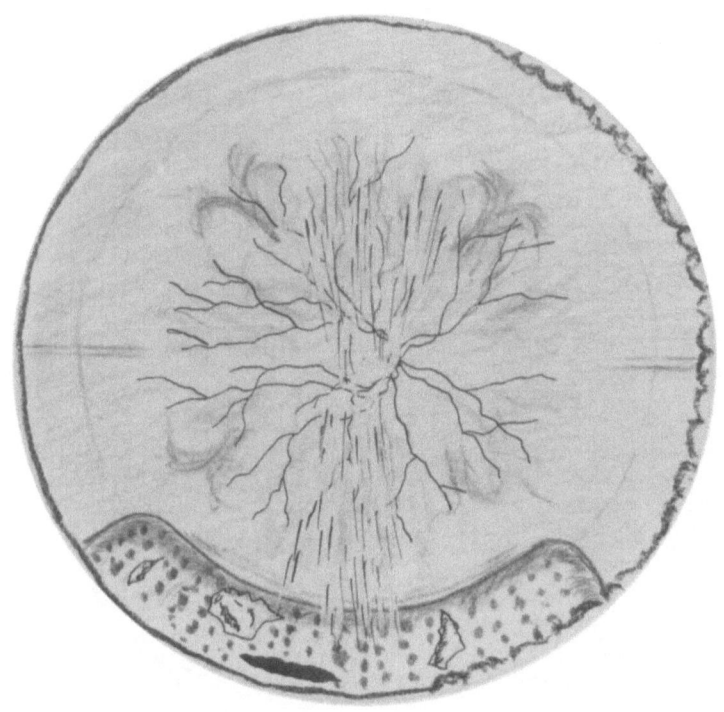

Fig. 2. (Case 1) Glass particles and retinal tear resting on inferior buckle. Note proliferation of vitreal fibers.

Comment

A piece of glass lacerated the retina and the resulting hole was responsible for a detachment of the retina. This case illustrates the hallmark of ocular perforation, vitreous fibrous proliferation from the site of perforation.

b. Retinal breaks due to vitreous fibrous contraction, occuring on the same side as the penetration.

Case 2. This 12 year old male sustained a lacerated left globe, in which a perforation occured through the limbus and iris. When he was examined three months later, a temporal retinal detachment with a large upper temporal dialysis was seen. Two masses of silvery vitreal fibrous tissue were seen in the lower temporal periphery; one extended superiorly towards the area of the break, and the other fanned out in a superior nasal direction (Fig. 3).

Comment

A large superior temporal retinal dialysis in this patient can be related to vitreal fibrous proliferation and contraction. The tear occured on the same

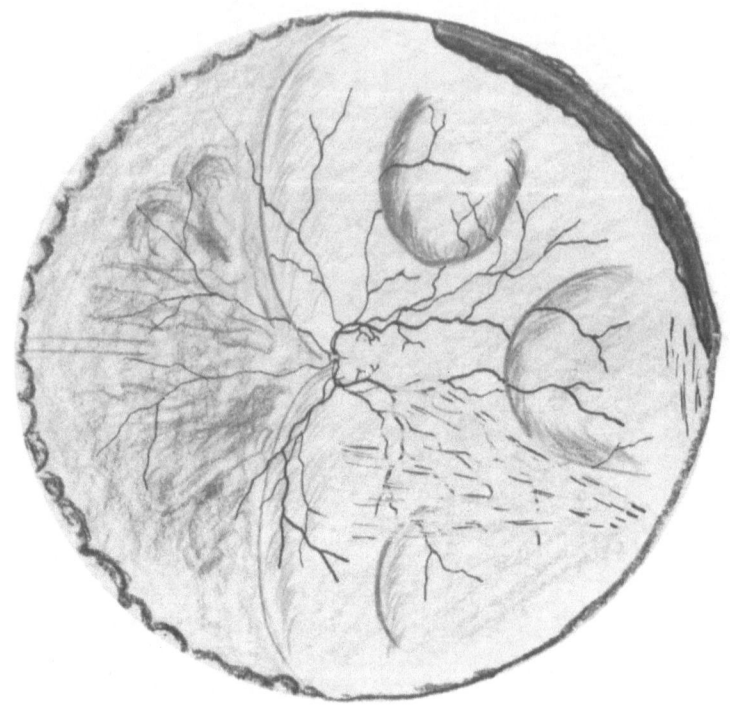

Fig. 3. (Case 2) Retinal detachment following penetration of globe. Fibrous tissue proliferates into the vitreous, and a superior retinal dialysis is seen on same side as perforation.

side as the ocular perforation but not due to direct retinal injury at the time of the accident.

c. Retinal break due to vitreous fibrous proliferation on the side contralateral to the point of penetration.

Case 3. A 13 year old boy was injured in a firecracker accident. The resulting rupture of the left globe was repaired surgically. He was seen three years later with a detachment of the retina. The fundus (Fig. 4) showed a chorioretinal defect in the nasal periphery corresponding to the site of choroidal rupture. Prominent silvery vitreal fibers radiated from this area towards the superior temporal retina, causing an upper temporal dialysis and a detachment of the retina. The presence of fixed retinal folds is suggestive of pathologic vitreoretinal adhesions.

Comment

In this patient a retinal break resulted from vitreal fibrous proliferation at a point opposite to the perforation site.

196

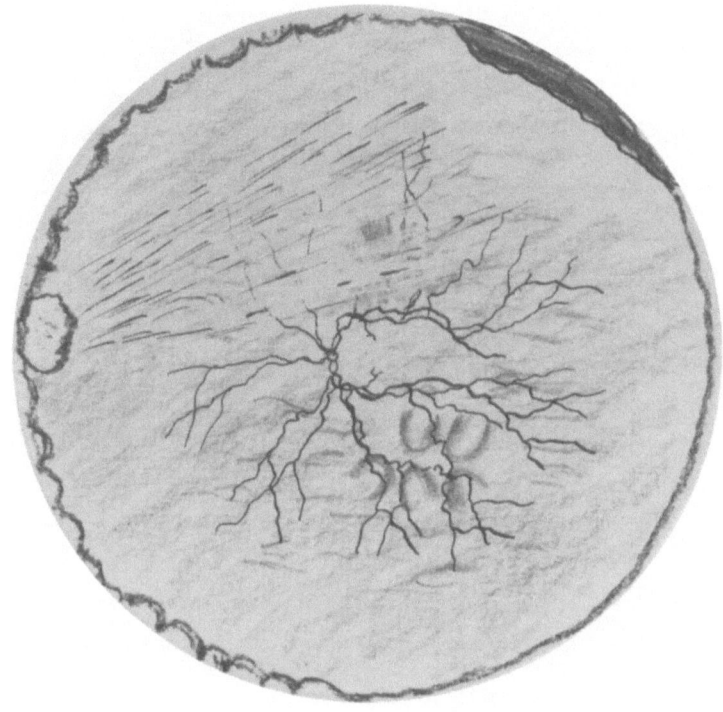

Fig. 4. (Case 3) Retinal detachment following perforating trauma. A retinal dialysis occured on the contralateral side due to traction by proliferating vitreous fibrils.

II. *Retinal detachment from blunt trauma to a healthy eye*
a. Vitreous base avulsion with retinal dialysis
Case 4. A 14 year old boy was struck in the right eye with a hard ball. This produced a hemorrhage into the vitreous. Three weeks later, settling of the blood in the inferior vitreous cavity permitted a view of the fundus periphery. A large tear in the pars plana epithelium was seen, associated with hemorrhages and pigment clumping. No retinal dialysis was seen, nor was there ophthalmoscopic evidence of a vitreous avulsion.
  Comment
This case illustrates the earliest and minimum result of an avulsed vitreous base. A severe vitreous hemorrhage was produced, but no retinal dialysis could be seen on follow-up examinations.
Case 5. A 13 year old boy was struck in the left eye with a tennis ball. At the time of examination, the globe was extremely soft. The macula was edematous and demonstrated radiating lines. A superior nasal dialysis of the retina was seen, associated with an irregular gray curvilinear 'bucket handle'

197

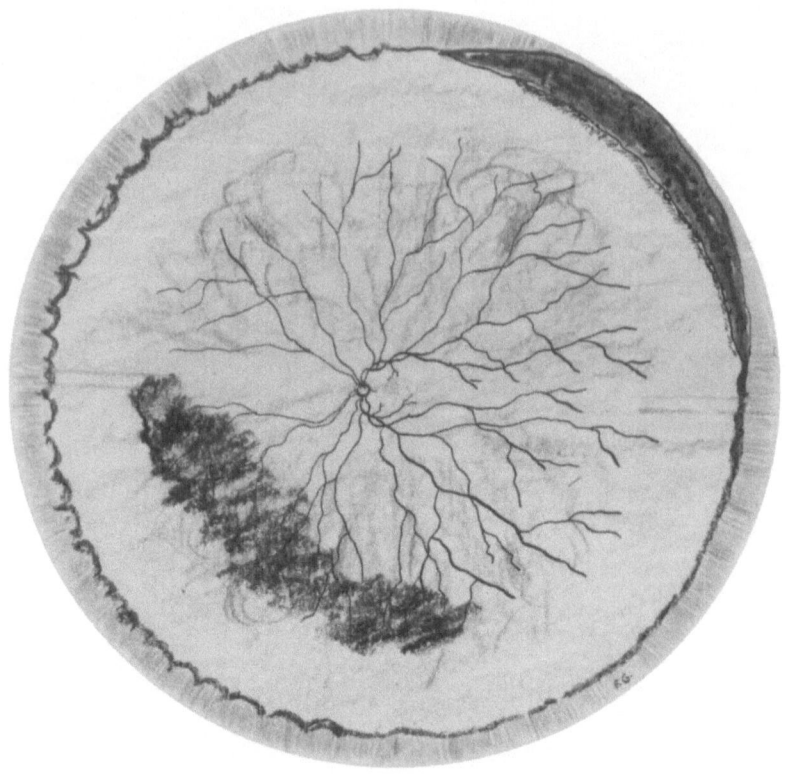

Fig. 5. (Case 4) Traumatic tear in pars plana epithelium upper temporally. Note hemorrhage into vitreous.

membrane projecting into the vitreous posteriorly. No detachment of the retina ensued.

Comment

A typical traumatic dialysis with an ophthalmoscopically visible avulsed vitreous base was produced by a contusion injury. Follow-up examinations showed no evidence of detachment of the retina.

Case 6. A 12 year old male was struck in the left eye by a belt six weeks before the examination. The retina was totally detached, and a large upper temporal dialysis was seen. The retinal tear extended across the ora serrata to involve the epithelium of the pars plana. A grayish membrane extended posteriorly at the site of dialysis.

Comment

This case demonstrates the hallmarks of contusion retinal detachment: a superior dialysis extending across the ora to involve the pars plana, and associated with an avulsed vitreous base.

198

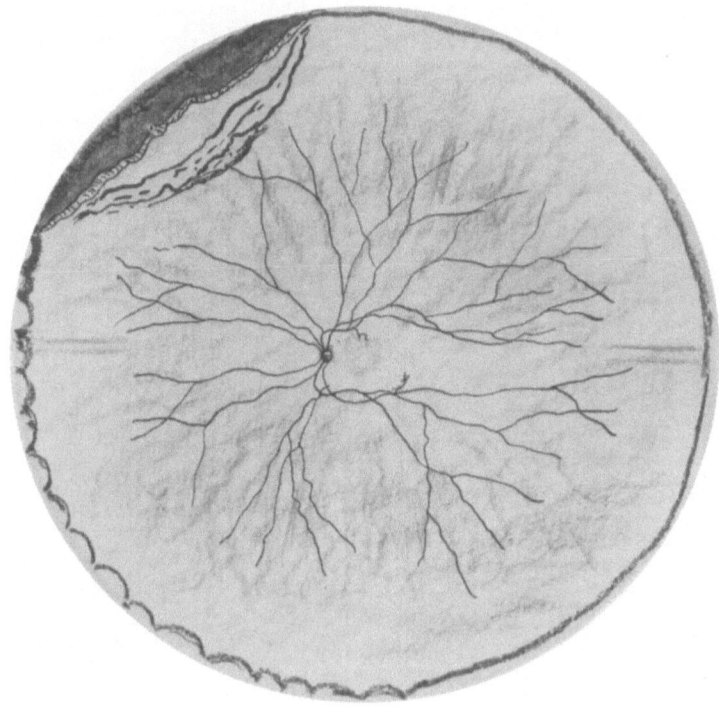

Fig. 6. (Case 5) Traumatic superior nasal retinal dialysis with 'bucket-handle' membrane representing avulsed vitreous base.

Case 7. An 18 year old male presented with a loss of vision in the left eye since three days. He had been struck in that eye with an ice ball seven years ago. Examination showed an inferior retinal detachment with an inferior temporal dialysis. In addition, a large strand of vitreous was seen hovering over the dialysis (Fig. 8).

Comment

This case illustrates a traumatic dialysis located inferiorly. It can be distinguished from the so-calles dialysis of the young by the clear history of trauma and the ophthalmoscopically visible vitreous base avulsion. The inferior location of the retinal break presumably caused a retinal detachment that was slow in developing, and did not become symptomatic until it reached the macula.

b. Equatorial breaks with retinal necrosis

Case 8. A boy was struck in the left eye with a rubber ball. Ophthalmoscopy showed an inferior retinal detachment with a large retinal tear. The edges

199

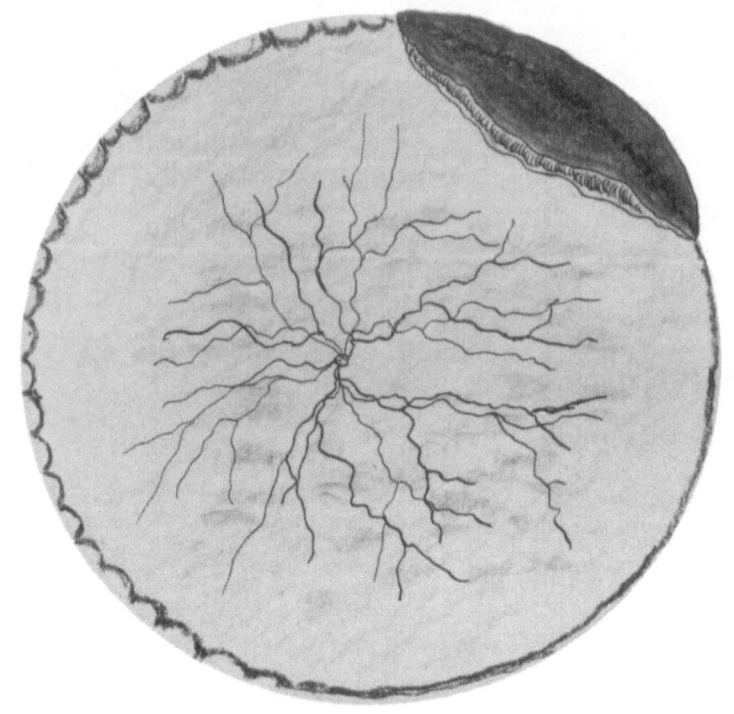

Fig. 7.

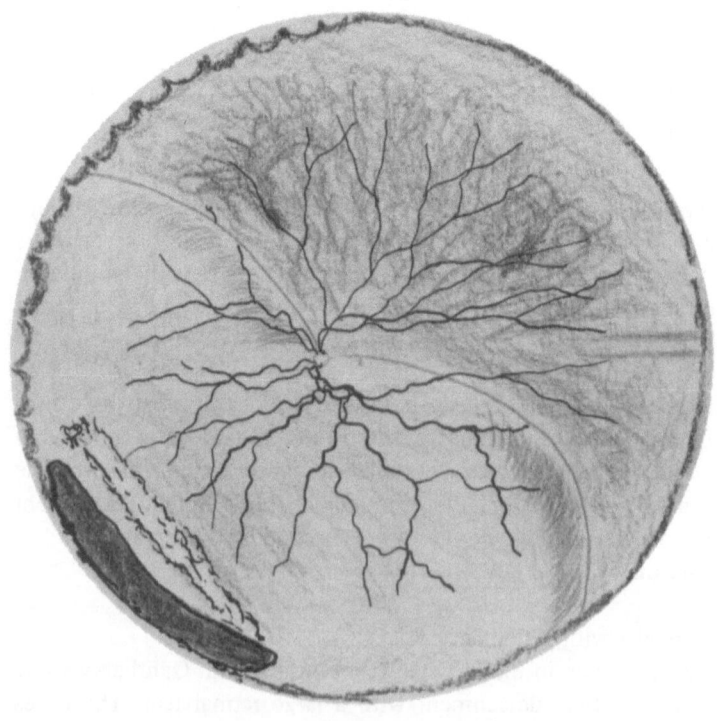

Fig. 8.

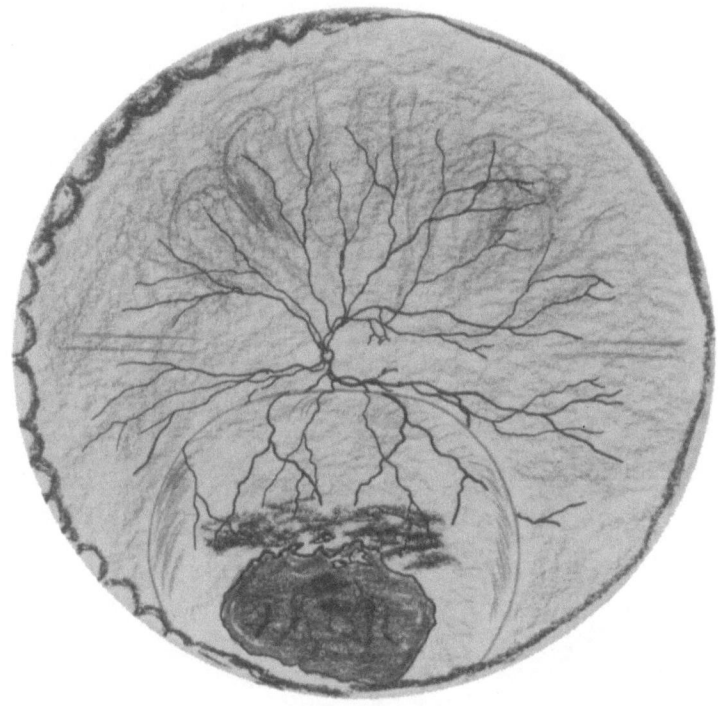

Fig. 9. (Case 8) Traumatic retinal necrosis and hemorrhage, with large equatorial tear and inferior retinal detachment.

appeared very jagged, and the presence of partially loose retinal tissue suggested local necrosis. There was much associated bleeding on the retina and in the vitreous (Fig. 9).

Comment

This large retinal break is suggestive of direct impact upon the sclera with a resulting 'explosion' of the retina. Such a hole is considered pathognomonic of retinal detachment due to contusion (Cox *et al.* 1966).

c. Traumatic giant tear

Case 9. This patient was struck in the left eye with a fist. Fundoscopy showed a giant retinal tear, with the superior retina everted inferiorly.

←

Fig. 7. (Case 6) Contusion retinal detachment with superior dialysis involving pars plana.
Fig. 8. (Case 7) Inferior traumatic dialysis and avulsed vitreous base.

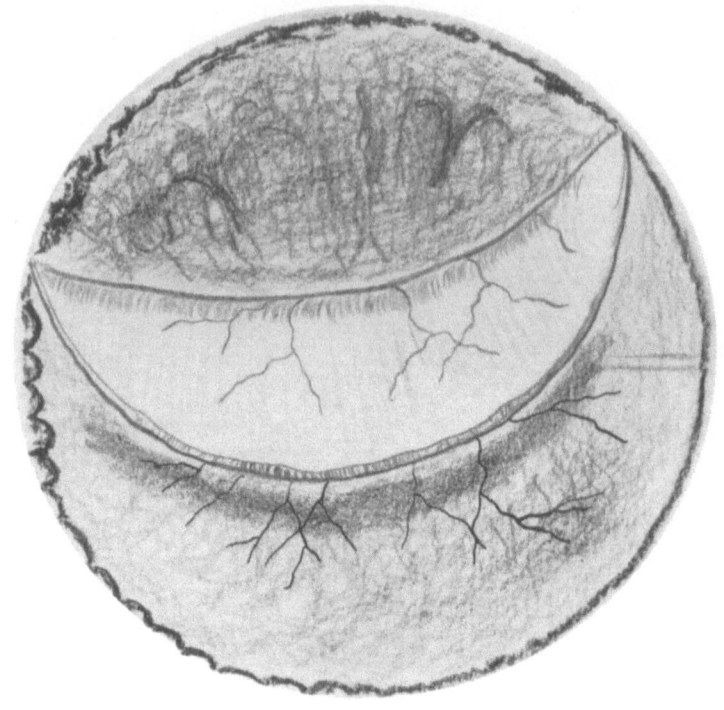

Fig. 10. (Case 9) Traumatic giant tear.

Gonioscopy showed a marked angle recession and a partial iris avulsion (Fig. 10).

Comment

This case illustrates a sequel of very severe contusion injury to the eye, a giant tear.

d. Traumatic macular hole

Macular holes result from atrophic changes following severe commotio retinae. They do not result in detachment of the retina (Eagling 1974).

III. *Retinal detachment due to blunt injury in predisposed eyes*

Case 10. A 26 year old black female was punched in the left eye and developed loss of vision one month later. The patient was highly myopic in both eyes and displayed lattice degeneration and a retinal tear in the right

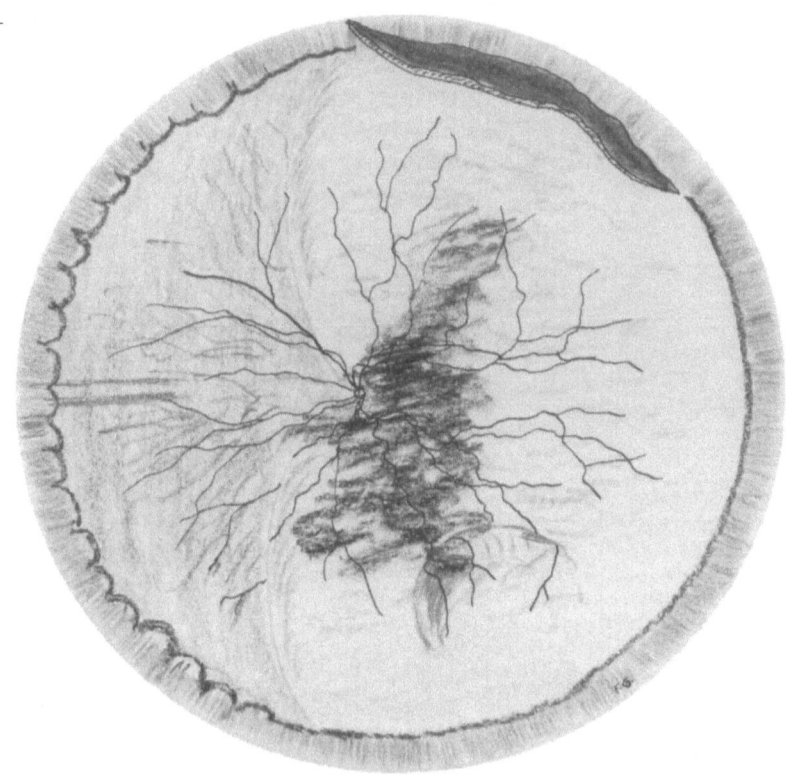

Fig. 11. (Case 10) Traumatic retinal dialysis extending across ora serrata. Hemorrhage in the vitreous and a subtotal retinal *detachment. Patient is a high myope.*

eye. The left eye had a subtotal retinal detachment with a superior temporal linear tear that extended across the ora serrata onto the pars plana ciliaris. Extensive hemorrhage into the vitreous was noted (Fig. 11).

Comment

This patient appears to have been predisposed to detachment of the retina because of her high myopia and the presence of lattice degeneration and a break in the fellow eye. The injury produced a retinal break pathognomonic of blunt trauma rather than equatorial degeneration.

Case 11. A 67 year old white male was injured when the blast of an air hose hit his right eye. He experienced flashes and floaters, and lost vision in that eye four days later. Examination revealed no objective signs of ocular trauma. The retina was subtotally detached and horseshoe tears were seen in the superior temporal equator and in the far temporal periphery. A prominent patch of lattice degeneration of the retina was seen in the superior equator

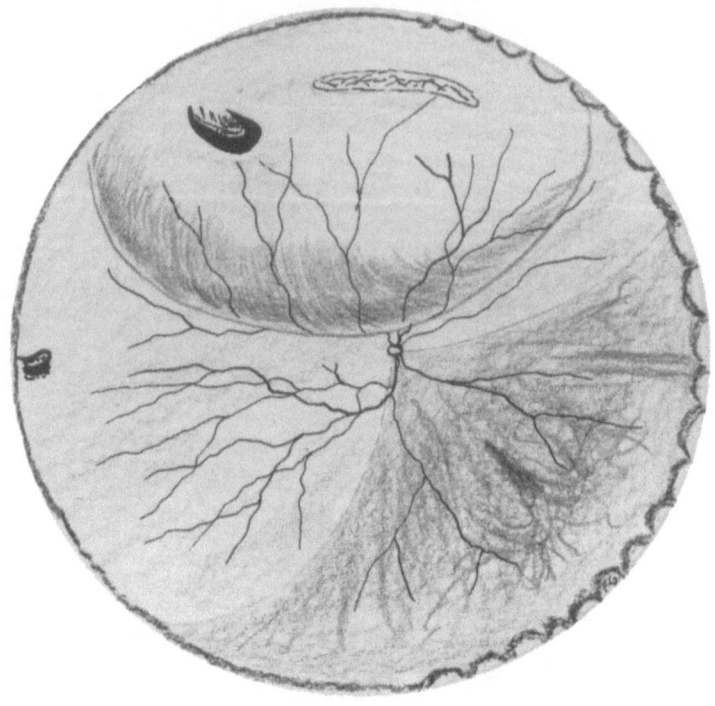

Fig. 12. (Case 11) Bullous retinal detachment with horseshoe tears and equatorial lattice degeneration.

(Fig. 12). Lattice degeneration was also observed in the fellow eye, which developed a spontaneous retinal detachment six years later.

Comment

The presence of an equatorial horseshoe tear and lattice degeneration of the retina, together with similar pathology and subsequent retinal detachment in the fellow eye clearly mark this patient as one predisposed to the development of spontaneous retinal detachment. In spite of the absence of objective signs of ocular injury, the close association in time between the onset of the detachment and a significant direct injury to the eye suggests a causal relationship of the two events.

Case 12. This patient had undergone a routine cataract extraction in the right eye, and was making a successful recovery. Five months after his surgery, he was struck in the right eye with a champagne bottle cork. A severe traumatic iritis with large subconjunctival hemorrhages were seen immediately after the injury. Ten days later, a retinal detachment developed. Ophthalmoscopy showed all of the temporal and portions of the nasal retina to be separated. In addition to a superior nasal horseshoe tear, multiple fine retinal breaks were seen superior temporally in association with retinal degeneration. A prominent vitreous hemorrhage had settled inferiorly (Fig. 13). The left eye displayed an area of lattice degeneration of the retina.

Comment

The combination of the aphakia and the lattice degeneration of the retina created an above-normal risk for detachment of the retina in this eye. The injury was of a violent nature and directly to the eye. Although the configuration of the detachment was not typical of what is seen in contusion retinal detachments, the etiologic association of the injury and the retinal detachment appears clear.

IV. *Spontaneous retinal detachment in a predisposed eye,*
preceded by indirect injury

Case 13. A 55 year old male developed a retinal detachment in the right eye with multiple retinal breaks in three quadrants (Fig. 14). Lattice degeneration of the retina was noted superiorly in the affected eye, as well as in the fellow

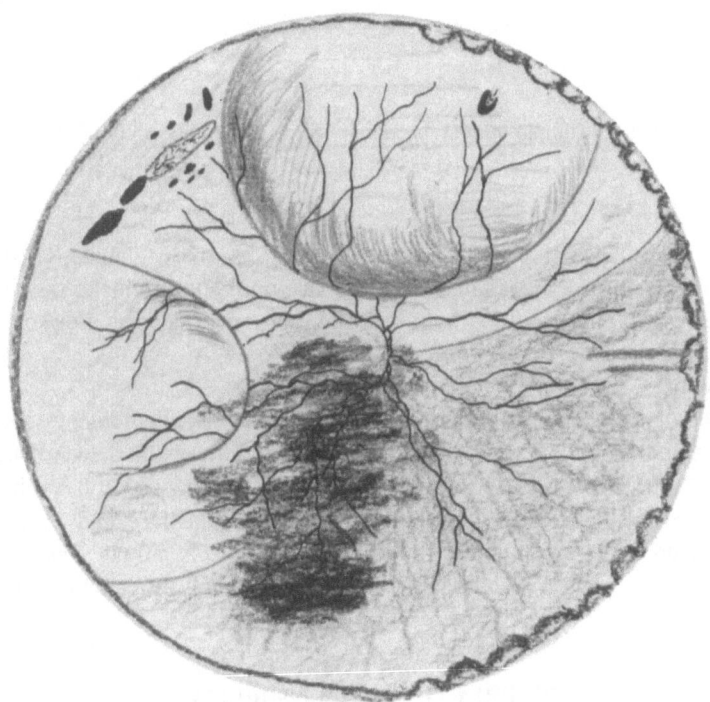

Fig. 13. (Case 12) Retinal detachment with vitreous hemorrhage. Multiple retinal tears in an area of lattice degeneration upper temporally.

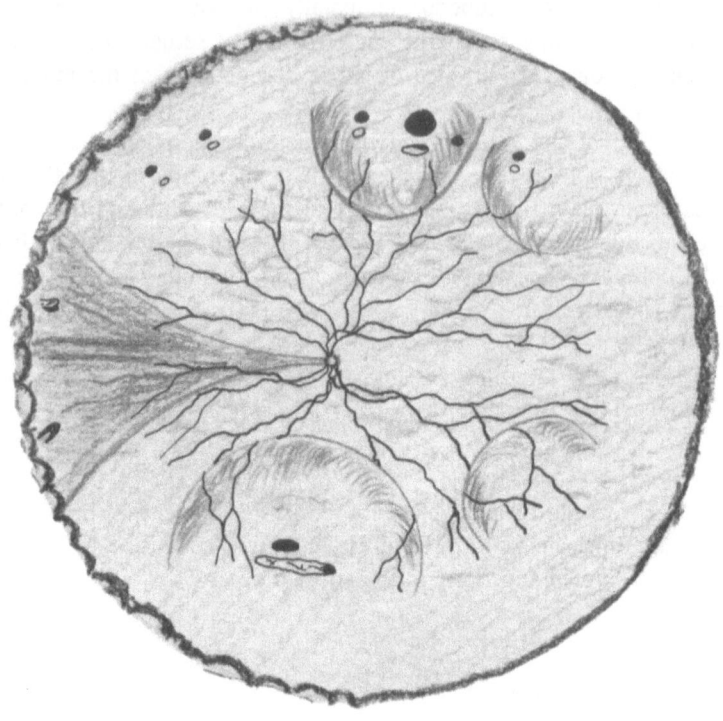

Fig. 14. (Case 13) Multiple retinal breaks in three quadrants and inferior lattice degeneration.

eye. Following successful reattachment of the retina, the patient reported an injury to the right eye and right part of the face one month prior to the onset of ocular symptoms. Sutures were required to repair a laceration of the eyebrow.

Comment

Both eyes of this patient appear predisposed to the deveopment of spontaneous rhegmatogenous retinal detachment. The pattern of the detachment in the right eye showed none of the stigmata of trauma described above. Although an injury clearly occured to that side of the face and eyebrow, there was no evidence of direct injury to the eye. This would suggest the absence of any causal relationship of the injury and the retinal detachment.

CRITERIA OF COMPENSIBILITY

The criteria in classifying a given retinal detachment as traumatic in origin have been outlined by Cox, Schepens, and Freeman (1972). They include a history of unilateral injury to the eye, objective signs of contusion, and an absence of visible vitreoretinal degeneration known to cause retinal breaks in the affected or fellow eye.

History

A history of direct injury to the eye should be an essential factor in arriving at a diagnosis of traumatic detachment. It is generally felt at this time that indirect trauma plays no role in the etiology of detachment of the retina (Gartner 1974). In a series of 140 eye combat injuries, 49 of which caused perforating wounds and 22 severe ocular concussions, only 2 developed detached retinas (Treister, 1969). Among 1,326 replies of patients with skull injuries following traffic accidents, no case of retinal detachment was reported (Liesenhoff & Plog 1972).

A major difficulty arises in the frequently long latent interval between the time of injury and the onset of symptoms related to the retinal detachment (Tasman 1972). In 50% of a series of 234 eyes with retinal detachment due to ocular contusion or ocular penetration 50% were diagnosed 8 months following the injury (Cox & Freeman 1979).

Objective Evidence of Ocular Injury

Blunt trauma to the eye can produce a large variety of ocular damage (Eagling 1974). The detection of such lesions may offer unequivocal evidence of past injury. This includes iridodialysis, subluxation of the lens, choroidal ruptures, and massive scarring at the posterior pole from a commotio retinae. Similarly a perforating scar through the cornea, iris, or lens leaves no doubt that the eye was injured.

Special significance must be attributed to the presence of traumatic angle recession, which is considered proof of previous ocular contusion (Syrdalen 1970). The reported correlation between angle recession and traumatic retinal dialysis varies among different observers (Tasman 1972). It is important to evaluate the angle in comparison with that of the fellow eye, especially since a wide open chamber angle is a usual finding among retinal detachment patients (Syrdalen 1970).

Retinal Signs

The ophthalmoscopic picture is often adequate in establishing a relationship between trauma and retinal detachment. A retinal dialysis, when associated with signs of vitreous base avulsion, is considered pathognomic of a contu-

207

sion retinal detachment (Weidenthal & Schepens 1966). Traumatic dialyses occur with greater frequency superiorly than inferiorly (Cox & Hagler 1966). It is important to distinguish an inferior traumatic dialysis from dialyses seen in young patients without a history of trauma. This difficulty is enhanced by the frequency with which both traumatic and spontaneously occuring retinal dialyses can remain asymptomatic for long periods of time. Young patients are inclined to forget or deny previous injury.

A certain number of patients exhibit a necrosis-type of retinal hole, presumably due to direct impact of the offending object (Cox, Schepens & Freeman 1966). This is much more likely to occur in the inferior temporal (exposed) quadrant of the globe. A jagged irregular hole without other signs of retinal degeneration, is rare in spontaneous rhegmatogenous retinal detachment.

Macular holes typically occur in the older population. When seen in younger patients, especially unilaterally and associated with chorioretinal atrophy and pigmentation, the likelihood is great that such a hole was induced by contusion. Traumatic macular holes do not usually cause a detachment of the retina (Eagling 1974).

Giant retinal tears occur as a result of very severe direct injury. The obvious history, the lack of lattice degeneration in the affected eye or the fellow eye usually establish the traumatic nature of such a detachment.

Retinal breaks can be caused by lacerations of the retina by foreign objects. In other cases of retinal detachment due to perforation of the globe, isolated vitreoretinal adhesions are a cause of retinal break formation (Ruiz 1969). The most characteristic sign of an eye that suffered a perforation is the presence of silvery, glistening vitreous fibers, usually emanating from the site of perforation and fanning out in all directions. These may be so delicate as to be visible with the slit lamp only. Usually they are easily recognized ophthalmoscopically, and are proof positive of a prior perforating injury.

Duration of Retinal Detachment

An important aspect in evaluating a given retinal detachment is to determine its age. The presence of demarkation lines, and intraretinal macrocysts are indications of a retinal detachment of long duration (Hagler & North 1967). These objective signs must be consistent with the reported time of injury in determining a time relationship between trauma and retinal detachment.

Case 14. A 32 year old black male suffered an injury to the left side of the head three months before examination. No direct injury to the eye was reported. Examination revealed a subtotal retinal detachment with an upper nasal dialysis. Prominent demarkation lines were seen at the temporal borders of the detachment, and several intraretinal macrocysts were observed. A more careful history of the patient brought out the fact that he had been an amateur boxer for a period of two years.

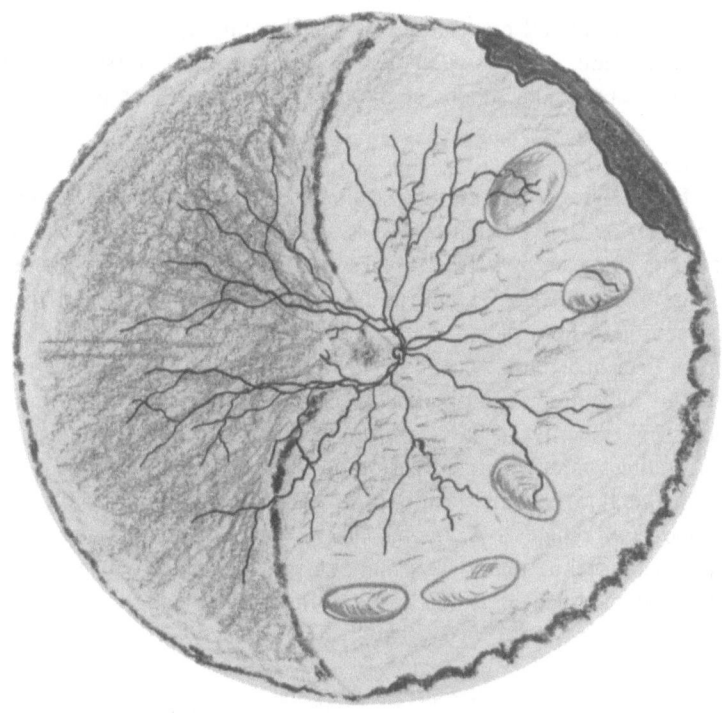

Fig. 15. (Case 14) Nasal retinal detachment with superior nasal dialysis. Note pigmented demarcation lines and intraretinal macrocysts.

Comment

This patient had a retinal detachment consistent with past blunt injury to the globe. However, he displayed demarcation lines which suggest a retinal detachment of at least 3 months' duration, and intraretinal cysts suggesting a detachment of at least 6 months' duration. The possibility is suggested that he was punched in the eye while boxing, and that the existing retinal detachment antedated the reported injury.

Predisposing Factors

A key judgment that an ophthalmologist must make is whether a given retinal detachment following injury would have occured spontaneously or whether trauma was a precipitating factor. The incidence of myopia among patients with contusion retinal detachment is somewhat larger than that in the general population, but significantly smaller than what is found in the idiopathic retinal detachment population (Witmer 1972). A highly myopic eye must be considered predisposed to detachment of the retina.

Since an aphakic eye has a chance of 2.2% (Scheie, Morse & Aminlari 1973) of developing detachment of the retina, an absent lens is a predisposing factor.

Multiple equatorial retinal breaks, in different quadrants, are highly suggestive of underlying vitreoretinal pathology, especially when associated with lattice degeneration. If the fellow eye is similarly involved, either by lattice degeneration alone or by retinal breaks, a predisposition to retinal detachment is assumed. Our case 11 illustrates this. The question of partial monetary compensation for a patient with pre-existing vitreoretinal pathology who develops a detached retina secondary to trauma is too difficult to generalize and must be judged on an individual basis. Dufour (1961) plotted graphically the increasing severity of injury (from rubbing of the eyes, to physical exertion, indirect injury, corneal perforation, contusion of the globe, to perforation of the globe) against factors of increasing disposition (from a normal eye to one with progressive myopia, lattice degeneration, familial disease, aphakia and horseshoe tears). The more severe the injury with a minimum of predisposition, the greater the chance of the trauma being the cause of the detachment.

SUMMARY

In evaluating a given case of reported trauma and retinal detachment, a judgment of compensibility must take into account multiple factors of history of injury, objective ocular signs of past trauma, and the typical picture of a contusion or perforation retinal detachment (Table 2).

Table 2. Evidence of causal relationships between injury and retinal detachment

1. History of direct contusion or perforating injury to affected eye.
2. Evidence of previous trauma to anterior segment, including angle recession.
3. Evidence of trauma to the posterior segment.
4. Vitreous base avulsion and retinal dialysis.
5. Proliferating intravitreal fibrous tissue.
6. Absence of predisposing vitreoretinal pathology in the affected eye and the fellow eye.

Where the history of direct trauma to the eye is nebulous and no objective signs of injury can be seen; where the retinal detachment shows no stigmata of past trauma, and where there is evidence of degenerative vitreoretinal disease in the affected eye as well as in the fellow eye; or where there is funduscopic evidence that the retinal detachment is old and preceded the time of reported injury – these factors suggest a lack of causal relationship between the trauma and the retinal detachment (Table 3).

Table 3. Factors suggesting lack of causal relationship between trauma and retinal detachment

---

1. Minimal injury to the eye, indirect injury, strain.
2. Absence of objective signs of ocular trauma.
3. Predisposing conditions, eg. high myopia, aphakia.
4. Degenerative vitreoretinal changes in both eyes.
5. Long standing retinal detachment.

REFERENCES

Cox, M.S. & H.M. Freeman. Traumatic Retinal Detachment 'Ocular Trauma' (H.M. Freeman, Ed). Appleton-Century-Crofts, New York 1979, p. 285.

Cox, M.S. C.L. Schepens & H.M. Freeman. Retinal Detachment Due to Ocular Contusion. Archives of Ophthalmology 56: 678 (1966).

Dufour, R. Evaluation of the Role of Traumatism in the Pathogenesis of Retinal Detachment. Ophthalmologica 141: 334-42 (1961); 262-67 (1961).

Eagling, E.M. Ocular Damage After Blunt Trauma to The Eye. British Journal of Ophthalmology 58: 126 (1974).

Gärtner, J. Über die Rolle des Traumas bei der Entstehung der Netzhautabhebung. Ophthalmologica 168: 1-12 (1974).

Hagler, W.S. & A.W. North. Intraretinal Macrocycts and Retinal Detachment. Transactions Am. Academy Ophth. and Otol. 71: 442 (1967).

Liesenhoff, H. & G. Plog. Concerning the Probability of Relationship between Indirect Trauma and Retinal Detachment. Modern Problems in Ophthalmology, Vol. 10, p. 474. S. Karger, 1972.

Ruiz, R.S. Traumatic Retinal Detachments. Br. J. Ophth. 53: 59 (1969).

Scheie, H.G., P.H. Morse & A. Aminlari. Incidence of Retinal Detachment Following Cataract Extraction. Archives of Ophthalmology 89: 293 (1973).

Syrdalen, P. Trauma and Retinal Detachment. Acta Ophthal. 48: 1006 (1970).

Tasman, W. Peripheral Retinal Changes Following Blunt Trauma. Tr. Amer. Ophthal. Soc. 70: 190 (1972).

Treister, G. Ocular Casualties in the Six-Day War. Am. J. Ophth. 68: 669 (1969).

Weidenthal, D.T. & C.L. Schepens. Peripheral Fundus Changes Associated with Ocular Contusion. Amer. Journal of Ophth. 62: 465 (1966).

Witmer, R. Traumatic Retinal Detachment. Modern Problems in Ophthalmology, Vol. 10. S. Karger, 1972.

Author's address:
Brookdale Hospital Medical Center
Brooklyn, New York 11212
U.S.A.

CRYOTHERAPY FOR TREATMENT
OF LATTICE DEGENERATION

ISAAC BONIUK

(St. Louis, MO., U.S.A.)

ABSTRACT

Cryotherapy is an effective means of treatment for lattice degeneration with a minimum of complications over a prolonged period.

INTRODUCTION

Photocoagulation and cryotherapy have both been employed in the prophylactic treatment of retinal detachment (Meyer-Schwickerath 1960; Pischel & Colyear 1960; McPherson 1968; Schafer 1967; Benson et al. 1977). In 1974, we evaluated xenon photocoagulation versus cryotherapy in the prevention of retinal detachment in 922 eyes; 367 of these eyes had lattice degeneration (Boniuk 1974). We found that while prophylactic treatment was favorable using either modality, the incidence of complications with photocoagulation was significantly greater than with cryotherapy. For this 1979 study, we evaluated 357 eyes in 318 patients treated with cryotherapy for lattice degeneration during the years 1965–1974; a number of these patients were included in the 1974 study, others are new to this study. The purpose of this study was to evaluate whether a longer follow-up would verify the high success rate with low incidence of complications using cryotherapy.

TECHNIQUE AND TREATMENT

In eyes with lattice degeneration, indications for treatment were as follows: (1) recent onset of photopsia and/or vitreous hemorrhage; (2) associated retinal tears; (3) fellow eyes of patients with retinal detachment, especially if the detachments were associated with similar pathology; (4) patients with a family history of lattice and retinal detachment; and (5) lattice in eyes soon to have cataract extraction performed. Eyes with associated horseshoe-shaped retinal tears with lattice degeneration were also included in this group.

213

Docum. Ophthal. Proc. Series, Vol. 25, ed. by H. Zauberman
© 1981, Dr. W. Junk bv Publishers, The Hague

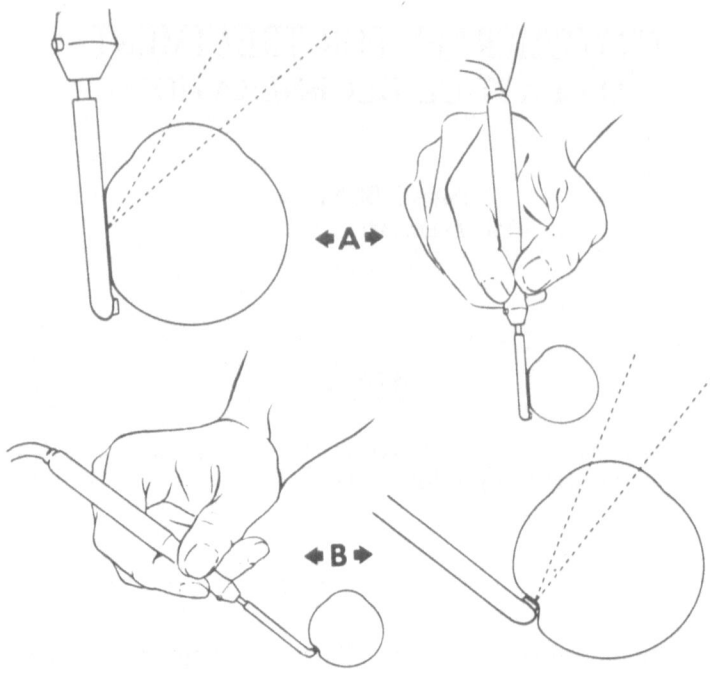

Fig. 1. When treating a zone of pathology, after any individual freeze one should immediately rotate the eye, note where the freeze occurred, and then place the probe in juxtaposition to the edge of the previous freeze thereby avoiding gaps in the treatment. The treater must be certain that the tip of the probe is in view rather than the shaft. © Retina Consultants, Ltd.

All areas of lattice were treated at one sitting (Burgess & Boniuk 1980). The conjunctiva was not opened unless the pathology in several quadrants could not be reached otherwise. In some cases where the pathology extended posteriorly in one area, the probe was punched through the conjunctiva to allow posterior treatment.

Under direct visualization with the indirect ophthalmoscope, cryo treatment was begun at the posterior edge of the lattice until a freeze was seen and had just begun to spread. The eye was then rotated, and the probe was replaced by external monitoring immediately adjacent to the previous freeze (Fig. 1). Thus, by this combination of internal and external monitoring, the area of pathology was completely and confluently covered. Meticulous attention to detail assured coverage of the pathology from back to front, and in its circumferential extent. If the lattice was relatively anterior, the treatment was carried out to the ora serrata in each meridion of treatment. If the lattice was more posteriorly located, treatment was carried out from its edges to the ora serrata, to wall off that zone. If two patches of lattice were close together,

214

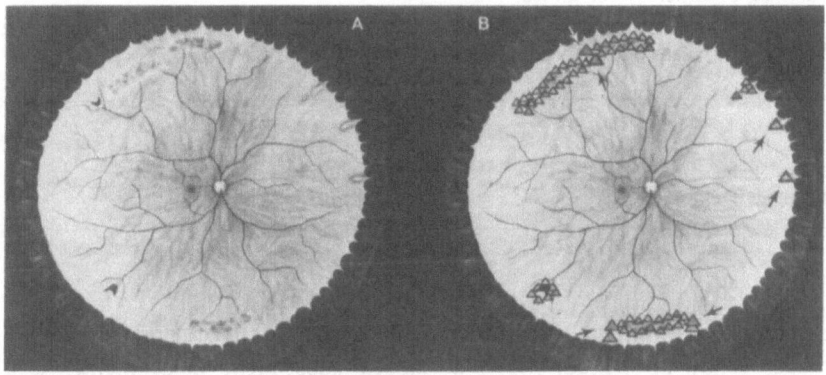

Fig. 2. A. Zones of lattice degeneration and holes are shown as well as vitreoretinal adhesions in the upper nasal quadrant; B. The small triangles show where cryo lesions should be placed. The larger triangles, also indicated by arrows, show where treatment is optional (to zones of vitreoretinal adhesion, to wall off lattice at its edges, or to a small space between two adjacent areas of lattice). (From Waltman-Krupin: *Complications in Ophthalmic Surgery, Lippincott, 1980.)*

this interval area was treated; if vitreoretinal adhesions were present, these were treated (Fig. 2). After covering all areas to be treated, the eye was re-examined with indirect ophthalmoscopy and scleral depression using either the cryo probe or a cotton-tipped applicator, and any gaps in the treatment were filled in.

RESULTS

In this study, 357 eyes were evaluated. These patients were selected consecutively from 1965 through 1974, and follow-up ranged from 3 years, to 12.8 years with an average of 5.8 years. 217 eyes (60%) were followed for a period or 3 years or longer. The patients ranged in age from 14 years to 79 years.

Table 1 shows the breakdown of the cases treated with photocoagulation and cryotherapy in our original study in 1974. The low complication rate of

Table 1. Prophylactic therapy, 1965–1972

Follow-up 6 months to 7 years, 796 eyes

	Photo	Cryo
Number of eyes	339	457
Subsequent detachment	16 (4.7%)	11 (2.4%)
New tears	43 (12.7%)	17 (3.7%)
Maculopathy	14 (4.1%)	9 (1.9%)

Table 2. Cryotherapy for lattice, 1965–1974

Follow-up 3 years to 12.8 years, 217 eyes

Subsequent detachment	9 eyes (4.1%)
'New' tears	16 eyes (7.3%)
Macular pucker	1 eye (0.5%)

cryotherapy is verified in this study and appears to be maintained over a longer follow-up period. 4.1% developed subsequent detachment, 7.3% 'new' tears, and the likelihood of macular pucker was 0.5% (Table 2).

In the nine eyes which subsequently detached, the location of breaks can be grouped into three areas: three developed in a new area; three developed at the edge of the old treated area; and three could be considered residual lattice, or occurred between treatment spots. Five of these eyes were successfully reattached with one procedure; eight eyes reattached and achieved vision equal to or greater than 20/30. The one failure had extensive vitreous hemorrhage, and detachment with massive periretinal proliferation (MPP) occurred from lattice underlying the vitreous hemorrhage which was not covered at the original treatment.

The interval from treatment to detachment ranged from three weeks to eight years. Symptoms were present in six, absent in three. In seven eyes, the macula was attached at presentation. Two eyes had cataract extractions at 3 months and 10 months before detachment.

Of the 16 eyes with 'new' holes, 11 of these occurred after three years. Only four had symptoms and these holes were away from previously treated zones. Seven eyes had new holes in an area of residual pathology, or where original pathology was not thoroughly covered. Such new holes could have been prevented by more meticulous coverage of the pathology. Two eyes had spontaneously sealed holes outside of treated areas.

DISCUSSION

Longer follow-up of eyes treated with cryotherapy for lattice degeneration yielded the following conclusions. The incidence of macular fibroplasia is less than 1%. When subsequent detachment develops, repair is almost always successful with good visual results. New symptoms or cataract surgery dictate early re-evaluation. Meticulous attention to detail at time of treatment may lower the incidence of 'new' hole formation and/or subsequent detachment (See Fig. 3 for illustrative case).

The results in our original study clearly indicated a lesser tendency for eyes treated with cryotherapy to subsequently detach, or develop new tears

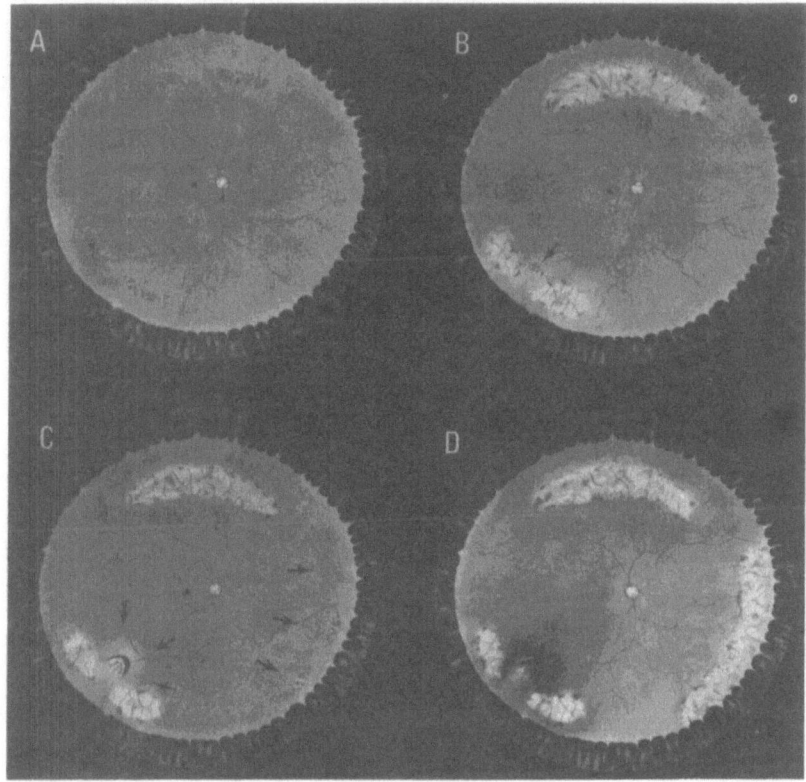

Fig. 3. A. Zones of lattice degeneration; B. Cryo scarring to the zones of lattice degeneration, but note tiny patch of lattice missed at original treatment (it was more subtle then); C. A horseshoe tear with small detachment (outlined by arrows) has occurred from this missed area. 'New' areas of lattice nasally (arrows); D. Detachment treated by cryotherapy and local plombage without drainage of subretinal fluid. Also confluent cryo treatment to nasal lattice. © Retina Consultants, Ltd.

or maculopathy when compared to photocoagulation. The natural history of lattice has not been well articulated (Hyams *et al.* 1974). But, on the basis of our studies, we feel that carefully performed prophylactic treatment for lattice degeneration is beneficial and results in few complications, and the beneficial effects of such treatment appear to be maintained.

REFERENCES

Benson, W. E., P. H. Morse & P. Nantawan. Late complications following cryotherapy of lattice degeneration. Amer. J. Ophthalmol. 84: 514-516 (1977).

Boniuk, I., E. Okun, G.P. Johnston & N. Arribas. Xenon photocoagulation vs. cryotherapy in the prevention of retinal detachment. Mod. Probl. Ophthalmol. 12: 81-92 (1974).

Burgess D. & I. Boniuk. Complications of photocoagulation and prophylactic cryotherapy. In Waltman S., Krupin, T. (eds): Complications in ophthalmic surgery. Lippincott. Philadelphia pp. 303-317, 1980.

Hyams, S.W., M. Ivry, D. Krakowski, *et al*. Chorioretinal lesions predisposing to retinal detachment. Amer. J. Ophthalmol. 78: 429-437 (1974).

Meyer-Schwickerath, G. Light coagulation; transl. by S. Drance. Mosby, St. Louis (1960).

McPherson, A. Cryosurgery in the prophylaxis and primary management of retinal detachment; in McPherson: New and controversial aspects of retinal detachment. Harper & Row, New York, pp. 186-201. (1968).

Pischel, D. K.& B. H. Colyear. Light coagulation therapy. Amer. J. Ophthalmol. 50: 590-595 (1960).

Shafer, D.M. Cryosurgery for retinal tears without detachment. Int. Ophthalmol. Clin. 7: 421-428 (1967).

Author's address:
Retina Consultants Ltd.
East Pavilion — Suite 17413
4949 Barnes Hosp. Plaza
St. Louis, MO., 63110
U.S.A.

FACTORS INFLUENCING THE FINAL VISUAL ACUITY FOLLOWING RETINAL DETACHMENT SURGERY

PINI D. GAISINER & TERESA BISO

(*Rosario, Argentina*)

ABSTRACT

The purpose of this study was to evaluate statistically the different factors influencing the final visual acuity following retinal detachment surgery. The material was derived from cases with a follow-up of at least six months, and anatomically cured. The variables were collected into three different levels: preoperative, operative and post-operative, which contained 25 categories and 57 subcategories. Twenty-three variables remained which were significant. The results of this study were considered taking into account previous visual acuity, patient age, symptoms, location and extension of detachment, condition of the macula, location of breaks, surgical technique, and postoperatory complications. Other factors, including sex, family history, aphakia, previous ocular tension, vitreous hemorrhage and shape of breaks, were discarded as they proved to yield no additional useful information related to the final visual acuity. A potentially important factor which could not be analyzed and included in this study owing to its subjective nature, is the duration of the preoperatory macular detachment.

INTRODUCTION

The ultimate aim of all retinal detachment surgery is the improvement and recovery of visual acuity. Thus, the purpose of this study is to determine which elements can help us to predict that aim taking into account the reduced number of reports available about this subject (see references).

MATERIAL AND METHODS

The material was obtained from 205 eyes anatomically cured out of a total of 237 consecutive cases (86%) with retinal detachments operated between January 1, 1974 and July 31, 1978. In all the cases the variables analyzed were grouped in three levels: Preoperatory – data for each patient, age and sex, family history, personal history, visual acuity, refractive error, extension and location of the detachment, status of the macula and breaks. Operatory – date of surgery, pre and post operatory rest, type of surgery, results after

219

Table 1. Distribution of 205 cases of retinal detachment surgery according to their initial visual acuity and their final visual acuity

Pre operative visual acuity	Post-operative visual acuity				
	up to 1/40	1/20 to 2/10	3/10 to 6/10	7/10 to 10/10	Total
Up to 1/40	9	66	55	12	142
1/20 to 2/10	1	5	19	10	35
3/10 to 6/10	—	2	6	10	18
7/10 to 10/10	—	1	1	8	10
Total	10	74	81	40	205

surgical procedure, complications. Postoperatory – anatomic results when discharged, visual acuity after six months.

In spite of considering of significant importance the period between the moment in which the patient noticed the loss of his central vision and the date of the operation as indicative of the duration of the macular detachment, its quantification was not possible owing to the considerable degree of subjective appreciation that such a perception involves.

Certain variables were normalized and standardized in order to improve their distribution.

This study includes frequency tables for determining the material to be analyzed.

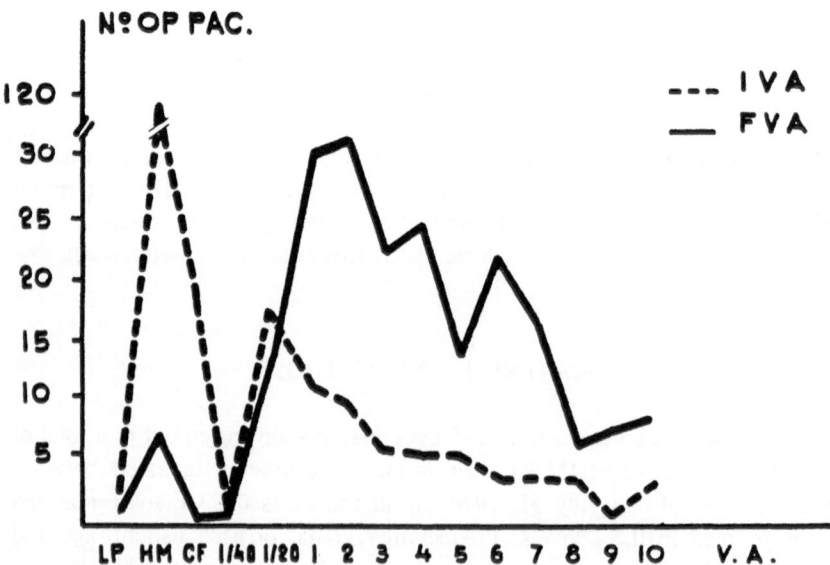

Fig. 1. Initial visual acuity (IVA) and final visual acuity (FVA) in 205 retinal detachment cases anatomically cured.

RESULTS

Pre and postoperatory visual acuity

Table 1 shows that four (1.9%) of the 205 eyes observed were affected by a lower visual acuity post-operatively. Twenty-eight eyes (13.6%) maintained the same level of visual acuity and the rest, 173 eyes (84.4%) were favorably affected. One hundred and six eyes out of the 173 previously mentioned recovered an acuity above 3/10 (Fig. 1).

Table 2. Percentual distribution of final visual acuity according to detached quadrant

Quadrant	Total %	Up to 1/40	1/20 to 2/10	3/10 to 6/10	7/10 to 10/10
UT – LT	21	5	23	49	23
UT – LT – UN – LN	14	10	55	28	7
UT – LT – LN	14	—	35	54	11
UT – LT – UN	12	8	38	38	16
UT – UN	7	—	42	29	29
UT	7	—	21	43	36
LT – ln	7	—	36	36	28
LT – UN – LN	6	23	54	23	—
UN – LN	4	—	13	37	50
UT – UN – LN	3	—	43	43	14
LT	3	16	50	—	34
LT – UN	1	—	—	100	—
UN	1	—	—	50	50
UT – LN	—	—	—	100	—

UT: Upper temporal; LT: Lower temporal; UN: Upper nasal; LN: Lower nasal.

Table 3. Final visual acuity and previous status of the macula

Status of the macula	Final visual acuity				
	up to 1/40	1/20 to 2/10	3/10 to 6/10	7/10 to 10/10	Total %
Detached	4.6	42.4	41.7	11.3	63.9
Attached	—	8.8	32.4	58.8	14.4
Pseudo-foramen	4.0	40.0	40.0	16.0	10.6
Hidden by overhanging fold	—	43.8	50.0	6.3	6.7
Not specified	25.0	37.5	25.0	12.5	3.3

221

Table 4. Type of surgery and final visual acuity (%)

	up to 1/40	1/20 to 2/10	3/10 to 6/10	7/10 to 10/10
With drainage	5	37	40	18
Without drainage	4	31	41	24
Encircling procedure	6	40	36	17
Segmental buckling	6	29	47	18
Segmental buckling plus encircling procedure	12	32	36	20
Diathermy	4	37	40	19
Cryotherapy	11	26	37	26

Detached quadrants

Sixty one per cent of the 205 operated eyes had both temporal quadrants detached and seventy eight per cent had the upper temporal detached (Table 2). Fifty eight per cent of the eyes with both temporal quadrants detached obtained a final visual acuity of 3/10 or more.

Previous status of the macula

Table 3 shows that the macula was detached in 63.9% of the eyes observed; 52.9% of them maintained a visual acuity of 3/10 or more. The macula was attached preoperatively in 14.4% of these eyes. In this group, 91.1% maintained a postoperative visual acuity of 3/10 or more.

Operative procedure

Non drained eyes obtained a slightly better final visual acuity than those in which subretinal fluid was released (Table 4). The same table shows that the percentage of better final visual acuity corresponds to those eyes operated on by segmental buckling while the chance of recovery is less favorable in the eyes operated on by encircling procedures and segmental buckling plus encircling procedures.

Eyes treated with cryotherapy had a better percentage of final visual acuity compared with the eyes treated with diathermy.

It is convenient to remark that non-drained eyes and those operated on with local indentation procedures presuppose less complex cases.

222

Statistical analysis

Statistical analysis of the material obtained was based on the model of a stepwise multiple regression analysis with the purpose of observing the successive influence of each of the variables introduced in the model. It is evident that the characteristic which is more significant in explaining the final visual acuity is the initial visual acuity followed by the location of the retinal detachment and the detached quadrant. The remaining variables successively introduced in the model become less significant with respect to the general equation.

The basis for this analysis was an initial equation of the following type: $Y = \beta_1 X_1 + \beta_2 X_2 \ldots + \beta_9 X_9$, in which Y is the dependent variable (final visual acuity) and β is the regression coefficient.

The following variables were taken into account: age, symptoms, initial visual acuity, detached quadrant, status of the macula, type of breaks, location of breaks, and type of surgery.

The total regression coefficient was 0.60 and the different values obtained for the successive variables considered, were: Table 5.

We have proved the validity of the stepwise multiple regression model and obtained a significant value (F = 15.9) $p < 0.01$.

Table 5. Variables with significant regression coefficients

Variable	Coefficient β
Initial visual acuity	0.5281
Localization of retinal detachment	0.1084
Detached quadrants	0.0856
Shape of breaks	0.0845
Age	0.0525
Type of surgery	0.0432
Number of breaks	0.0220

REFERENCES

Burton, T.C. & R.W. Lambert. A predictive model for visual recovery following retinal detachment surgery. Ophthalmology 85: 619-625 (1978).

Chisholm, I.A., E. McClure & W.S. Foulds. Functional recovery of the retina after retinal detachment. Transactions of the Ophthalmological Societies of the United Kingdom 95: 167-172 (1973).

Grupposo, S.S. Visual results after scleral buckling with silicone implant, in Schepens, C.L., Regan, C.D.J. (eds): Controversial aspects of the management of retinal detachment. Boston, Little Brown & Co, 1965, pp. 354-363.

Grupposo, S.S. Visual acuity following surgery for retinal detachment. Arch. Ophtalmol. 93: 327-330 (1975).

Gundry, M. F. & E. W. G. Davis. Recovery of visual acuity after retinal detachment surgery. Am. J. Ophtalmol. 77: 310-314 (1974).

Jay, B. The functional cure of retinal detachments. Transactions of the Ophtalmological Societies of the United Kingdom 85: 101-110 (1965).

Authors' address:
Paraguay 1394
2000 Rosario
Argentina

SURGICAL MANAGEMENT OF RETINAL DETACHMENT WITHOUT INDUCING CHORIORETINAL SCARS

R. AXER-SIEGEL, Y. YASSUR & I. BEN-SIRA

(Tel-Aviv, Israel)

INTRODUCTION

Surgical management of retinal detachment without inducing chorioretinal scars was introduced in 1975 by H. Zauberman who performed surgery on 37 cases of retinal detachment without inducing chorioretinal lesions, and suggested that in phakic patients this procedure is superfluous if vitreous traction is successfully counteracted with scleral buckling procedure.

We have attempted to conduct a prospective study in order to test the efficacy of the above-mentioned technique.

MATERIALS AND METHODS

Seventy cases with detached retinae were operated upon in our department during the period of January 1975 to May 1976.

The test group included 41 eyes which were operated upon by scleral buckling with a good alleviation of vitreo-retinal traction without inducing chorioretinal lesions. This group was composed of 30 phakic and 11 aphakic eyes with retinal detachment. In ten of the eyes, the operation was due to recurrent retinal detachment following a previous operation. In five of the eyes no retinal tear was found.

The control group consisted of 29 eyes with retinal detachment which were operated upon by scleral buckling and cryoapplications. This group was comprised of 22 phakic and 7 aphakic eyes. In five of the eyes the operation was due to recurrent retinal detachment after a previous surgery. In four of the eyes no retinal tear was noticed.

RESULTS

In the test group, an immediate post-operative reattachment of the retinae was obtained in 37 out of 41 cases (90%) – 28/30 phakic and 9/11 aphakic. However, after a mean follow-up period of three years, reattachment of the

225

Docum. Ophthal. Proc. Series, Vol. 25, ed. by H. Zauberman
© *1981, Dr. W. Junk bv Publishers, The Hague*

retinae was observed in only 19 out of 38 eyes (50%) which remained under our follow-up control (15/27 phakic and 4/11 aphakic eyes).

In the control group, an immediate post-operative reattachment of the retinae was obtained in 27 out of 29 cases (90%) – 20/22 phakic and 7/7 aphakic – and after a mean follow-up period of three years, there were still 18 out of 24 eyes (75%) with attached retinae (13/18 phakic and 5/6 aphakic).

There were no differences between the two groups in the late postoperative complication of macular pucker.

DISCUSSION

It is difficult to draw definite conclusions as to the importance of cryotherapy in retinal detachment surgery, as the present study was non-randomized. However, it seems that scleral buckling alone may counteract vitreous traction during the short post-operative period, but it is not sufficient to keep the retina from re-detaching later.

It is therefore suggested that the better anatomical results which were obtained by buckling procedures with cryoapplication and the lack of difference in the post-operative complications sometimes attributed to cryopexy like macular pucker advocate the induction of cryogenic chorioretinal lesions during retinal detachment surgery.

REFERENCES

Zauberman, H. et al. Treatment of retinal detachment without inducing chorioretinal lesion. Tr. Am. Acad. Ophthalmol. and Otol. 79: 835 (1975).

Authors' address:
Department of Ophthalmology
Beilinson Medical Center
Tel-Aviv University
Sackler School of Medicine
Tel-Aviv, Israel

226

PIGMENT EPITHELIUM AND ROD OUTER SEGMENT CELL-SURFACE INTERACTIONS IN NORMAL AND RCS RATS

IZHAK NIR

(*Haifa, Israel*)

INTRODUCTION

Phagocytosis of rod outer segment tips by the pigment epithelium (PE) is required for normal development of retinal photoreceptors (Young 1976). In RCS rats with retinitis pigmentosa, the balance between membrane renewal and removal is disturbed due to a defective phagocytosis process. This leads to accumulation of rod outer segment (ROS) membrane debris in the sub-retinal space and to subsequent retinal dystrophy (Bok & Hall 1971).

Phagocytosis is a complex series of events which includes recognition, adhesion and internalization (Stossel 1976). The internalization of inert particles by the PE in RCS rats (Custer & Bok 1975) suggests that cellular components associated with this activity are functioning properly. Further attention should be focused, therefore, on the recognition and adhesion between ROS and PE cells.

In the present study I employed cytochemical procedures in order to evaluate the attachment between ROS and PE plasma membranes. Exclusion of markers from the PE-ROS interface as observed by electron microscopy was used as a measurement for intercellular adhesion.

MATERIAL AND METHODS

New born RCS and normal albino rats were raised for 7–25 days under 12 hours dark, 12 hours light cycle. Animals were sacrified 60 minutes after the onset of light. Under these illumination condition accelerated disk shedding and phagocytosis can be expected (LaVail 1976).

Eye cups were isolated, fixed with glutaraldehyde and incubated with cationized ferritin or ferritin labelled concanavalin A (500 μg/ml in 0.1 M phosphate buffer pH–7.0) for 45 minutes at room temperature. After incubation, the tissue was post-fixed with O_sO_4 and prepared for electron microscopy.

This work was supported by a grant from Israel Ministry of Health (180–156).

227

Docum. Ophthal. Proc. Series, Vol. 25, ed. by H. Zauberman
© 1981, Dr. W. Junk bv Publishers, The Hague

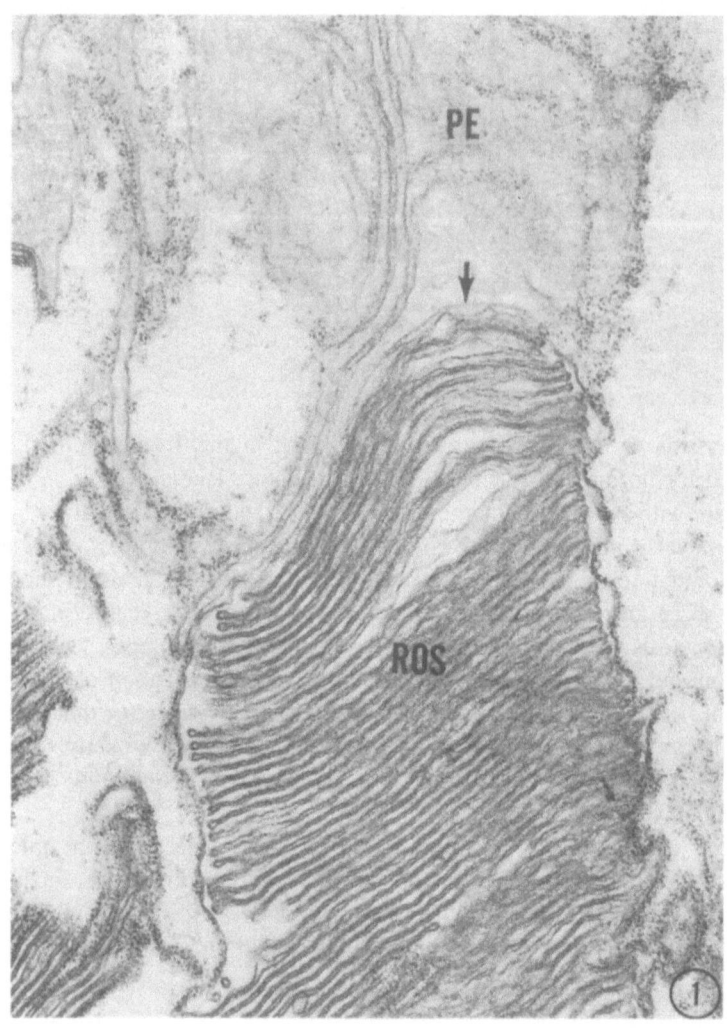

Fig. 1. Binding of cationized ferritin to a rod outer segment (ROS) and pigment epithelium (PE) microvilli in 21 days old normal rat. Note that the PE-ROS interface (arrow) is devoid of ferritin particles. ×69,000

RESULTS AND DISCUSSION

Positively charged cationized ferritin reacts with anionic sites on cell membranes (Danon *et al.* 1972). In glutaraldehyde fixed retina, cationized ferritin binds intensively to both photoreceptor and pigment epithelium cell surface. The marker is expected, however, to be excluded from regions of close contacts between the plasma membranes of these cells. This can be clearly

228

seen in normal rats which are actively phagocytizing ROS tips. In Fig. 1, adhesion between PE cells and ROS tips in normal rats, 60 minutes after the onset of light, is demonstrated. The free surface of the ROS plasma membrane and the PE microvilli are covered with numerous ferritin particles. The ROS tip is partially engulfed by a PE microvilli. The microvilli in this region were tangentially sectioned so that a sheet-like structure is seen in close proximity to a ROS tip. In this area the PE-ROS interface is devoid of ferritin particles (arrow).

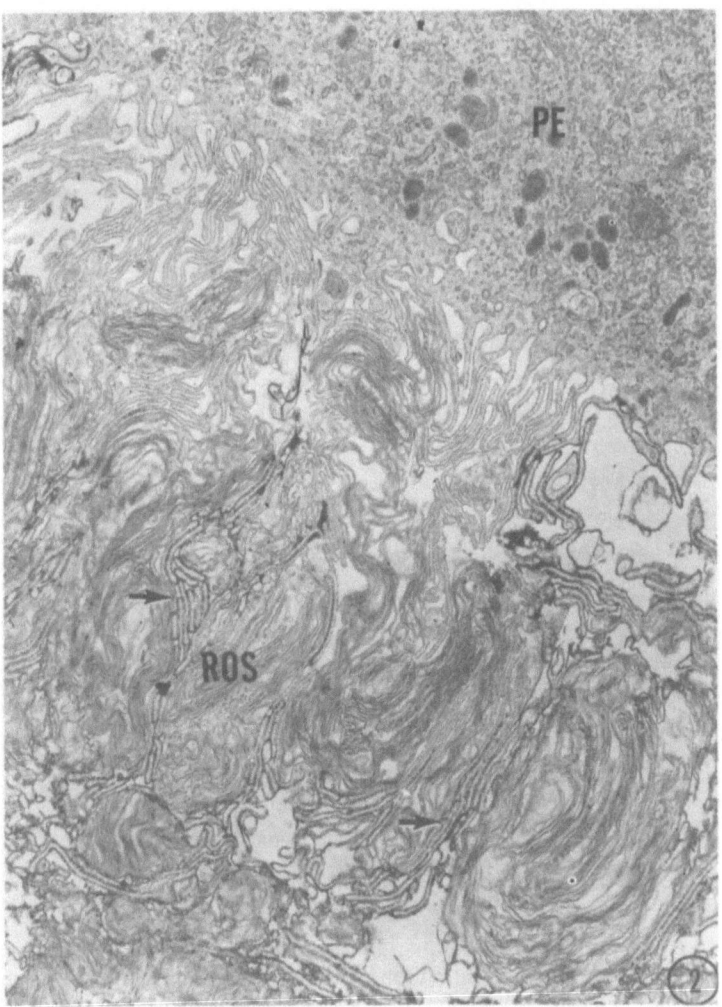

Fig. 2. Pigment epithelium (PE) and rod outer segments (ROS) in 21 days old RCS rat. Clusters of PE microvilli (delineated by electron dense ferritin particles) can be observed between ROS debris (arrows). ×12,000

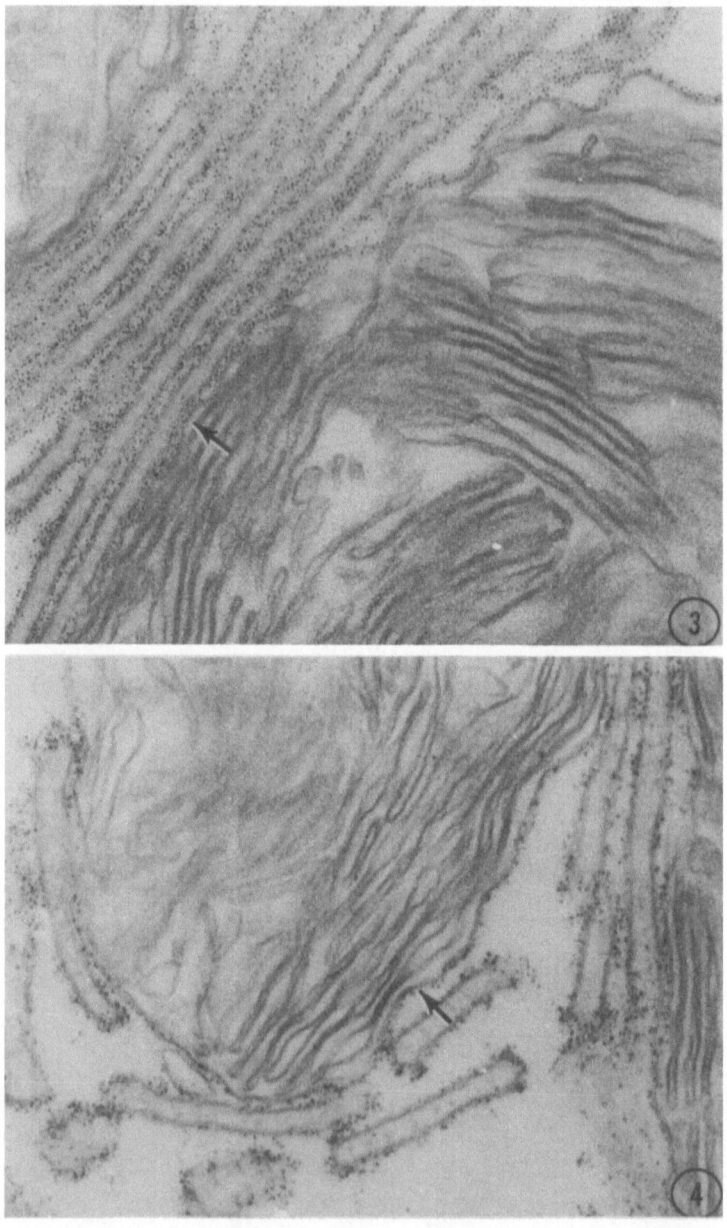

Fig. 3. Binding of cationized ferritin to the surface of ROS debris (arrow) and adjacent PE microvilli. ×70,000

Fig. 4. Binding of ferritin labelled concanavalin A to the surface of ROS debris (arrow) and adjacent PE microvilli. ×96,000

230

In 21 days old RCS rats, substantial accumulation of ROS membrane debris in the subretinal space can be seen (Fig. 2). Numerous PE microvilli are observed between the ROS structures. Some of the microvilli are situated in close proximity to the ROS plasma membrane (Fig. 2). In detailed examination, however, binding of cationized ferritin to both PE and ROS plasma membranes can be clearly identified (Fig. 3). This suggests that in the RCS rat, the distance between the PE and ROS plasma membranes is large enough to enable the cationized ferritin to reach its binding sites on membrane surfaces. This observation is not specific only to cationized ferritin. Similar results were obtained also with ferritin labelled concanavalin A which binds to sugar moieties on ROS and PE surfaces (Hall & Nir 1976). In Fig. 4, the binding of concanavalin A to the surface of ROS debris and to adjacent PE microvilli is demonstrated. It can be concluded, therefore, that under conditions which induce phagocytosis in normal rats, close contacts are being established between the PE and ROS tips to such an extent as to prevent cationized ferritin and ferritin labelled concanavalin A from penetrating between the closely apposed membranes. In RCS rats under the same conditions, similar attachment between the PE microvilli and ROS is not observed.

These results lend support to the suggestion that the absence of phagocytosis in RCS rats is due to a malfunction in the recognition and adhesion processes.

REFERENCES

Bok, D. & M. O. Hall. The role of the PE in the etiology of inherited retinal dystrophy in the rat. J. Cell Biol. 49: 664 (1971).

Custer, N. V. & D. Bok. Pigment epithelium photoreceptor interactions in normal and dystrophic rat retina. Exp. Eye Res. 21: 153 (1975).

Danon, D., L. Goldstein, Y. Marikovsky & E. Skutelsky. Use of cationized ferritin as a label of negative charges on cell surfaces. Ultras. Res. 38: 500 (1972).

Hall, M. O. & I. Nir. The binding of concanavalin A to the rod outer segment and pigment epithelium of normal and RCS rats. Exp. Eye Res. 22: 469 (1976).

LaVail, M. M. Rod outer segment disk shedding in rat retina: Relationship to cyclic lighting. Science 194: 1071 (1976).

Stossel, T. P. The mechanism of phagocytosis. J. Reticuloendothelial Soc. 19: 237 (1976).

Young, R. W. Visual cells and the concept of renewal. Invest. Ophthalmol. 15: 700 (1976).

Author's address:
Technion —
Faculty of Medicine
Haifa, Israel

THE METABOLIC AND CELLULAR BASIS OF GYRATE ATROPHY OF THE CHOROID AND RETINA

S. MERIN, S. YATZIV, M. STATTER & Y. SHAPIRO

(*Jerusalem, Israel*)

ABSTRACT

Biochemical abnormalities in form of hyperornithinemia, hypolysinemia, and hyperornithinuria are constant findings in gyrate atrophy of the choroid and retina. We found, in addition, a high concentration of ornithine in the aqueous of one patient. His cataractous lens had more than a 10 times higher concentration of ornithine than in a senile cataract, and undetectable lysine levels.

Patients with gyrate atrophy show muscular wasting and by electron microscopy degenerated myofibers, dysmorphic mitochondria and tubular aggregates. One patient showed numerous nemaline rods.

It is possible that the low levels of lysine are the cause of the chorioretinal atrophy.

INTRODUCTION

Gyrate atrophy of the choroid and retina is a rare hereditary disease of the eye. It causes progressive functional loss of vision, mainly in the form of visual field loss. The disease was regarded an isolated ocular affection since its first description in the 19th century (Cutler 1895; Fuchs 1896), until Simmell & Takki (1973) proved that abnormal biochemical findings in the plasma and urine are a consistent finding of this disease.

Recently we studied five patients with gyrate atrophy and described their biochemical abnormalities in blood and urine and their abnormal metabolic response to loading doses of amino acid and diet supplementation (Yatziv *et al.* 1979).

The present study describes some additional metabolic abnormalities, the main findings of the previous study and some new findings about abnormal cellular changes in the muscles. The clinical, biochemical and cellular abnormalities of gyrate atrophy combine to form a picture of a systemic disease, affecting, among other tissues, the eye.

This work was supported (in part) by the Mayer H. Lebenson Fund for Ophthalmic Research.

233

Docum. Ophthal. Proc. Series, Vol. 25, ed. by H. Zauberman
© *1981, Dr. W. Junk bv Publishers, The Hague*

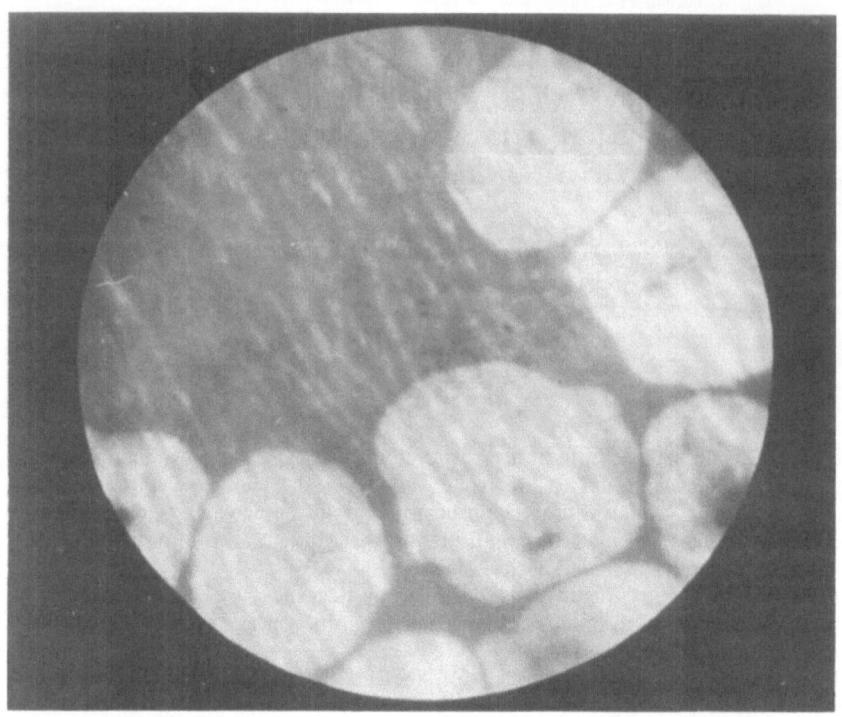

Fig. 1. The fundus of a patient with gyrate atrophy of choroid and retina.

OCULAR FINDINGS

Patients with gyrate atrophy of choroid and retina begin to complain of night blindness towards the end of the first decade of life or during the second decade. When the child is old enough to have visual fields reliably measured, a constriction of these visual fields is noted. The peripheral loss of the visual fields is progressive, similar to many cases of retinitis pigmentosa. Myopia is common, part of it of lenticular origin. Cataractous changes in the lens can be found early in life. A 25 year old patient was operated by us for a mature cataract.

The vitreous shows cells and 'debris' similar to retinitis pigmentosa. The fundus shows circumscribed areas of chorioretinal atrophy, growing in size and number, from the periphery to the center (Fig. 1). In the posterior pole atrophy of the pigment epithelium and pigmentary stippling can be noted. The electroretinogram is subnormal, diminishes progressively and rapidly till extinction early in life.

Table 1. Plasma ornithine and lysine levels in patients, heterozygotes and controls

| | Plasma levels (micromol/L) | |
	Ornithine	Lysine
5 patients	571–883	40– 89
4 obligatory heterozygotes	84–156	117–240
Controls	30– 90	120–215

BIOCHEMICAL FINDINGS

Patients with gyrate atrophy show consistently hyperornithinemia and hypo-lysinemia. Obligatory heterozygotes have plasma levels of ornithine some-what intermediate between controls and patients, with the lowest values overlapping highest control values. Plasma lysine values of heterozygotes are normal (Table 1). Ornithine tolerance tests cause in patients a great increase in the hyperornithinemia and in the existing basal hyperornithinuria. Contra-ry to controls and heterozygotes, patients have no rise in plasma glutamic acid and proline following a loading dose of ornithine (Yatziv et al. 1979), a fact which could be expected in patients with low activity of OKA (ornithine ketoacid aminotransferase) (Trijbels et al. 1977; O'Donnell et al. 1978; Arshinoff et al. 1977; Valle et al. 1977).

Lysine loading causes in patients a small increase in plasma lysine and increased both hyperlysinuria and hyperornithinuria.

The aqueous in patients with gyrate atrophy has a higher than normal concentration of ornithine. In one patient we found an ornithine concentra-tion of 320 micromole/L. Although this is a high figure, it is still only half of the ornithine concentration in plasma, in the same patient.

The ornithine concentration in a cataractous lens in a patient was more than 10 times that of a control lens, the lysine concentration is undetectable,

Table 2. The concentration of some amino acids in the cataractous lens of a patient with gyrate atrophy and a patient with senile cataract, in micromoles/100 mg net weight *

	Ornithine	Lysine	Phenylalanine and tyrosine
Patient	0.028	not detectable	0.017
Control	0.002	0.008	0.015

* Methods of measurement: The lenses were kept at $-80\,^\circ$C until processed. Each was weighed, homogenized in 1–2 ml of 5 % sulfosalicylic acid, centrifuged at refriger-ated centrifuge at 30,000 for 30 minutes and the supernatant was used for amino acid estimation in a Beckman Unichrom Amino Acid Analyzer.

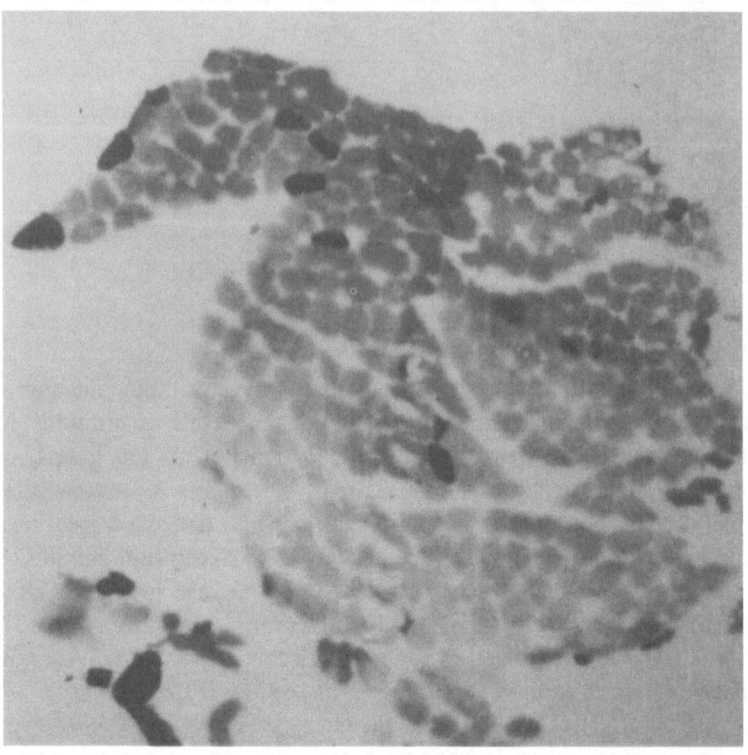

Fig. 2. Muscle biopsy in a patient with gyrate atrophy of choroid and retina. Light microscopy shows very marked reduction in type 2 myofibers (dark staining). Type 1 fibers (light staining) are preponderant and normal (myosin ATPase staining at pH 9.4).

while some other amino acids are found in normal concentration (Table 2).

MUSCULAR ATROPHY

Patients with gyrate atrophy of the choroid and retina have a typical appearance. They are thin, due to both general muscular wasting and loss of subcutaneous fat. The proximal muscles are affected more than the distal. A muscle biopsy, using the percutaneous needle technique, showed abnormal muscle fibers in a patient with gyrate atrophy. Light microscopy revealed fewer type 2 fibers (Fig. 2) and basophilic 'specks' in many myofibers. Electron microscopy indicates that many myofibers are degenerated and have dysmorphic mitochondria and tubular aggregates. In one patient nemaline rods were found (Fig. 3). Most of these findings are similar to the recently

236

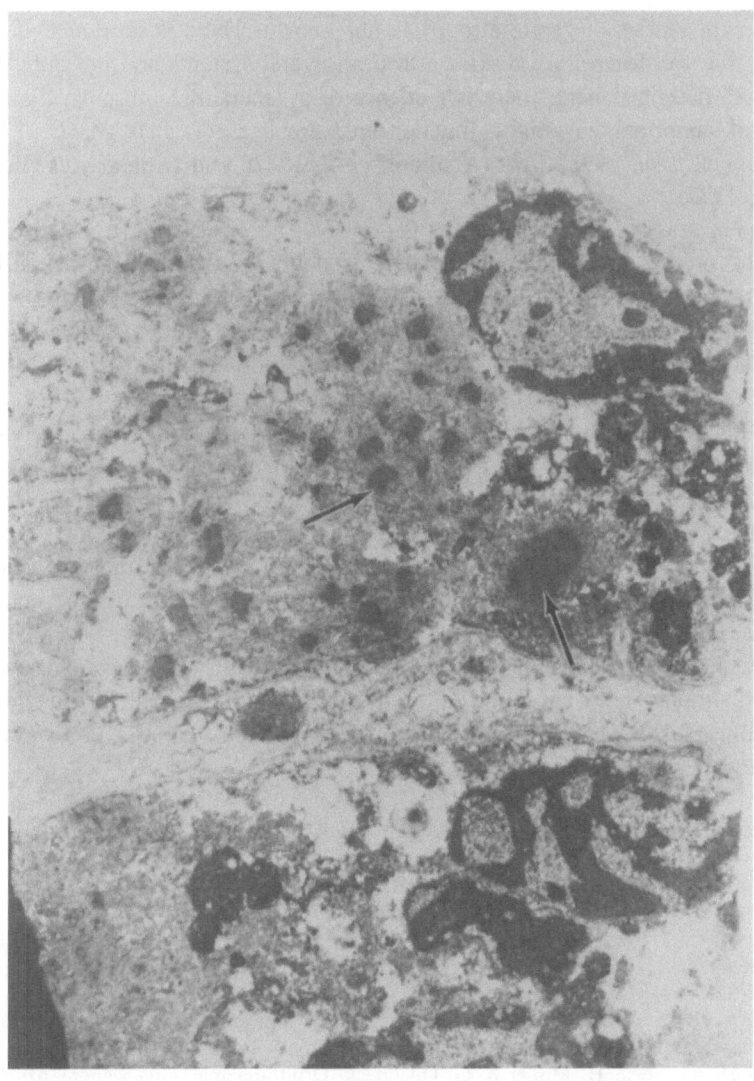

Fig. 3. Same patient. Electronmicroscopy shows numerous nemaline rods among degenerated myofibers. Arrows point to some rods. (Subsarcolemmial area, ×20,000).

described structural muscle abnormalities by Sipila *et al.* (1979) and to the findings in five patients with gyrate atrophy by our group (Shapira *et al.* in prep.). Abnormal tubular aggregates within type 2 fibers were previously mentioned (McCullock and Marliss 1975).

DISCUSSION

The pathogenesis of gyrate atrophy is not known. There is no doubt, however, that we deal with a disease affecting several systems and not only the eye. As described here, there is evidence of a generalized muscular disease and of abnormal enzymatic function in fibroblasts (Trijbels et al. 1977; O'Donnell et al. 1978), liver (Arshinoff et al. 1977), and lymphocytes (Valle et al. 1977).

The increase in plasma ornithine is probably the most striking biochemical finding of the disease. However, there is doubt of the importance of the hyperornithinemia in the pathogenesis of the ocular disease. Patients with hyperornithinemia do not necessarily show gyrate atrophy. Two such patients described by Bickel et al. (1968) and another patient described by Shih et al. (1969) had normal fundi. The low plasma levels of lysine are probably a result of the high ornithine and an abnormal renal tubular reabsorption (Yatziv et al. 1979). All our patients and four out of five patients described by Berson et al. (1976) had low levels of plasma lysine. Obligatory heterozygotes have normal levels of lysine and usually high levels of plasma ornithine. All these facts indicate that it is possible that low levels of lysine and not high levels of ornithine may be the cause of the ocular disease.

Nemaline rods were not previously described in muscles of patients with gyrate atrophy. They are found in a rare hereditary disease called 'congenital nemaline rod myopathy.' Occasionally, these rods are seen as a non-specific finding in various myopathies.

REFERENCES

Arshinoff, S., J.C. McCulloch, J.A. Parker, M. Philips & E.B. Marliss. Ornithine metabolism and liver pathology in hyperornithinemia and gyrate atrophy. Clin. Res. 25: 321 A (1977).

Berson, E.L., S.Y. Schmidt & A.R. Rabin. Plasma amino acids in hereditary retinal disease: ornithine, lysine and taurine. Brit. J. Ophthalmol. 60: 142-147 (1976).

Bickel H., D. Feist, H. Muller & G. Quadbeck. Ornithinaemie, eine weitere Aminosäurenstoftwechselstörung mit Hirnschädung. Dtsch. Med. Wschr. 93: 2247-2251 (1968).

Cutler, C.W. Drei ungewöhnliche Fälle von retino-choroidal Degeneration. Arch. Augenheilk. 30: 117-122 (1895).

Fuchs, E. Ueber zwei der Retinitis pigmentosa verwandte Krankheiten (Retinitis punctata albescens und Atrophia gyrata choroideae et retinae). Arch. Augenheilk. 32: 111 (1896).

McCulloch, C. & E.B. Marliss. Gyrate atrophy of the choroid and retina with hyperornithinemia. Am. J. Ophthalmol. 80: 1047-1057 (1975).

O'Donnell, J.J., R.P. Sandman & S.R. Martin. Gyrate atrophy of the retina: Inborn error of L-ornithine: 2-oxoacid aminotransferase. Science 200: 200-201 (1978).

Shapira, Y., S. Yatziv, S. Merin, M. Statter & R. Yarom. The myopathy of hyperornithinemic gyrate atrophy of choroid and retina (in prep.).

Shih, V. E., M. L. Efron & H. W. Moser. Hyperornithinemia, hyperammonemia and homocitrullinemia. A new disorder of amino acid metabolism associated with myoclonic seizures and mental retardation. Am. J. Dis. Child. 117: 83-92 (1969).

Simell, O. & K. Takki. Raised plasma ornithine and gyrate atrophy of the choroid and retina. Lancet 1: 1031-1033 (1973).

Sipilä, I., O. Simell, J. Rapola, K. Sainio & L. Tuuteri. Gyrate atrophy of the choroid and retina with hyperornithinemia: Tubular aggregates and type 2 fiber atrophy in muscle. Neurology 29: 996-1005 (1979).

Trijbels, J. M. F., R. C. A. Sengers, J. A. J. M. Bakkeren, A. F. M. de Kort & A. F. Deutman. L-ornithine-ketoacid-transamidase deficiency in cultured fibroblasts of a patient with hyperornithinemia and gyrate atrophy of the choroid and retina. Clin. Chim. Acta 79: 371-377 (1977).

Valle, D., M. I. Kaiser-Kupfer & L. A. Del-Valle. Gyrate atrophy of the choroid and retina: deficiency of ornithine amino-transferase in transformed lymphocytes. Proc. Natl. Acad. Sci. U.S.A. 74: 5159-5161 (1977).

Yatziv, S., M. Statter & S. Merin. Metabolic studies in two families with hyperornithinemia and gyrate atrophy of choroid and retina. J. Lab. Clin. Med. 93: 749-757 (1979).

Authors' addresses:

A. Merin (requests for reprints)
Department of Ophthalmology
Hadassah University Hospital
Ein Kerem and Mt. Scopus
Jerusalem, Israel

S. Yatziv, M. Statter & Y. Shapiro
Department of Pediatrics
Hadassah University Hospital
Ein Kerem and Mt. Scopus
Jerusalem, Israel

MANAGEMENT OF PATIENTS
WITH CONGENITAL CONE DEFICIENCY
(ACHROMATOPSIA WITH AMBLYOPIA)

S. MERIN, S. RONEN & I. NAWRATZKI

(*Jerusalem, Israel*)

ABSTRACT

Twenty patients with congenital cone deficiency were treated by pilocarpine 2%. All had low visual acuity, photophobia, nystagmus and a severe color vision defect up to total color blindness. Most had squint, hyperopic astigmatism and some had retinal changes. The visual acuity improved in 11 out of 17 patients. In 16 out of 17 patients there was an objective improvement in the photophobia and the nystagmus together with a clear subjective improvement in vision.

A follow up of ten patients who were up to four months on this treatment indicated that pilocarpine may be a valuable treatment of congenital cone deficiency.

INTRODUCTION

Hereditary diseases of the retina, of a functional nature, are usually considered untreatable. We examine the patients and their families, we test their retinal functions, establish a diagnosis, but rarely is any treatment prescribed except for low vision aids and for treatment of complications. Congenital cone deficiency is such a hereditary retinal disease of a functional nature. Treatment usually included prescription of sunglasses, but these are of little help. In 1973, Schachar *et al.* suggested treatment by miotics and reported good results in five patients.

In the present study we treated 20 patients with congenital cone dysfunction by Pilocarpine. Short-term results are reported and indicate that Pilocarpine is a valuable treatment in patients with cone deficiency.

PATIENTS AND METHODS

Twenty patients with congenital cone deficiency were examined in the Genetic Clinic. All had the four typical findings of this disease: low visual acuity, severe color vision defects, photophobia and nystagmus. Most, but not all had squint, high astigmatism, usually hyperopic – astigmatism and retinal-macular changes. The low visual acuity included poor day vision,

241

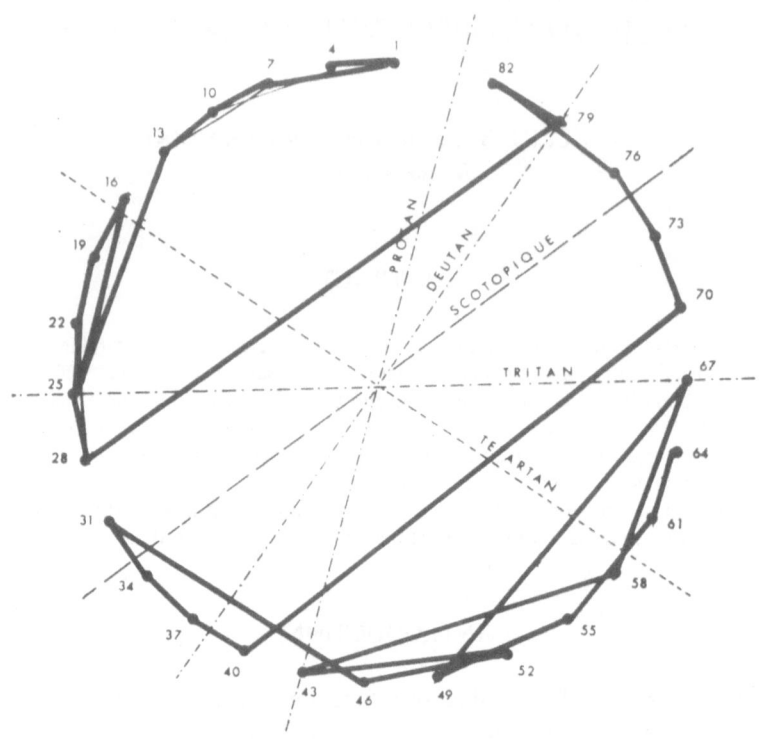

Fig. 1. 'Scotopic' lines in a 14-year-old patient with congenital cone deficiency

poor near vision, normal night vision. Typically patients had better visual acuity in mesopic light than in photopic light. The electroretinogram was abnormal in all cases, showing poor or absent cone function as described by Auerbach and Merin (1974). Color vision was severely defective and most patients could not read the Ishihara charts. Farnsworth 28-hue test showed in some a scotopic line (Fig. 1) and in others a completely confused pattern (Fig. 2). The hereditary transmission of the disease was clearly autosomal recessive in most patients, as indicated in one family (Fig. 3).

The age of the patients varied from one year in the youngest to 31 years in the oldest. Three patients were under five years old.

Visual acuity for distance and near was examined under ordinary conditions. The diameter of the pupillary aperture, the nystagmus and photophobia were estimated. Then patients were given in both eyes one drop of pilocarpine hydrochloride 2%. All examinations were repeated about one

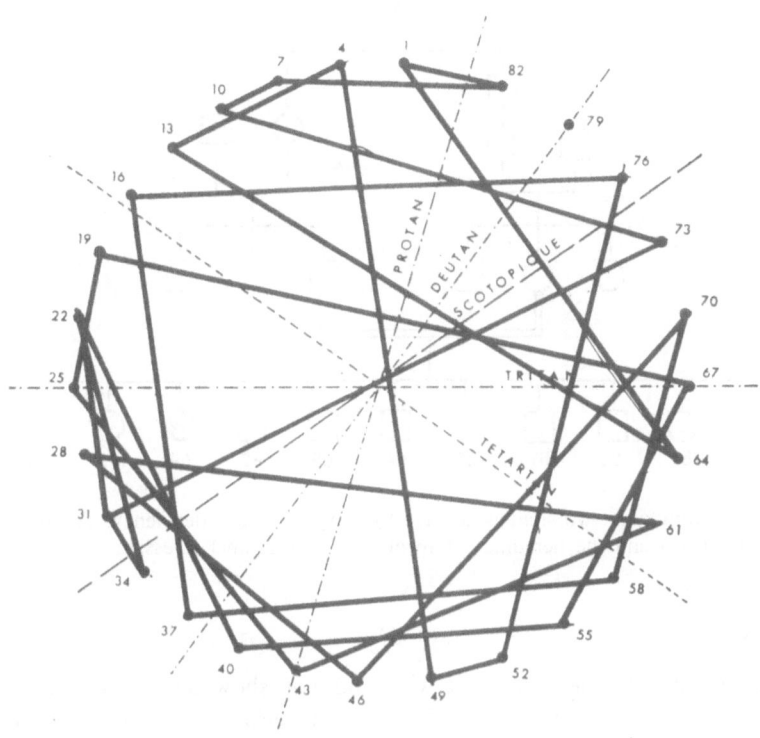

Fig. 2. Complete confusion of line in a 13-year-old patient with congenital cone deficiency

hour after the pilocarpine, and their subjective response was assessed. Ten patients were treated twice daily by pilocarpine 2% and followed up for periods between one and four months. In eight patients the subjective response to ordinary sunglasses and to 10% transmission dark glasses ('NOIR'® glasses) was compared to the subjective response to pilocarpine.

RESULTS

The visual acuity improved by one or two lines on the Snellen visual acuity chart or similar on a special children box in 11 out of 17 patients. Photophobia and nystagmus improved objectively in 16 out of 17 patients. Subjectively all these 16 patients improved. The one patient who claimed no

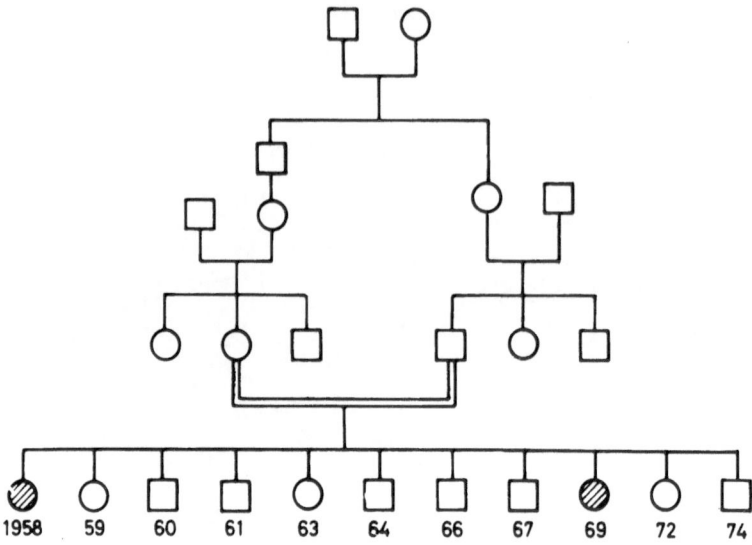

Fig. 3. A family with two siblings affected by congenital cone deficiency. The parents are first cousins and the hereditary transmission is autosomal recessive

improvement was the same one who did not show any change in the nystagmus and photophobia. Pupillary aperture decreased from 3.5–5.0 mm before the pilocarpine to 2.0–3.5 mm after it.

In a ten-year-old patient the visual acuity improved from 6/120 to 6/30 one hour after pilocarpine. The best visual acuity obtained in any patient was 6/30. In another, 22-year-old patient there was no change in the visual acuity. This was in spite of a remarkable subjective improvement. The patient claimed, that for the first time in his life he started to cross roads without help.

In the rather short follow up only one of ten patients stopped the treatment as he did not feel any improvement.

All examined patients felt that pilocarpine 2% heips more than ordinary sunglasses or the 10% transmission glasses.

DISCUSSION

Patients with congenital cone deficiency have their best visual acuity at luminance levels between 0.0 log mL and 1.0 log mL, which is equivalent to feeble interior lighting (Schachar et al. 1973). As most of the day the lighting is beyond this range, patients see worse. The rationale of using pilocarpine is to reduce the total amount of light which reaches the retina and especially to reduce the scattered light. This reduction of light has two effects: (1) it reduces the lighting to the range of maximal visual acuity possible in these patients, and (2) it decreases the dazzling of the rhodopsin-containing retina in achromats. This dazzling is, most probably, responsible for the photophobia and nystagmus. It was this second mechanism which seemed to us the more important result of pilocarpine treatment.

Accommodative spasm as a result of using pilocarpine was not a serious problem. None of the patients complained of pain. As most patients were hyperopic-astigmatic, the resultant myopia and pin-hole effect of the pupil could also be helpful in the good subjective results.

REFERENCES

Auerbach, E. & S. Merin. Achromatopsia with amblyopia. I. A clinical and electro-tetinographical study of 39 cases. Doc. Ophthalmol. 37: 79 (1974).
Schachar, R. A., J. Pokorny & A. E. Krill. Use of miotics in patients with cone degenerations. Am. J. Ophthalmol. 76: 816 (1973).

Authors' address:
The Genetic Clinic
The Jerusalem Institute for Prevention of Blindness
Jerusalem, Israel

CLASSIFICATION AND PROGNOSIS
IN RETINITIS PIGMENTOSA

MICHAEL F. MARMOR

(*Stanford and Palo Alto, Calif., U.S.A.*)

ABSTRACT

A series of consecutive patients with retinitis pigmentosa was reviewed. Roughly 20% of the cases were distinguished by relatively strong ERG signals (scotopic b-wave $\geq 100\,\mu V$, flicker b-wave implicit time $\leq 32\,msec$) and relatively mild symptoms. These cases, which may be described as having 'delimited retinitis pigmentosa,' have a better-than-average visual prognosis. Similarities between delimited and sectorial retinitis pigmentosa are pointed out: both represent mild disease whose recognition has important implications for the patient. Among conventional cases, visual loss may commence at any age, and once it begins will typically progress from 20/40 to 20/200 in about 6 years. Intermediate levels of acuity appear to be unstable. By age 50, roughly 25% of retinitis pigmentosa patients retain good acuity, but more than 50% have acuity of 20/200 or worse.

INTRODUCTION

Retinitis pigmentosa (RP) is not a homogeneous disease, but surprisingly little information is available to distinguish subgroups of the disease on the basis of electrophysiological findings or clinical symptoms. Many patients with the disease have poor acuity, but little is known about whether vision is lost gradually, in step-wise fashion or abruptly, or whether the onset of visual loss can be related to age or other clinical findings.

I have reviewed more than 100 consecutive cases of retinitis pigmentosa, and compared them with respect to ERG findings, visual function, and – by retrospective investigation – the natural history of visual loss (Marmor 1979; 1980a). The results define a major subgroup of RP which has a relatively favorable prognosis and is similar in many respects to sectorial RP, and show that visual loss in RP is step-like and unpredictable.

SUBJECTS AND METHODS

The population studied comprises patients examined personally by the author over a five-year period and given a diagnosis of either RP or sectorial

Supported in part by National Eye Institute Grant EYO1678.

Docum. Ophthal. Proc. Series, Vol. 25, ed. by H. Zauberman
© *1981, Dr. W. Junk bv Publishers, The Hague*

RP. Variants such as cone dystrophy, centro-peripheral retinitis pigmentosa or Leber's amaurosis congenita were excluded, as well as any cases in which the pigmentary degeneration was suspected of being acquired.

The probable mode of inheritance for each patient was determined by the family history and classified as recessive (including sporadic), dominant or x-linked. The visual history was investigated for all eyes with corrected acuity (at the time of my latest examination) of 20/40 or worse. Hospital charts, physicians' records, and optometry records were examined or reviewed by telephone, until a best corrected acuity of 20/30 or better could be documented or until no further information about the patient could be located.

The techniques for recording the ERG have been described previously (Marmor 1979). A Grass photostimulator was used to illuminate a fullfield dome; signals were picked up with Burian-Allen electrodes and displayed on an oscilloscope. Four stimulus conditions were used: (1) Photopic (cone): strong white flash (Grass intensity 8) over a 15 ft-lambert background (*normal* $\geq 95\ \mu V$). (2) Flicker (cone): 30 Hz train of strong flashes (*normal b-wave implicit time* $\leq 32\ msec$). (3) Rod: weak white flash (2 log units less intense) after 10–15 min dark adaptation (*normal* $\geq 195\mu V$). (4) Scotopic (mixed cone and rod): strong flash after 15 min dark adaptation (*normal* $\geq 290\mu V$).

RESULTS

Electroretinogram vs. Age

ERG records were available for a total of 78 patients. Fig. 1 shows b-wave amplitudes from the recessive (and sporadic) cases, plotted against age. The ERGs have been segregated into two groups, those with normal and abnormal flicker b-wave implicit time, which stand apart in terms of b-wave amplitude. Signals with normal timing comprise 17% of the sample and, with few exceptions, had a photopic amplitude $\geq 70\ \mu V$ and a scotopic amplitude $\geq 100\ \mu V$. Data from dominant and x-linked cases were plotted in similar fashion, and showed a similar division between the majority of patients who had abnormal flicker b-wave implicit time and the minority (18–20%) who had normal timing.

Fig. 2 shows scotopic b-wave amplitudes and flicker b-wave implicit time from the patients with sectorial retinitis pigmentosa. Both photopic and scotopic amplitudes were generally larger than those with diffuse RP (and abnormal timing), but showed a marked diminution with age. The flicker b-wave implicit time was well within the normal range for the younger patients with sectorial RP, but with age it increased to borderline levels.

248

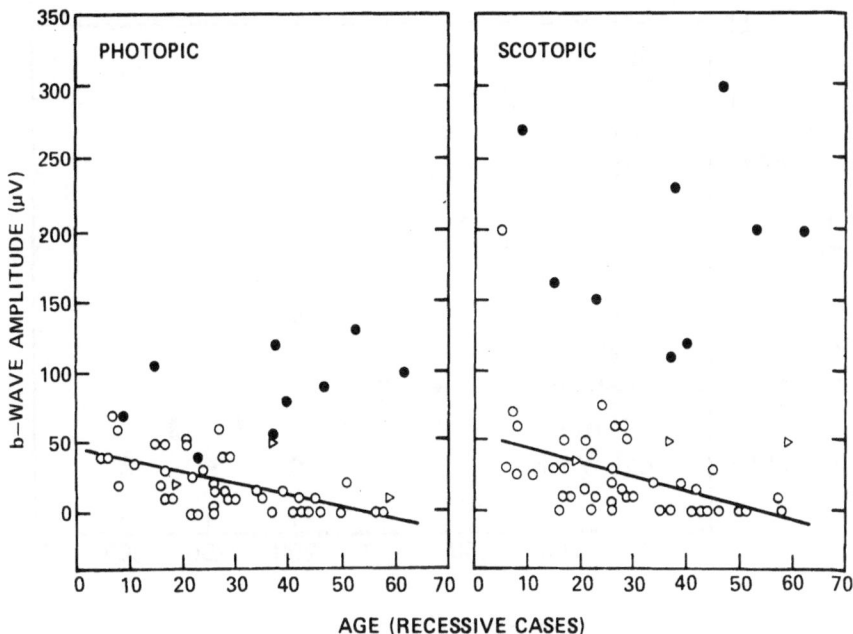

Fig. 1. B-wave amplitude in recessive RP. Symbols refer to flicker b-wave implicit time: closed circles, ≤ 32 msec (normal); triangles 33-34 msec (borderline); open circles ≥ 35 msec (prolonged). Each point represents one patient. Lines were drawn by method of least squares from open symbols only.

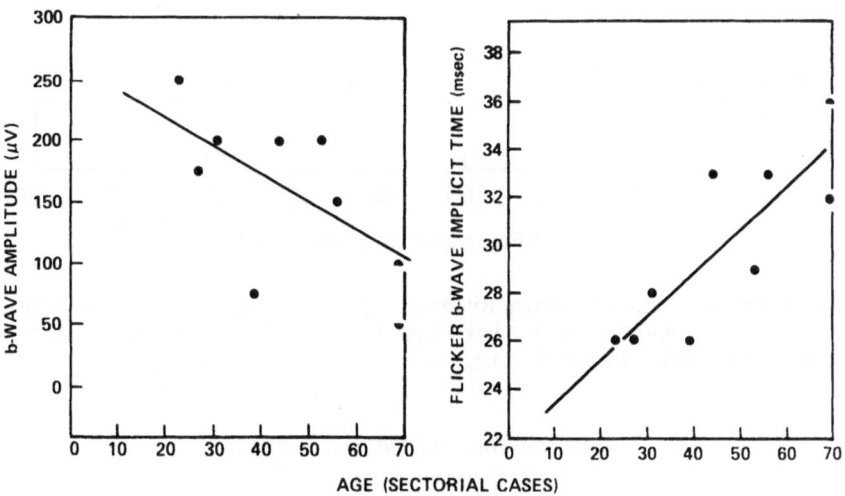

Fig. 2. ERG parameters in sectorial RP. Each point represents one patient; half circles are used where the two eyes differed significantly. Lines were drawn by method of least squares.

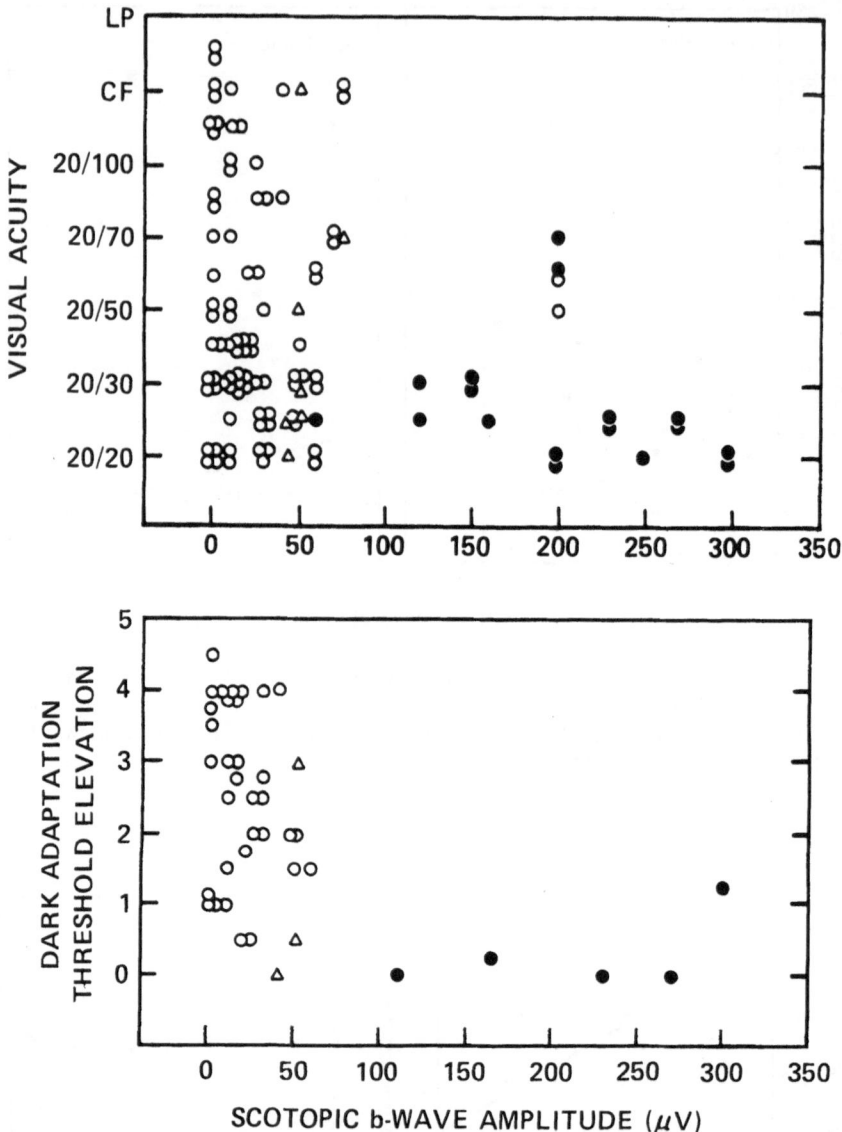

Fig. 3. Visual function in recessive RP, relative to b-wave amplitude. For visual acuity each point represents one eye; for dark adaptation threshold, each point represents one patient. Threshold is measured in log units.

Visual Function vs. Electroretinogram

Fig. 3 shows the visual acuity and dark adaptation threshold of patients with recessive RP, plotted against b-wave amplitude. Patients with low amplitude ERGs and abnormal b-wave timing showed varying degrees of visual loss and threshold elevation, and the correlation wiht b-wave amplitude was

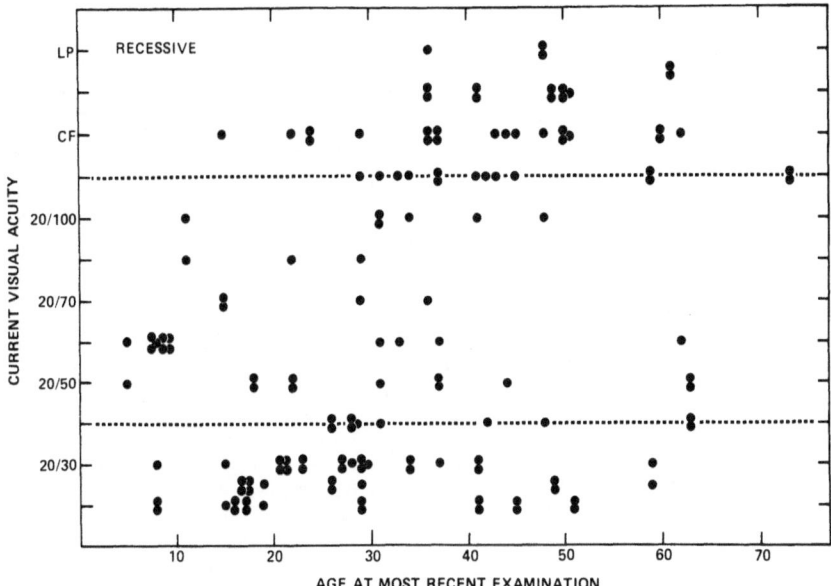

Fig. 4. Visual acuity in recessive RP. Each point represents one eye. The divisions of acuity are 20/30, 20/40, 20/50, 20/60, 20/70, 20/80, 20/100, 20/200, CF (counting fingers), HM (hand movements), LP (light perception).

minimal. In contrast, the patients with normal ERG timing stand out in having uniformly good acuity and only mild deficiency in dark adaptation. Only two eyes among the sporadic and recessive cases had acuity worse than 20/30, and those still possessed reading vision. The results were similar among dominant and recessive cases. The sectorial retinitis pigmentosa patients behaved similar to those with normal ERG timing. Out of 16 eyes with sectorial RP, 14 had an acuity of 20/30 or better, 1 was 20/50, and 1 was 20/200.

Visual Acuity vs. Age and Time

Visual acuity is generally well preserved among RP patients with normal ERG timing, but the situation is different for the patient with conventional RP. Fig. 4 shows a scattergram of the visual acuity at latest examination as a function of age, for eyes with recessive or sporadic RP. Note that most eyes have either very good vision (20/40 or better) or very poor vision (20/200 or worse), and relatively few have intermediate levels of vision. These results showed little correlation with visible ocular pathology: a few patients with poor acuity had atrophic macular scars, but all of the patients with good acuity showed abnormal foveal reflexes or architecture and only two patients had cataracts of possible visual significance.

251

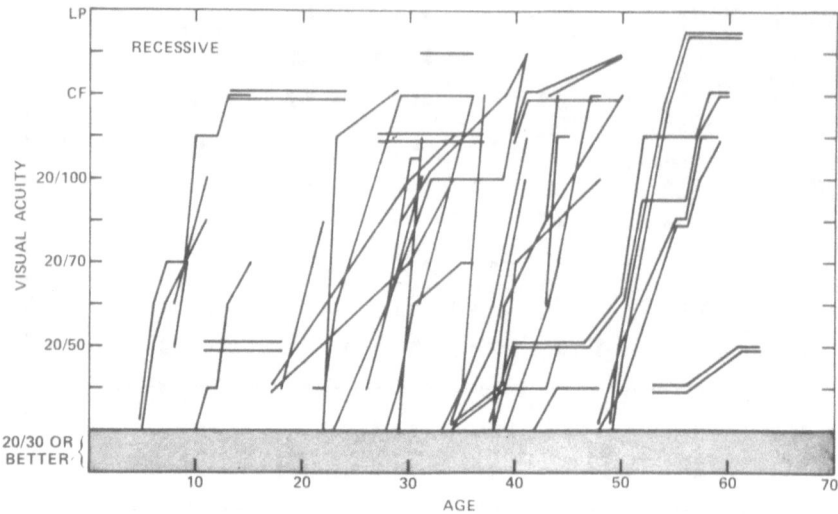

Fig. 5. Visual history of eyes with recessive RP which could be traced over at least 5 years or a 3-line change in acuity. Each line connects all recorded acuities for one eye. Acuities of 20/30 or better are not discriminated.

Fig. 5 shows that visual acuity can fail rather unpredictably at any age in RP, and that once an eye begins to fail (i.e., drops below 20/40) the acuity will usually drop all the way to 20/200 or worse within 4–10 years (the median slope of these lines is approximately 6 years). The limited data available from dominant and x-linked cases was consistent with these observations, but the numbers were too few to judge whether or not inheritance affected the pattern of visual loss. Among patients for whom a progressive loss of acuity could be documented, roughly 40% showed significant asymmetry of acuity (more then two lines) for five or more years. Thus, the loss of visual acuity in RP is most often bilateral, but a loss of acuity in one eye does not automatically mean that it will be lost in the second eye.

Using the cumulative information from this retrospective study of visual acuity, the relationship of visual acuity to age can be shown with reasonable accuracy. Fig. 6 shows the proportion of recessive cases which had 'good,' 'intermediate,' or 'poor' levels of acuity within each decade of age. Indeterminate cases result because the known information about older cases was incorporated into the statistics for younger ones. Thus, a 50 year old patient with good acuity, was assumed to have good acuity in younger years; however, a 50 year old patient with 20/200 vision, about whom no further information could be obtained, was classed as having indeterminate vision (20/20 to 20/200) in his younger years. Note that the number of patients with mid-range acuity was relatively small (about 10%) throughout the plot. The distribution of acuity among dominant cases was similar (Fig. 7), except

252

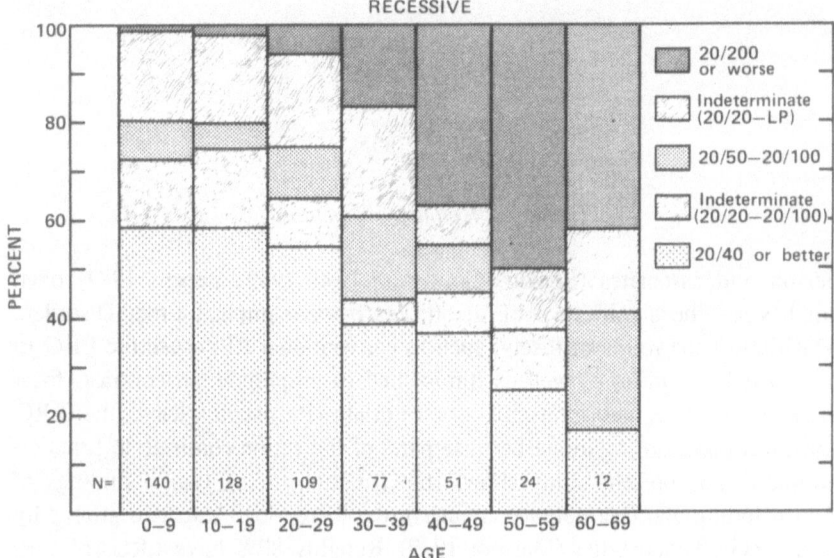

Fig. 6. Prevalence of different levels of acuity, at different ages, in recessive RP. Acuity is divided into good, mid-range and poor categories as shown. The indeterminate categories represent eyes whose earliest recorded acuity in an older age group was mid-range or poor. The data cumulate from older to younger age groups to incorporate all available information about each eye. N = number of eyes.

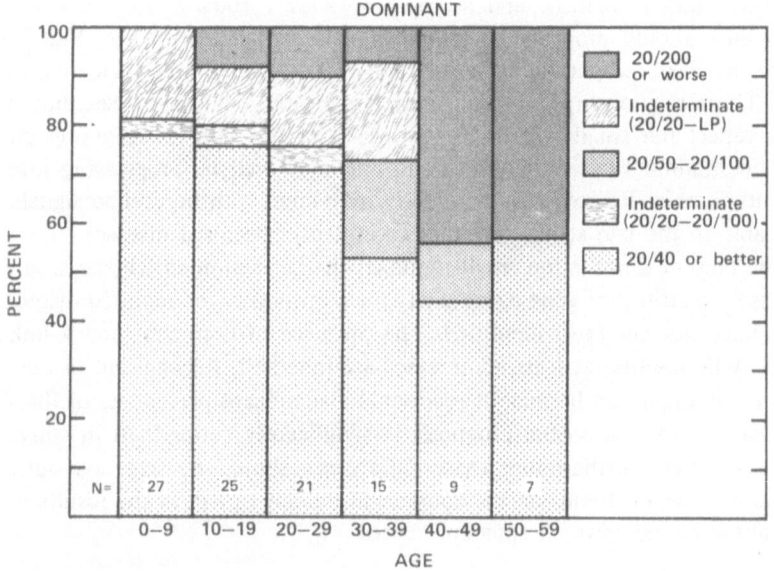

Fig. 7. Prevalence of different levels of acuity, at different ages, in dominant RP.

253

that a slightly larger percentage of patients retained good acuity at any given age.

DISCUSSION

Delimited Retinitis Pigmentosa

Berson and associates (Berson, Gouras & Hoff 1969; Berson 1972) have emphasized the significance of the flicker b-wave implicit time. Disorders which affect the retina diffusely, such as conventional RP, cause the ERG to be delayed in timing as well as diminished in amplitude. In contrast, focal diseases, such as chorioretinitis or sectorial RP, usually leave the ERG wave-form and timing intact because parts of the retina continue to function normally. The present study shows that patients having typical findings of RP (including 360° pigmentary changes) may be divided into two groups by their ERG characteristics (Marmor 1979). Roughly 80% have ERGs of very low amplitude and prolonged b-wave implicit time; the remaining 20% have ERGs of moderate amplitude and normal b-wave timing, as well as unusually mild symptoms and a good visual prognosis. These latter individuals behave, from a functional standpoint, as if their disease were of limited extent within the fundus. Thus, the term *delimited RP* is suggested to describe them.

The ERG dividing line between conventional and delimited RP is relatively sharp: the patients with mild disease are set apart by flicker b-wave implicit times ≤ 32 msec and scotopic b-waves $\geq 100 \mu V$. However, these guidelines should probably be tempered in accordance with age. Figs. 1–3 show that ERG amplitude decreases, and flicker b-wave time increases, with age. These relationships were not clear among the delimited cases, but this may reflect the small size or heterogeneity of the sample. A young child with borderline ERG amplitude or timing may well be progressing into a serious form of RP, whereas an elderly individual with borderline signals is probably in the late stages of either delimited or sectorial disease.

The present series is too small to judge whether delimited RP is a separate disease, an artifact of gene expressivity, or a misnomer for acquired disorders that have not yet been identified. The presence of dominant and x-linked cases indicates that at least some cases are inherited. Recognition of delimited RP is important because it represents a significant percentage of the RP population, and the visual prognosis is significantly better than in conventional disease. Furthermore, these mild cases should be screened out, or accounted for, in studies on the course and therapy of RP, or the results may be falsely biased towards apparent success.

Visual acuity was almost uniformly good among patients with delimited or sectorial RP, i.e., those with ERGs of large amplitude and normal timing. However, among patients with conventional RP, the size of the ERG showed little correlation with acuity which ranged from 20/20 to light perception. The present data (Marmor 1980a) show that in conventional RP acuity may be lost at any age, and once acuity begins to fail (i.e., drops below 20/40) it will drop to 20/200 or beyond within 4 to 10 years (the median being near 6). Visual loss is generally bilateral, but one eye may be spared for 5 or more years in a significant minority of cases. An interesting implication of the data is that the midranges of acuity (20/50 to 20/100) appear to be unstable and to indicate a guarded prognosis for central vision over the ensuing few years. Thus, patients with intermediate levels of acuity may be good subjects for the evaluation of therapeutic measures.

The cumulative statistics confirm the general findings of others (Arakawa *et al.* 1975; Pearlman 1979; Fishman 1978) that good acuity becomes less prevalent with age in RP. Patients should be apprised of these results to be aware not only of possible loss of vision, but of the hopeful aspects of the prognosis. For example roughly 25% of RP patients will retain good reading vision throughout life, and the longer that good vision is retained the better the chances of keeping it.

The etiology of visual loss in RP has not been determined. Some degree of foveal pathology was evident in all of my patients, as well as the majority of RP patients examined by others (Francois & Verriest 1962; Fishman, Maggiano & Fishman 1977). Since foveal changes may be present while central acuity is still good, it is difficult to judge whether an individual's loss of acuity is a result of primary damage to the photoreceptors or a secondary degenerative phenomenon such as cystoid edema. Current histologic (Szamier *et al.* 1979) and physiologic (Ripps, Brin & Weale 1978) evidence suggests that cone and rod outer segments shorten progressively in RP. Since our data show that visual acuity in RP does *not* diminish gradually over a lifetime, visual acuity is probably related to the number and arrangement of functioning outer segments rather than to cone outer segment length. Clearly, we need more subtle tests than Snellen acuity to evaluate and follow the early stages of RP when cellular damage is just beginning. Color vision and contrast sensitivity may both be abnormal in RP while acuity remains good (Marmor 1980b), but these tests are not refined enough, as yet, to stage the disease or predict when visual loss might be imminent.

Hereditary Influences

Dominant RP has often been described as milder than recessive or x-linked disease in its clinical and electrophysiological manifestations (Tanino & Ohba

1976a, 1976b; Fishman 1978), although one recent survey (Pearlman & Saxton 1979) minimizes these differences. In the present study, the three genetic types showed similar ERG amplitudes, but at any given age, the dominant cases appeared to have slightly better acuity than recessive cases. However, the numbers of dominant and x-linked cases were too small to draw any firm conclusions.

Berson (1972) has suggested that dominant RP *with complete penetrance* is characterized by a normal cone b-wave implicit time, whereas recessive and x-linked RP, and dominant RP *with incomplete penetrance* show prolonged cone b-wave timing. However, only 18% of the dominant cases in the present study showed normal ERG timing, and only 1 of 9 cases with prolonged timing had a family history suggestive of reduced penetrance. Furthermore, normal ERG timing was also found in 17–20% of the patients with recessive and x-linked disease. Thus, the present study suggests that the typical RP patient, regardless of inheritance, has abnormal ERG timing, and that individuals with delimited disease may be found in every hereditary group. The discrepancy between Berson's data on dominant cases and my own may depend in part on the patient population, since there are only 6 or 7 families in each study.

Sectorial vs. delimited retinitis pigmentosa

A comparison between delimited and sectorial RP is inevitable since both represent limited and slowly progressive disease, neither is confined to a single mode of inheritance (Bisantis 1971), and both are characterized by normal flicker b-wave implicit time (except possibly in some older cases). The fundus pigmentation in sectorial disease is generally limited to symmetric regions in the two eyes, whereas the delimited cases mostly had 360° involvement. However, there is increasing evidence that sectorial disease is slowly progressive and may functionally involve larger areas of the fundus than are affected visibly (Bisantis 1971; Hellner & Rickers 1973; Abraham 1975; Abraham, Ivry & Tsvieli 1976). Note, incidentally that the ERG in sectorial and probably delimited disease may be almost of normal size in very young children (in contrast to the situation in conventional RP). If the sectorial nature of sectorial RP can be minimized, then the clinical differences between sectorial and delimited RP are small. The question of importance for the physician is not whether to call a patient delimited or sectorial, but to make the distinction between the severe forms of RP, and the milder and more slowly progressive forms which have happier implications for the patient.

REFERENCES

Abraham, F. A. Sector retinitis pigmentosa. Electrophysiological and psychophysical study of the visual system. Doc. Ophthalmol. 39: 13-28 (1975).

Abraham, F. A., M. Ivry & R. Tsvieli. Sector retinitis pigmentosa: a fluorescein angiographic study. Ophtalmologica 172: 287-297 (1976).

Arakawa, T., M. Nishimura, H. Inomata, T. Nabeshima & K. Ohshio. Pigmentary retinal dystrophy, the statistical studies of 572 cases. F. Ophthal. Jpn. 26: 1036-1044 (1975).

Berson, E. L. Electroretinographic testing as an aid in determining visual prognosis in families with hereditary retinal degenerations. In: Retinal Congress. Eds. R. C. Pruett and C. D. J. Regan. New York: Appleton-Century Crofts, 1972, pp. 41-54.

Berson, E. L., P. Gouras & M. Hoff. Temporal aspects of the electroretinogram. Arch. Ophthalmol. 81: 207-214 (1969).

Bisantis, C. La rétinopathie pigmentaire en secteur. Contribution à la connaissance de ses divers aspects cliniques. Ann. Oculist. 204: 907-954 (1971).

Fishman, G. A. Retinitis pigmentosa. Visual loss. Arch. Ophthalmol. 96: 1185-1188 (1978).

Fishman, G. A., J. M. Maggiano & M. Fishman. Foveal lesions seen in retinitis pigmentosa. Arch. Ophthalmol. 95: 1993-1996 (1977).

Francois, J. & G. Verriest. Etude biométrique de la retinopathie pigmentaire. Ann. d'Oculist. 125: 937-951 (1962).

Hellner, K. A. & J. Rickers. Familiary bilateral segmental retinopathia pigmentosa. Ophthalmologica 166: 327-341 (1973).

Marmor M. F. The electroretinogram in retinitis pigmentosa. Arch. Ophthalmol. 97: 1300-1304 (1979).

Marmor, M. F. The natural history of visual loss in retinitis pigmentosa. Amer. J. Ophthalmol. 89: 692-698 (1980a).

Marmor, M. F. Contrast sensitivity: a subtle test for retinal disease. Ann. Ophthalmol. In press (1980b).

Pearlman, J. T. & J. Saxton. A mathematical model of retinitis pigmentosa. In: Proceedings of the XVIth Symposium of the International Society for Clinical Electrophysiology of Vision. Ed. Y. Tazawa. Tokyo: Japanese Journal of Ophthalmology, 1979, pp. 307-314.

Ripps, H., K. P. Brin & R. A. Weale. Rhodopsin and visual threshold in retinitis pigmentosa. Invest. Ophthalmol. Vis. Sci. 17: 735-745 (1978).

Szamier, R. B., E. L. Berson, R. Klein & S. Meyers. Sex-linked retinitis pigmentosa: ultrastructure of photoreceptors and pigment epithelium. Invest. Ophthalmol. Vis. Sci. 18: 145-160 (1979).

Tanino, T. & N. Ohba. Studies on pigmentary retinal dystrophy. I. Age of onset of subjective symptom and the mode of inheritance. Jpn. J. Ophthalmol. 20: 474-481 (1976a).

Tanino, T. & N. Ohba. Studies on pigmentary retinal dystrophy. II. Recordability of electroretinogram and the mode of inheritance. Jpn. J. Ophthalmol. 20: 482-486 (1976b).

From the Division of Ophthalmology, Stanford University School of Medicine and the Ophthalmology Section, Veterans Administration Medical Center, Palo Alto, Calif.

Author's address:
Ophthalmology Section (112B1)
Veterans Administration Medical Center
3801 Miranda Avenue
Palo Alto, California 94203
U.S.A.

REFERENCES

CHARACTERIZING THE C-WAVE
OF THE ELECTRORETINOGRAM

MICHAEL F. MARMOR & MARK LURIE

(*Palo Alto, California, U.S.A.*)

ABSTRACT

The c-wave of the electroretinogram is a slow cornea-positive response which must be recorded by d.c.-amplification. It is generated in part by the pigment epithelium but also by the Müller cells and inner retina. The amplitude and waveform of the c-wave are quite variable which complicates its definition for clinical use. Both c-wave amplitude and time-to-peak increase with stimulus energy, and the c-wave can integrate stimulus energy over several seconds. For every light intensity there is a critical duration beyond which integration no longer takes place. If the c-wave is to be used as a clinical measure of pigment epithelial function, the techniques for human recording must be improved, and recording protocols must be devised which selectively emphasize the pigment epithelial components of the response.

INTRODUCTION

The retinal pigment epithelium (RPE) is important to the physiology of the retina: it participates in the metabolism of photoreceptors, the phagocytosis of photoreceptor outer segments, the visual pigment regeneration cycle and the maintenance of retinal adhesion. However, there is no clinical test available to demonstrate the functional status of the RPE (Marmor & Lurie 1979). The light response of the standing potential, measured as the clinical electrooculogram, is often interpreted as a test of RPE function, but this is not accurate. The light response is abolished by central retinal artery occlusion (Thaler, Heilig & Lessel 1977), and thus depends upon inner retina as much as RPE.

The c-wave of the electroretinogram is a slow cornea-positive response which occurs, typically, a few seconds after the b-wave. The major positive component is generated by the RPE (Noell 1953; Steinberg, Schmidt &

From the Division of Ophthalmology, Stanford University School of Medicine and the Ophthalmology Section, Veterans Administration Medical Center, Palo Alto, Calif.

This study was supported in part by National Eye Institute Grant EYO1678 and by the Medical Research Section of the Veterans Administration.

259

Brown 1970), so that the c-wave offers promise as a clinical test for RPE function. However, the c-wave is technically difficult to record in man (Knave, Nilsson & Lunt 1973; Täumer *et al.* 1976; Marmor, Pockrand & Lurie 1979) and the corneal response is a composite of signals produced by retinal as well as RPE structures (Noell 1953; Faber 1969; Lurie & Marmor 1979a). If the c-wave is to measure the status of the RPE, recording protocols must be developed which are clinically feasible and which will emphasize and normalize the RPE components of the response. This report summarizes some of our recent work defining the components and the response characteristics of the c-wave (Marmor, Pockrand & Lurie 1979; Lurie & Marmor 1979, 1980).

METHODS

Our recording techniques have been described in detail elsewhere (Lurie & Marmor 1980). Experiments on Dutch rabbits were mostly performed with urethane anesthesia, but occasionally pentobarbital, ketamine or a surgical section of the midbrain was used. Most c-waves were recorded from the cornea of eyes dilated with 1% cyclopentolate and 10% neosynephrine; in a few experiments c-waves were recorded from the vitreous using an opened-eye preparation. A silver-silver chloride amalgam provided non-polarizable contact with the tear film or vitreous, and the signals were recorded differentially by d.c. amplification.

Human recordings were made from the cornea by a similar technique, except that only topical anesthesia was used. Specially designed contact lenses held a silver-silver chloride electrode in contact with the tear film, with a minimum of discomfort. Voluntary fixation was sufficient in cooperative subjects to produce stable recordings for the duration of the c-wave.

RESULTS

An initial problem in studying the c-wave is the lack of unanimity about how to measure it. For example, the waveform is variable among different individuals. The response may commence from near the b-wave peak, near the baseline, or from a deep trough negative to the baseline (Fig. 1); arbitrarily, we shall use the baseline in this report. Regardless of how the c-wave is measured, it shows wide variation in waveform and amplitude among different individuals. In fact, some normal individuals appear to lack a c-wave (Täumer *et al.* 1976b; Marmor, Pockrand & Lurie 1979).

The c-wave is much slower than the a- and b-waves, but also differs in another important respect; as stimulus intensity or duration are increased, the c-wave grows not only in amplitude but in time-to-peak. This is illus-

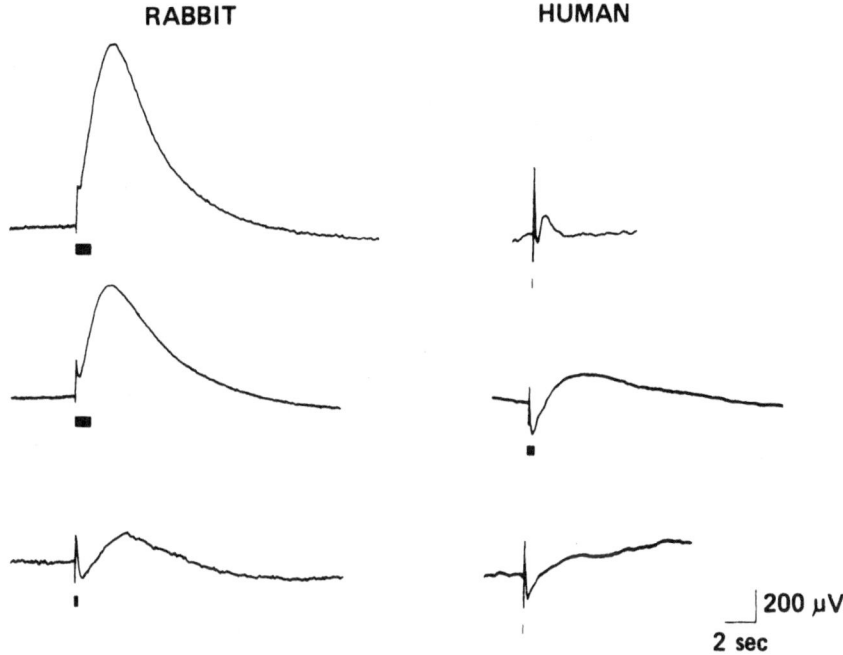

RABBIT   **HUMAN**

|_ 200 μV

2 sec

Fig. 1. Rabbit and human c-waves, from different individuals.

trated in Fig. 2 which shows families of c-waves produced by stimuli of constant duration or intensity. Note that for all but the longest stimuli, the c-wave does not reach its peak until well after the stimulus has ended. This means that the c-wave can integrate stimulus energy over several seconds, a remarkably long time by retinal standards. This integration is quite precise, as illustrated by the family of responses in Fig. 2 produced by stimuli of

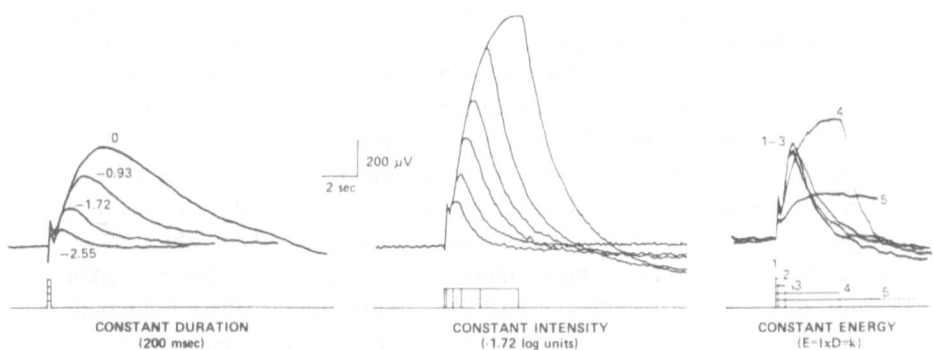

CONSTANT DURATION
(200 msec)

CONSTANT INTENSITY
(-1.72 log units)

CONSTANT ENERGY
(E=IxD=k)

Fig. 2. Rabbit c-waves to sets of stimuli having constant duration, intensity, and energy. Intensity is indicated in relative log units. The constant energy stimuli are shown accurately with respect to duration but schematically with respect to intensity.

261

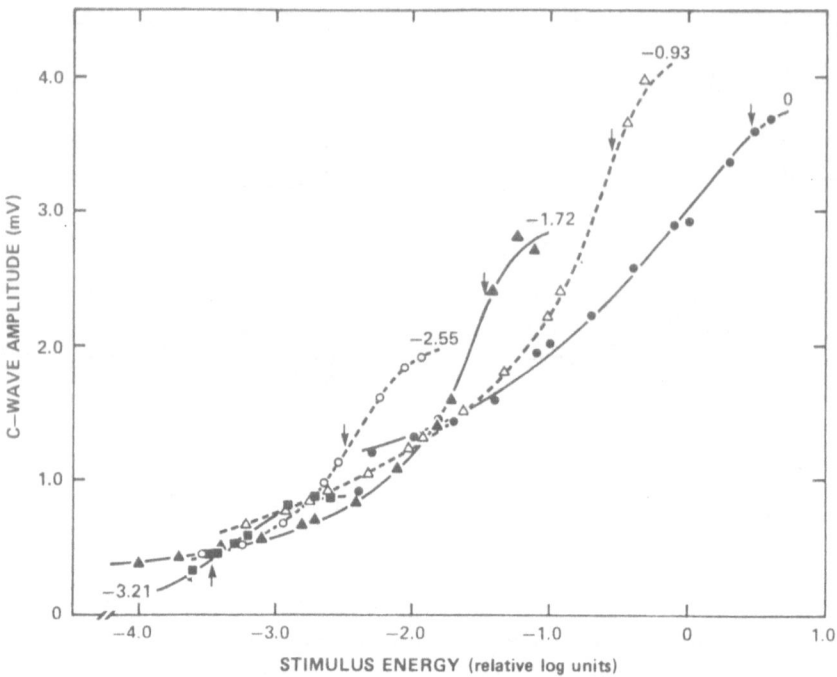

Fig. 3. Rabbit c-wave amplitude vs. log stimulus energy (intensity × duration). A common symbol identifies responses to each stimulus intensity (indicated as relative log units), and arrows show the critical durations (see Fig. 4).

constant energy. The first three of these responses virtually superimpose, because the stimulus energies were identical despite large differences in duration and intensity. However, for each stimulus intensity that may be chosen there is a limit (called the *critical duration*) to how long the c-wave can integrate energy: the last two responses of the figure did not superimpose because the stimuli were either too weak or too prolonged. If a stimulus exceeds the critical duration, the c-wave will fall immediately when the light goes off (as in the fourth response) unless the light is so prolonged that the wave falls spontaneously (as in the fifth response).

Fig. 3 shows a plot of rabbit c-wave amplitude against the log relative energy of the stimulus. Note that the responses do not cluster neatly along a single line, but separate into a set of sigmoid curves, each of which represents the responses to a single intensity of stimulus. In contrast, when c-wave time-to-peak is plotted against log stimulus energy (Fig. 4), the bulk of the responses fall along a single line. Thus, within a broad range of stimulus intensities and durations, stimuli of the same energy will always produce responses with the same time-to-peak. This relationship is often called the 'reciprocity law' since stimulus energy = intensity × duration, which requires intensity and duration to vary reciprocally when energy is

262

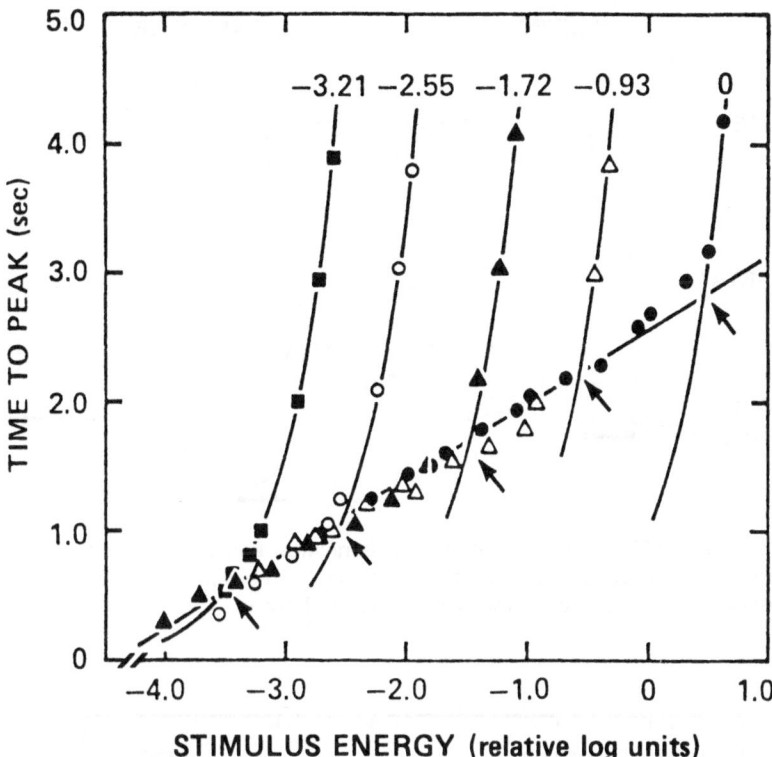

STIMULUS ENERGY (relative log units)

Fig. 4. Rabbit c-wave time-to-peak vs. log stimulus energy (intensity x duration). Same animal and same symbols as in Fig. 3. Most of the points fall along a common line, which satisfies the reciprocity law; however, the responses deviate at the critical duration for each intensity (arrows).

constant. The reciprocity law fails, of course, when stimuli exceed the critical duration for each stimulus intensity (arrows in Fig. 4). Time-to-peak then follows the vertically oriented curves which represent the condition: time-to-peak = stimulus duration.

These stimulus-response and temporal characteristics of the c-wave must ultimately be correlated with the different cellular component of the response. Pharmacologic agents can help to accomplish this. For example, sodium iodate selectively poisons the pigment epithelium, and changes the c-wave from a cornea-positive response to a large cornea-negative wave of similar time course (Fig. 5), which is often termed the slow PIII. The normal c-wave must actually be a composite of this negative-going slow PIII and a positive-going signal produced by the RPE. Perhaps this explains some of the variability in c-wave amplitude: animals or individuals having a strong slow PIII may appear to have a small c-wave, even though their RPE is healthy. Sodium aspartate is another agent which helps to analyze the components of the c-wave. It blocks synaptic transmission between the

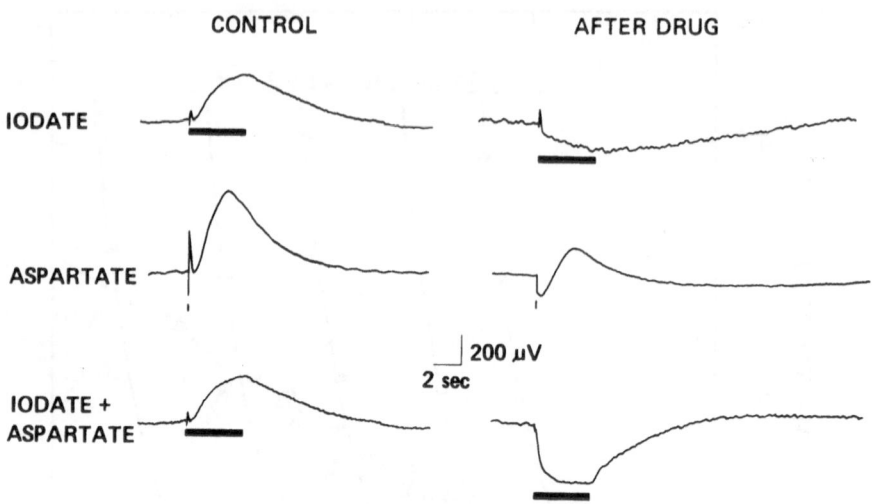

Fig. 5. Effects of intravenous iodate and/or intravitreal aspartate on the d.c. electro-retinogram of the rabbit. Bars indicate the duration of the stimulus. Note that iodate abolishes the c-wave, whereas aspartate blocks the b-wave.

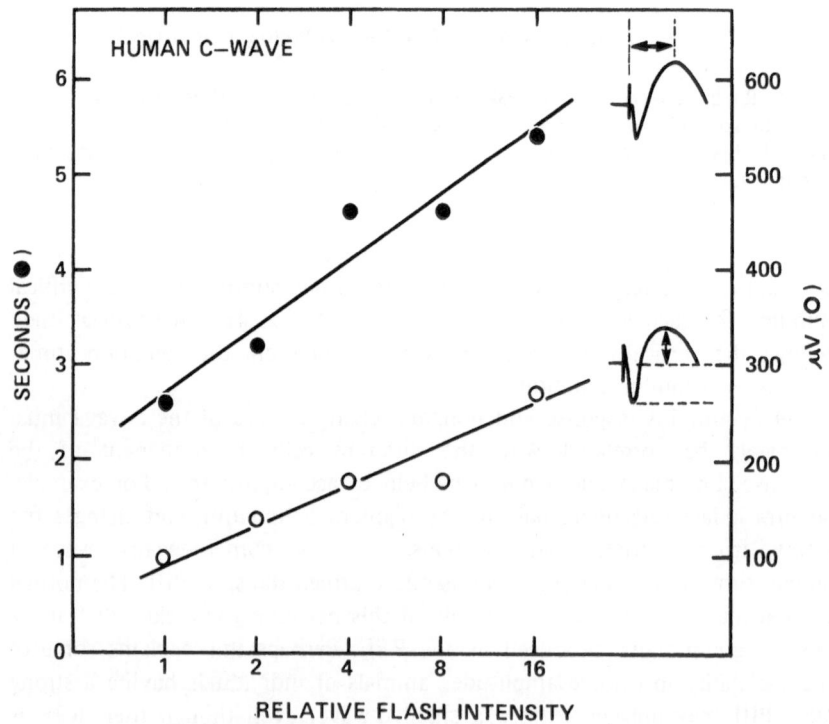

Fig. 6. Human c-wave amplitude and time-to-peak vs. log stimulus intensity (all flashes 10 μsec in duration).

photoreceptors and the inner retina, so that the b-wave and any other inner retinal signals are eliminated, while the c-wave remains relatively unaffected (Fig. 5). The administration of aspartate in addition to iodate shows that the slow PIII after iodate is itself a composite of signals originating in inner and outer retina.

These various c-wave components do not necessarily show the same variation with stimulus intensity or duration, but we do not have sufficient data, as yet, to recommend a specific range of stimuli as optimal for reflecting the status of the RPE. In preliminary experiments (Marmor, Pockrand & Lurie 1979) we have found that both the amplitude and time-to-peak of the human c-wave shows a roughly logarithmic relationship to stimulus energy over a short range of stimuli (Fig. 6). But our rabbit data cautions that wider ranges of stimuli must be explored.

DISCUSSION

The pigment epithelial response to light – which produces the major positivity of the c-wave – has been shown to be a passive reaction by the RPE cells to a fall in potassium concentration within the subretinal space, which occurs as a consequence of photoreceptor activation (Oakley & Green 1976). Thus, the c-wave is unquestionably dependent upon the integrity of the RPE. However, the c-wave also includes a summation of signals produced by neural and glial (Müller cell) elements. Most prominent is the slow PIII which appears to be largely a passive response by the distal parts of the Müller cells to the same light-induced change in extracellular potassium which induces the RPE response (Faber 1969). One reason for the variability in c-wave waveform and amplitude from individual to individual may be differences in the relative strength of the various c-wave components.

Our data suggest that c-wave time-to-peak may be more predictable than c-wave amplitude, and that temporal characteristics or light-integrating capacity may be useful parameters to measure in a clinical setting. However, one should keep in mind that some kinds of RPE disease or pathology might not alter the time-to-peak since it is primarily determined by the time course of extracellular ionic changes (Oakley & Green 1976).

Another problem to be solved before the c-wave can be used clinically is that of finding a comfortable and stable means of recording the c-wave from ordinary subjects. The c-wave is slow enough to require d.c. amplification which is especially subject to artifacts from electrode drift, eye movements or involuntary blinks. Several investigators have succeeded in recording c-waves from awake individuals (Knave, Nilsson & Lunt 1973; Täumer et al. 1976a; Marmor, Pockrand & Lurie 1979), but the quality of these recordings is not optimal, and the techniques are not yet suited to widespread use with unselected subjects. Our own experiments show that the c-wave appears to behave similarly in man as in the rabbit, but we have not been able to explore as wide a range of stimulus conditions as we would like.

The RPE is intimately involved in many disorders of the ocular fundus, but at present we only recognize such involvement when the cell become sufficiently damaged to show hyper- or hypo-pigmentation. We believe that the c-wave may ultimately provide a more sensitive test of RPE function than the ophthalmoscope.

REFERENCES

Faber, D. S. Analysis of the slow transretinal potentials in response to light. PH.D. Thesis. State University of New York at Buffalo, 1969.

Knave, B., S. E. Nilsson & T. Lunt. The human electroretinogram: DC recordings at low and conventional stimulus intensities. Acta Ophthalmol. 51: 716-726 (1973).

Lurie, M. & M. F. Marmor. Light-induced electrical responses of the retinal pigment epithelium. In: XXIII Concilium Ophthalmologicum, Kyoto, 1978, Acta. Ed. K. Shimizu. Amsterdam: Excerpta Medica, (1979) pp. 646-648.

Lurie, M. & M. F. Marmor. Analysis of the response properties and light-integrating characteristics of the c-wave in the rabbit eye. Exp. Eye Res. In Press (1980).

Marmor, M. F. & M. Lurie. Light-induced electrical responses of the pigment epithelium. In: The Retinal Pigment Epithelium. Ed. K. Zinn and M. F. Marmor. Cambridge: Harvard University Press, 1979, pp. 226-244.

Marmor, M. F., P. Pockrand & M. Lurie. Experiments toward the development of a clinical c-wave test. In: Proceedings of the XVIth Symposium of the International Society for Clinical Electrophysiology of Vision. Ed. Y. Tazawa. Tokyo: Japan Journal of Ophthalmology, 1979, pp. 107-111.

Noell, W. K. Studies on the electrophysiology and metabolism of the retina. U.S.A.F. School of Aviation Medicine, Randolph Field, Texas, Project Number 21-1201-0004, 1953.

Oakley, B. II & D. G. Green. Correlation of light-induced changes in retinal extracellular potassium concentration with c-wave of the electroretinogram. J. Neurophysiol. 39: 1117- 1133 (1976).

Steinberg, R. H., R. Schmidt & K. T. Brown. Intracellular responses to light from cat pigment epithelium: origin of the electroretinogram c-wave. Nature 227: 728-730 (1970).

Täumer, R., N. Rohde, W. Wichmann & J. Rover. A method for DC-ERG recording of alert humans. Albrecht von Graefes Arch. Klin. Ophthalmol. 198: 45-55 (1976a).

Täumer, R., W. Wichmann, N. Rohde & J. Rover. ERG of humans without c-wave. Albrecht von Graefes Arch. Klin. Ophthalmol. 198: 275-289 (1976b).

Thaler, A., P. Heilig & M. R. Lessel. Ischemic retinopathy: reduced light peak and dark trough amplitudes in electrooculography. XIV ISCERG Symposium, Louisville, 1976. Doc. Ophthal. Proc. Series 13: 119-121 (1977).

Authors' address:
Ophthalmology Section (112B1)
Veterans Administration Medical Center
3801 Miranda Avenue
Palo Alto, California 94304
U.S.A.

THE ULTRASTRUCTURE OF FENESTRATIONS IN ENDOTHELIAL CHORIOCAPILLARIES OF THE RABBIT
A freeze-fracturing study

S. MELAMED, I. BEN-SIRA & Y. BEN-SHAUL

(*Petah-Tikva, Israel*)

ABSTRACT

Replicas of freeze-fractured endothelial cells of normal rabbits choriocapillaries were studied. Differences in fenestral appearance on E-face and P-face could be detected. E-face pores appeared as circular craters containing particulate material arranged at the pores' rim and a central diaphragm. Mean pore diameter was 785 Å, average diaphragm size 300 Å and peripheral particle size 123 Å. In several pores, possible radiating connections between diaphragm and peripheral particles could be observed. Pores in P-face appeared as vallate papillae, with circular, particulate elevated rim surrounding a shallow surface and a central accumulation of particles resembling the diaphragm. P-face pore diameter was found to be 765 Å with a diaphragm size of 237 Å and peripheral particle size of 127 Å. The calculated space between peripheral particles and diaphragm was 120 Å for E-face and 127 Å on P-face. Using the Markham method, a regular pattern of eight peripheral particles at the pores' rim was shown for both E-face and P-face. A possble tridimensional model of the choriocapillary endothelial fenestration is presented. This assumed model consists of eight peripheral particles which are connected with a central diaphragm, creating a space of 120–127 Å between them. This sieve-like structure and the calculated passage size fit well with the 'small pore' theory of molecular permeability.

INTRODUCTION

The knowledge of the structural and physiological aspects of the choroidal endothelial fenestration is essential to the understanding of macromolecular permeability to the external retina. In the choriocapillary endothelium, transmission electron microscopy studies disclosed a diaphragm in the center of the pore in cross and tangential sections (Garron 1970; Matsusaka 1970; Hogan *et al.* 1971; Spitzans 1974). This finding was reconfirmed by other investigators using the freeze-fracture technique (Spitzans & Reale 1975; Raviola 1977). More thorough ultrastructural studies of the pores were carried out on fenestrae in other organs, such as kidney, pancreas and intestinal tract (Friederici 1962, 1969; Simionescu *et al.* 1974; Maul 1971). Maul (1971), studying the rat kidney, suggested an octagonal shape for the pores'

267

rim, and assumed the central diaphragm to consist of two rings. Clementi and Palade (1969), demonstrated that peroxidase molecules, about 50 Å in size, could pass more freely through the intestinal fenestrae than ferritin molecules, 110 Å in size. Bill (1968), showed that uveal capillaries are more permeable to myoglobin (40 Å than to albumin (70 Å) and to albumin more than to gammaglobulin (110 Å). The aim of this study was to determine whether the intra-fenestral ultrastructure can be correlated with the special permeability properties of the choriocapillaries.

MATERIALS AND METHODS

Four Albino rabbits of 2.5–3.0 kg body weight were anesthesized with 30 mg/kg Nembutal injected intravenously. After deep anesthesia was achieved one eye of each rabbit (4 eyes) were enucleated (other eyes were used for another study). The enucleated globes were cut in 0.1 M cacodylate buffer. The retina was gently stripped from the choroid and then the choroid was carefully removed from the sclera. The choroidal tissue was immediately immersed in a solution of 2.5% glutaraldehyde in 0.1 M cacodylate buffer and fixed at 4 °C overnight. After fixation, samples of tissue were washed several times with cacodylate buffer and suspended overnight in 30% glycerol at the same buffer at 4 °C. Samples, 2–3 mm in size, were frozen in freon 22, transferred immediately to liquid nitrogen, and freeze-fractured in a Balzer's freeze-etching unit, according to the standard procedures (Moor an Mühletaler 1963). All preparations were examined and photographed in a Jeol-100B electron microscope at 80 kv.

RESULTS

In the replicas of freeze-fractured tissue the choriocapillaries were easily identified because of their proximity to Bruchs' membrane and the characteristic appearance of the fenestrae. In enface view of the endothelial cell, groups of closely packed fenestrations are separated by non-fenestrated, relatively smooth, cytoplasmic areas. Most of the fenestrae observed were circular – some, which were cleaved obliquely, had an oval rather than circular shape (Fig. 1).

At higher magnifications, the differences among fenestrae exposed in different split membranes are more emphasized. On the E-face (Branton *et al.* 1975), the pores appear as circular craters containing particulate material arranged at the pores' rim and a central diaphragm. The diaphragm appeared either as a smooth face or as a cluster of small particles, presumably depending on the cleavage plane. The peripheral particles seem to be regularly

268

arranged close to the rim in many fenestrae, especially in those cleaved tangentially. Structures which look like radiating rays, could be observed in some pores, connecting the peripheral particles with the central diaphragm (Fig. 2). On the P-face, the fenestrae appear as vallate papillae, they seem to be protruded, with a circulate, elevated particulate rim surrounding a more shallow surface. In the crater, a cluster of particles resembling the diaphragm could frequently be observed (Fig. 3).

A histogram of 120 pores has been drawn, measuring the fenestral diameter, peripheral particle size and the diameter of the diaphragm. The measurement of the diaphragm diameter presented some difficulty because of the inconsistency in appearance of the diaphragms due to differences in the cleavage plane. Therefore, the measurements were either of the smooth central area or of the diameter of clustered particles. Of the 120 pores measured, 48 were on E-face and 72 on the P-face. Only circular, regular tangentially cleaved pores were selected for measurement. Measurements of the fenestrae and their sub-structures on both fractured faces are shown (Fig. 4). For uniformity, prints were enlarged to give 1 mm = 96 Å. The calculated average diameter of the pores on E-face is 785 Å. That of the central diaphragm is 300 Å, and the size of each peripheral particle is approximately 120 Å. Thus, the calculated average space between the peripheral particle and the diaphragm is about 120 Å. On the P-face, the average diameter of the fenestration was found to be 765 Å, the diaphragm 237 Å and that of the peripheral particles 138 Å, thus leaving a space of 127 Å. Details are summarized in Table 1.

Table 1. Average size of pores and their sub-units on E- and P-face

	Size (Å)	
	E-face	P-face
Pore diameter	785	765
Diaphragm diameter	300	237
Size of a peripheral particle	123	138
Calculated space between diaphragm and peripheral particles	120	127

Using the Markham technique (Markham *et al.* 1963), pores were rotated on a printing stage. Ten circular, tangentially cleaved fenestrae on E-face and seven on P-face were selected and printed in different number of rotations (n = 3,4,5,7,8 and 10). Enhancement of peripheral particles was maintained in all pores when they were rotated 8 times. It is therefore assumed that there is a regular structural pattern of 8 particles at the pore's rim on both E-face and P-face (Fig. 5).

269

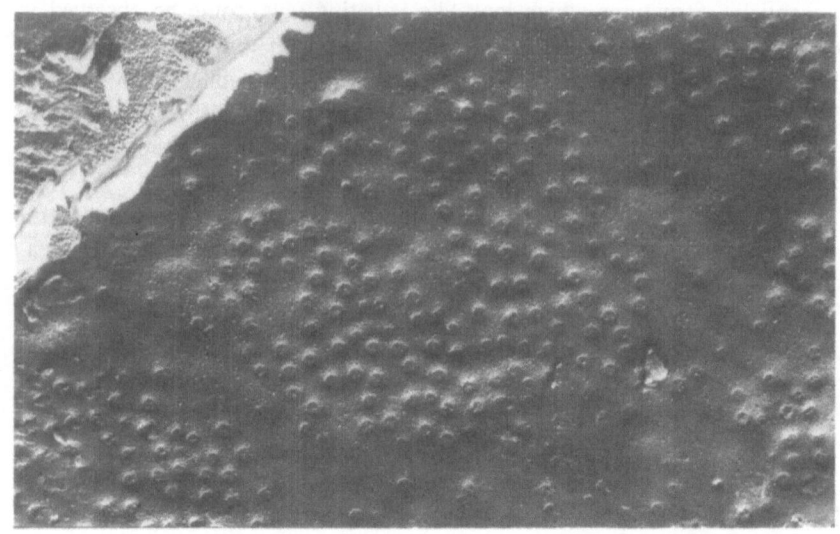

Fig. 1. Freeze-fractured replica of endothelial cell membrane showing groups of fenestrations separated by smooth cytoplasmic areas. ×24,000.

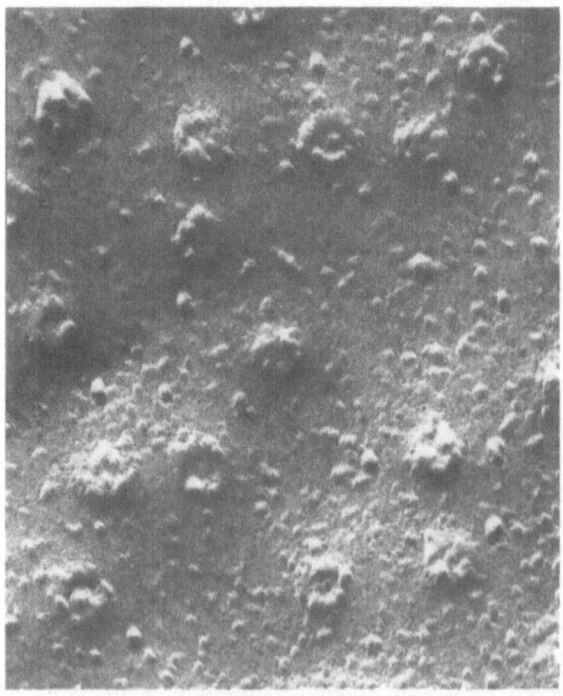

Fig. 3. P-face of a cleaved endothelial cell membrane. Note the elevated particulate rim and central clusters of particles representing the diaphragm. ×105,600.

270

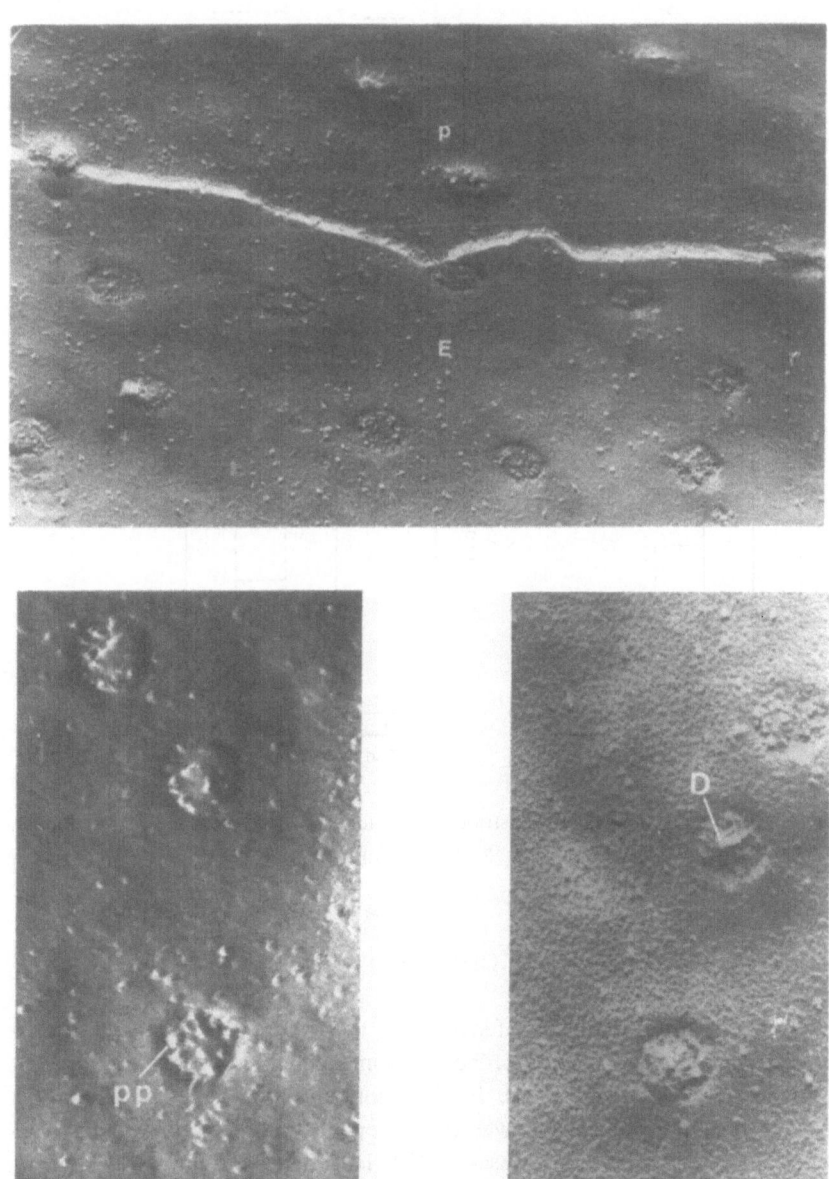

Fig. 2. Replica showing both E-face (E) and P-face (P) of a cleaved endothelial cell membrane.

The arrow indicates possible connections between diaphragm and peripheral particles.

2a and 2b show peripheral particles (PP) and diaphragm (D). ×132,000.

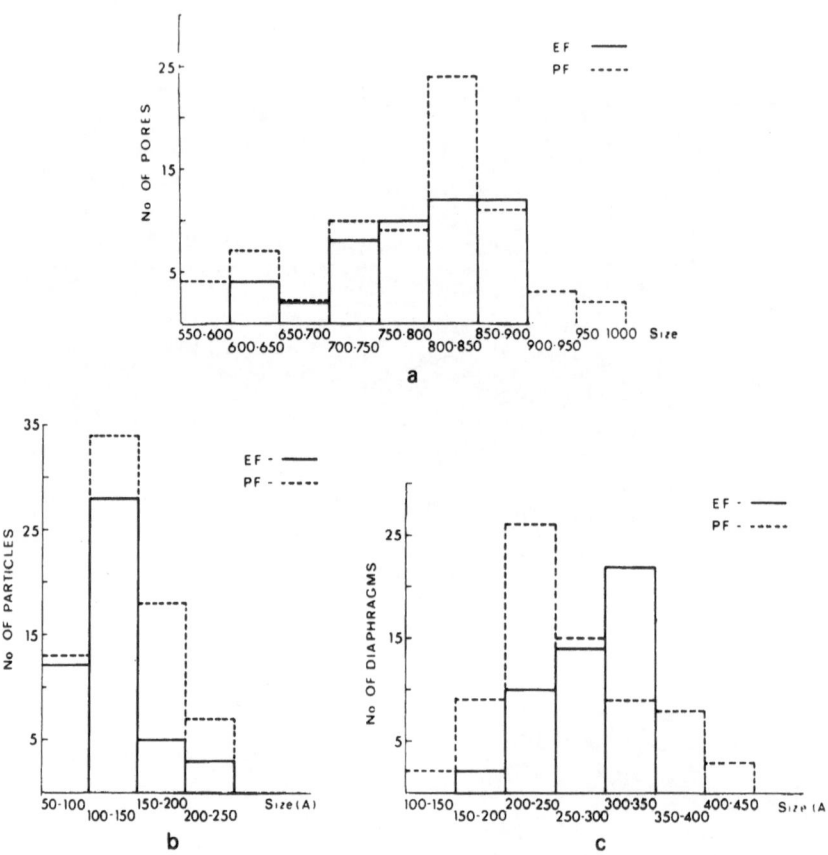

Fig. 4. Histograms showing size distributions of fenestral elements. a. Pore's diameter, b. Diameter of diaphragm, c. Size of peripheral particles.

DISCUSSION

The ultrastructure of capillary fenestrae in the kidney, pancreas and intestinal tract has already been described in some detail (Friederici 1962, 1969; Simionescu 1974; Maul 1971). In the choriocapillaries, the existence of a diaphragm or central density was confirmed by thin sectioning and freeze-fracturing (Garron 1970; Matsusaka 1970; Hogan 1971; Spitzans 1974; Spitzans & Reale 1975; Raviola 1977). Spitzans & Reale (1975) have described the diaphragm as a central thickening measuring approximately 300 Å while fenestral diameter in their material was found to be 600 Å. Raviola (1977), has also described a central diaphragm in freeze-fractured replicas of choriocapillary fenestrations, but no measurements were carried out. Hogan *et al.* (1971), describing thin sections of pores, found their diameter to be about 800 Å. Our study reconfirms the random distribution of fenestrae interrupted by cytoplasmic areas as described by Friederici (1962) in the mouse renal

272

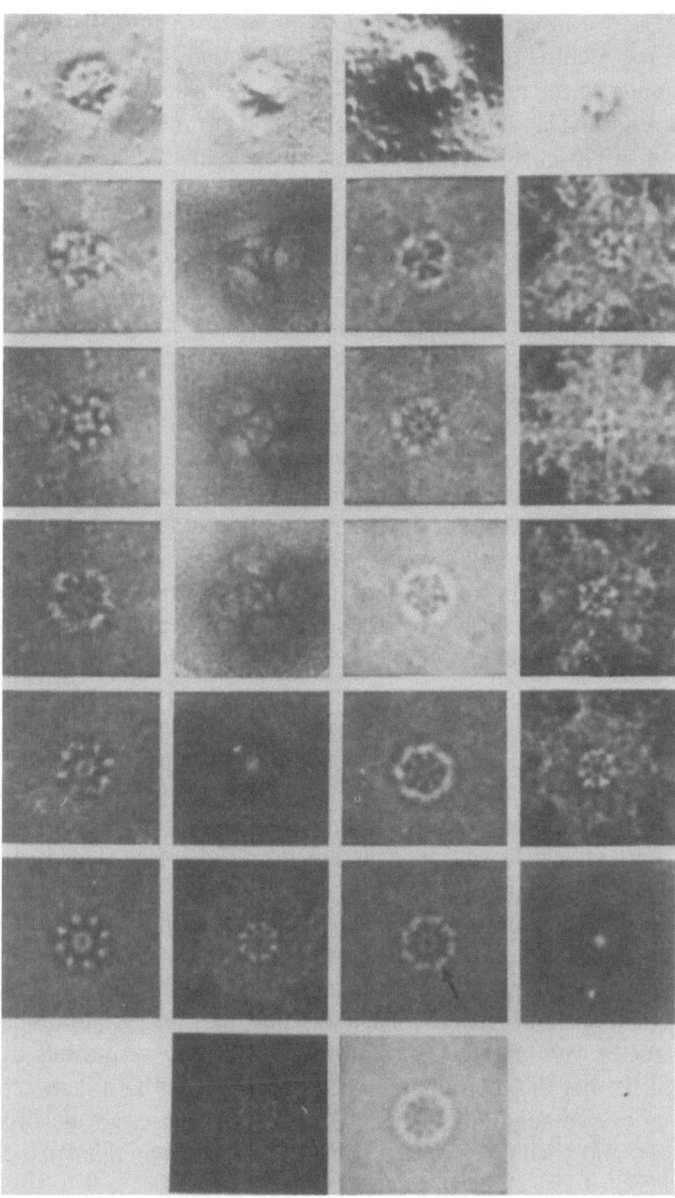

Fig. 5. Rotation of pores according to the Markham method. Top row shows the unrotated prints. The two on the left side are pores on E-face, the two on the right are on P-face. Rows 2, 3, 4, 5, 6, 7 represent rotations of n = 3, 4, 5, 7, 8, and 10 respectively. Marked enhancement results at n = 8 rotations. Note (arrow) that occasionally enhanced P-face particles looked as if composed of two sub-units.

papilla, and by Spitzans and Reale (1975) for the human choriocapillaries. In addition, our finding of mean pore diameter is closer to that found by Hogan *et al.* (1971). We found the pore diameter to be 785 Å on E-face and 765 Å on the P-face. Central diaphragm diameter was found to be around 300 Å on E-face (similar to the reported size of 300 Å by Spitzans & Reale (1975), and 237 Å on P-face. The difference between diaphragm measurement on E-face and P-face is attributed mainly to difficulties in measurements, as stated above.

In our study we have postulated the existence of peripheral particles at the pore's rim. Eight regularly arranged particles were shown and their octagonal pattern was enhanced repeatedly using the Markham method (Markham *et al.* 1963) in different pores, implying a consistent sub-structure. In occasional pores, fine radiating rays could be observed connecting the peripheral particles with the diaphragm. The existence of such connections raises the possibility that these intra-fenestral structures may be involved in the control of macromolecular leakage by active stretching and relaxing of the diaphragm, thus changing the diameter of the passages available for macromolecular permeability from the choroid to the retina. This study was not aimed to investigate the occurrence of contractile elements associated with the peripheral particles. The possibility that the intra-fenestral system acts as a sieve-like mechanism can not be excluded and deserves a further study.

The calculated space of 120–127 Å between diaphragm and peripheral particles corresponds well with the 'small pore' theory, enabling small molecules such as peroxidase (50 Å) to pass through the pores, while larger molecules like ferritin (110 Å) cannot pass freely (Clementi & Palade 1969). If, as suggested by Maul (1971), the pore is created by fusion of the two adjacent membranes, one has to presume that the appearance of the fenestrae on P-face should fit with its counterpart on the E-face. This is true to a limited extent. The pattern of practically all pores on P-face, when compared to each other, was found to be similar; the same applies to those observed on E-face. However, it would be expected that if the peripheral particles on one face are protruding, the other fractured face will show their imprints, namely, small shallow 'craters'. That was not the case, as protruding peripheral particles were observed on both fractured faces. A possible explanation might be that the protruding particles observed on both faces represent two halves or two sub-units of integral proteins which cross the two fused membranes, and that the cleavage plane passed through them rather than around them.

The possible cleavage planes within the fenestral elements are schematically depicted (Fig. 6). A possible cleavage plane sparing the diaphragm (above it or below it), thus creating a smooth face inside the pore, is also included. Several such manifested pores were encountered. Considering the pore elements to be formed as a result of adhesion or fusion of endothelial cell membranes, the P-faces should be adjacent to the center of the pore, while E-faces are external. The similarity of practically all E-face pores and P-face

274

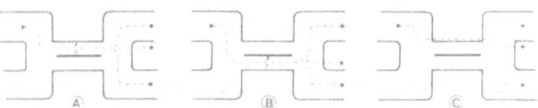

Fig. 6. Schematic drawing of possible cleavage planes within the fenestrae. A. Cleavage plane splitting the Bruch's membrane oriented side. B. Cleavage plane splitting the scleraloriented side. C. Cleavage plane passing by the fenestral elements.

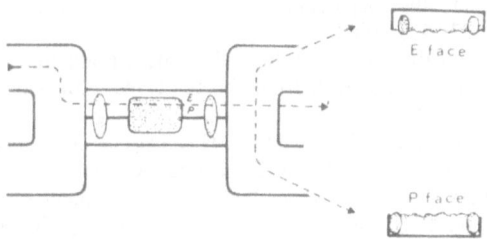

Fig. 7. Schematic presentation of possible integral proteins crossing the fused membranes which form the fenestration. Possible cleavage planes through these integral proteins are also depicted.

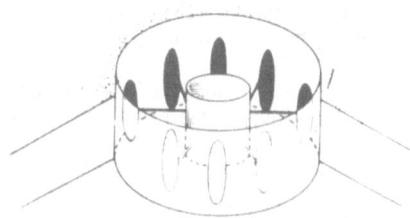

Fig. 8. A possible tri-dimensional model of a choriocapillary endothelial fenestration. The calculated space between diaphragm and peripheral particles was found to be 120-127 Å.

pores favours the possibility of a symmetrical arrangement at the width of the pores' element.

Fig. 7 shows schematically why the repeatedly protruding particles on both E-face and P-face might be explained by the passage of the cleavage plane through the postulated integral proteins. Having stated the regularity of the 8 peripheral particles with their average size and possible connections with the diaphragm, we suggest a possible tri-dimensional model of the fenestration in the choriocapillary (Fig. 8).

275

REFERENCES

Bill, A. Capillary Permeability to and Extravascular Dynamics of Myoglobin, Albumin and Gammaglobulin in the urea. Acta Physiol. Scand. 73: 204 (1968).

Branton, D., S. Bullivant, J. B. Gilula, M. J. Karnovsky, H. Moor, K. Mühlethaler, D. H. Northcote, L. Packer, B. Satir, V. Speth, L. A. Staehlein, R. L. Steere & R. S. Weinstein. Freeze Etching Nomenclature. Science 190: 54 (1975).

Clementi, F. & G. E. Palade. Intestinal capillaries – Permeability to Peroxidase and Ferritin. J. Cell Biol. 41: 33 (1969).

Friederici , H. H. R. The Tridimensional ultrastructure of fenestral capillaries. J. Ultrastruct. Res. 6: 171 (1962).

Friederici, H. H. R. On the diaphragm across ferestrae of capillary endothelium. J. Ultrastruct. Res. 27: 373 (1969).

Garron, L. K. The ultrastructure of the Retinal Pigment Epithelium with observations on the choriocapillaries and Buch's membrane. Trans. Am. Ophthalmol. Soc. 61: 545 (1970).

Hogan, M. J., J. A. Alvarado & J. E. Weddell. Histology of the Human Eye. An Atlas and Textbook, Philadelphia, 1971. W. B. Sahnders Co. p. 370.

Markham, R., S. Frey & B. J. Hills. Methods of Enhancement of Image detail and accentuation of Structure in Electron Microscopy. Virology, 20: 88 (1963).

Matsusaka, T. Ultrastructural differences between the choriocapillaries and Retinal Capillaries on the Human Eye. Jap. J. Ophthalmol. 14: 59 (1970).

Maul, G. G. Structure and formation of pores in fenestrated capillaries. J. Ultrastruct. Res. 36: 768 (1971).

Moor, H. & K. Mühlethaler. Fine structure in frozen-etched yeast cells. J. Cell Biol. 17: 609 (1963).

Raviola, G. The structural basis of the blood-ocular barriers. Exp. Eye Res. (Suppl.) p. 27 (1977).

Simionescu, M., N. Simionescu & G. E. Palade. Morphometric data on the endothelium of blood capillaries. J. Cell Biol. 60: 128 (1974).

Spitzans, M. The fine structure of the chorioretinal border tissues of the adult human eye. Adv. Ophthalmol. 28: 78 (1974).

Spitzans, M. & E. Reale. Fracture faces of fenestrations and junctions of endothelial cells in human choroidal vessels. Invest. Ophthalmol. 14: 98 (1975).

Authors' addresses:

S. Melamed and I. Ben-Sira
Department of Ophthalmology
Beilinson Medical Center
Tel-Aviv University
Petah-Tikva, Israel

Y. Ben-Shaul
Department of Microbiology
The George S. Wise Faculty of Life Sciences
Tel-Aviv University
Tel-Aviv, Israel

SUBRETINAL FAT AND COATS' DISEASE

L. MISSOTTEN & L. MACKEN

(*Leuven, Belgium*)

INTRODUCTION

Clinical observation of Coats' Disease suggests that the fatty deposits are a residue of plasma transudate in the subretinal space. Farkas *et al.* (1973) substantiated this hypothesis by chemical analysis of the proteins, sugar, and iron in th subretinal fluid. Analysis of the triglycerides ad fatty acids in these deposits, however, shows that their origin may be more complex.

PATIENT AND METHODS

A 12-year old girl with Coats' Disease was referred to us. Fundus examination showed three areas of vascular abnormalities in the upper, lower, and temporal peripheral areas. There were fatty deposits in each of these sectors, and a large mass of retroretinal fat was situated in the upper temporal quadrant. The macular area was relatively free of fatty deposits, and the vision was 6/12.

The abnormal vessels were cryocoagulated and some of the subretinal fat was removed through an incision in the sclera and the choroid for histologic and chemical analysis. The lipid fraction was analyzed by means of gas chromatography.

RESULTS

Histologic analysis showed a few lymphocytes and plasmocytes in a mass of foam cells containing lipid-filled vesicles and a few phagosomes with degenerated cellular constituents or photoreceptor segments. Cholesterol slits were not observed.

The distribution of triglycerides and fatty acids is given on Tables 1 and 2.

277

Docum. Ophthal. Proc. Series, Vol. 25, ed. by H. Zauberman
© *1981, Dr. W. Junk bv Publishers, The Hague*

Table 1. Distribution of the triglycerides in plasma, subretinal fat in Coats' disease and subdermal fat measured by gaschromatography

	Triglyceride composition (Weight percent)		
	Plasma	Subretinal fat	Subdermal fat
C 44 + odd.	0	7.7	4
C 46	0	21.9	7.9
C 48	5	63.3	16.1.
C 50	18	7.1	26.5
C 52	48	1	31.5
C 54	28	0	14
C 56	1	0	0
C 58	0	0	0

Table 2. Distribution of methylated fatty acids in plasma, subretinal fat and subdermal fat measured by gas chromatography

	Fatty acids (methylated) (weight percent)		
	Plasma	Subretinal fat	Subdermal fat
12:0	0	0.4	2.3
14:0	0.6	1.3	6.6
14:1	0	0.8	0.2
16:0	22.5	19.1	28.4
16:1	2.8	6.5	9.2
18:0	12.5	15.8	3.9
18:1	21.7	15.8	29.2
18:2	33.1	11.5	9.8
18:3	0	2.5	1.5
20:0	0	2.2	0.5
Odd and branched	0	18.7	8.4

DISCUSSION

The absence of free cholesterol in the subretinal space in our patient agrees with the observations of Tripathi and Ashton (1971), but not with those of other authors (Duke 1963; Farkas et al. 1973; Yeung & Harris 1976). The literature and our own observations suggest that cholesterol appears at a later stage of the disease after the subretinal deposits have produced a *complete* detachment of the retina.

The amounts of triglycerides and fatty acids in the subretinal mass differed markedly from those of the plasma lipids. In the fatty residues, stearic acid (18:0) was in slight excess, while palmitic acid (16:0), oleic acid (18:1), and especially linoleic acid (18:2) were less abundant. Propionic acid and other odd or branched fatty acids that were almost undetectable in the plasma constituted a major component of the subretinal fat. Selective absorption of a subretinal plasma transudate cannot explain this difference. Either the foam cells metabolize the triglyceride extensively before storage or cellular debris from photoreceptors and pigment epithelium contribute substantially to the subretinal fat that is deposited in Coats' Disease.

REFERENCES

Duke, J. R. The role of cholesterol in the pathogenesis of Coats'Disease. Tr. Am. Ophth. Soc. 61: 492-544 (1963).
Farkas, T. G., A. M. Potts & C. Boone. Some pathologic and biochemical aspects of Coats' Disease. Am. J. Ophthal. 75: 289-301 (1973).
Tripathi, R. & N. Ashton. Electron microscopical study of Coats' Disease. Brit. J. Ophthal., 55: 289-301 (1971).
Yeung, J. W.-S. & G. S. Harris. Coats' Disease: A study of cholesterol transport in the eye. Cand. J. Ophthal. 11: 61-68 (1976).

Authors' address:
Department of Ophthalmology
K.U. Leuven
Leuven
Belgium

BINOCULAR DIPLOPIA ASSOCIATED WITH SUBRETINAL NEOVASCULAR MEMBRANES

DEAN BURGESS, GILL ROPER-HALL & RONALD M. BURDE

(*St. Louis, Missouri, U.S.A.*)

ABSTRACT

A group of patients with subretinal neovascularization, whose major complaint was binocular diplopia are reported. The underlying pathophysiologic mechanism is presumed to be a minute, but real, shift in the photoreceptor array toward the subretinal neovascular membrane producing a rivalry between central and peripheral fusional mechanisms.

INTRODUCTION

Binocular diplopia as a presenting or major symptom of patients wih subretinal neovascular membranes has not, to our knowledge, been reported in the literature. Subretinal neovascular membranes typically may produce blurred vision, micropsia, metamorphopsia, and a positive scotoma. This report discusses the presumed pathophysiology producing the symptom of diplopia.

PATIENTS

Eleven patients were studied from June of 1974 through February of 1978. There were five males and six females; the age range was from 20 to 54 years. Eight patients had the classic triad of the presumed ocular histoplasmosis syndrome, and one patient had senile macular choroidal degeneration with a pigment epithelial detachment. All nine of these patients demonstrated a subretinal neovascular membrane, documented by fluorescein angiography. Two additional patients had subretinal neovascular membranes of unknown etiology.

Supported in part by a grant from Research To Prevent Blindness, Inc., New York, New York.

This paper was originally submitted in part for publication to the *Archives of Ophthalmology* and will be published by them some time before this symposium appears in *Documenta Ophthalmologica Proceedings Series*.

281

OPHTHALMIC EXAMINATION

General

All patients had a manifest and cycloplegic examination, as well as an Amsler grid chart recording distortion, micropsia or scotoma. Patients had a pupillary examination with particular attention paid to the presence of an afferent pupillary defect. All patients had kinetic visual fields performed on a Goldmann 940 bowl perimeter, and individual patients had static perimetry done on an adapted Goldmann 940 bowl perimeter using selected cuts to follow their scotomata.

Ocular motility examination included prism measurements for the deviation and fusion range, Worth stereoscopic test, Hess screen, and synoptophore evaluation including deviation, fusion range, stereopsis, and superimposition slides. These special superimposition slides were prepared so that central fixation objects could be compared simultaneously with objects at 5 and 10 degrees peripherally (Fig. 1).

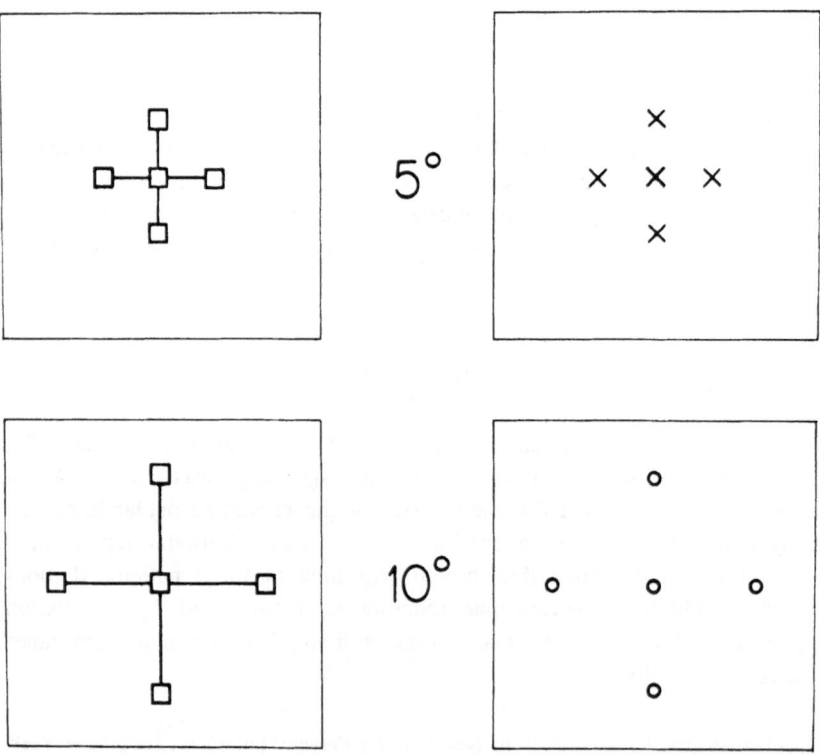

Fig. 1. Special experimental slides were designed for use in the synoptophore to compare superimposition of central targets simultaneously with peripheral targets placed either 5 or 10 degrees from the center.

All patients had their visual acuities recorded in the same setting on multiple visits with standard Snellen chart letters. Slit lamp and dilated direct and indirect ophthalmoscopic examinations were carried out routinely. The central area was evaluated with either the Hruby lens or a contact lens. Fundus photography and fluorescein angiography utilizing a 10 percent fluorescein solution were performed on all patients with a fundus camera (Zeiss Fundus III unit).

CLINICAL FINDINGS AND CASE REPORTS

Objective findings on the eleven patients studied are summarized in Table 1. Two cases are reported in detail in order to emphasize the clinical presentation.

Case 2: A 38-year old woman had a four-month history of diplopia and metamorphopsia. She had been treated with systemic corticosteroids, in spite of which, her vision continued to deteriorate eventually becoming 6/60 in the right eye. The vision in her left eye was 6/6. Ophthalmoscopic examination at this time revealed many peripheral punched-out chorioretinal scars in both eyes and a large grayish subretinal lesion with fluid extending into the fovea from below in the right eye.

Fluorescein angiography demonstrated a neovascular membrane just below the avascular zone (Fig. 2), and subsequently Argon laser treatment was used to obliterate the membrane. The patient's visual acuity stabilized at a 6/15 level, but the diplopia persisted. A small, concomitant right hypertropia was found on orthoptic evaluation, which could not be isolated to any particular paretic muscle. In addition, the patient noted micropsia of the image of the right eye. A 4 diopter basedown prism in front of the right eye neutralized the deviation only for a few minutes. Synoptophore examination, using the experimental slides, demonstrated a definite discrepancy between foveal and peripheral superimposition (Fig. 3).

Case 10: A 20-year-old woman was referred to the Neuro-Ophthalmology Service at Washington University Medical Center because of the sudden onset of vertical diplopia that appeared to be worse in down and left-gaze. Her visual acuity at the time of initial examination was $6/7\frac{1}{2}$ in each eye. A minimal, but slightly incomitant, left hypertropia was detected that appeared to be maximum in left downgaze. A left inferior rectus muscle palsy was suspected, and a Hess chart documented a left hypertropia with a subtle limitation of the left inferior rectus muscle. Ophthalmic and neuro-ophthalmic examination at this time, including a dilated fundus examination, was considered to be entirely normal except for the muscle findings. A 3 diopter Fresnel prism was applied to the patient's left spectacle lens. On the next visit, the patient reported no improvement with the use of the Fresnel prism,

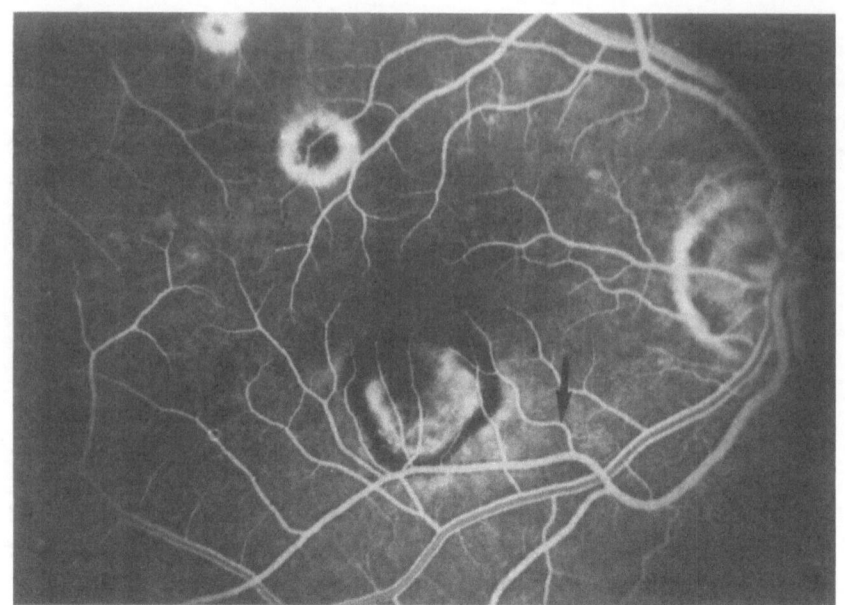

Fig. 2a

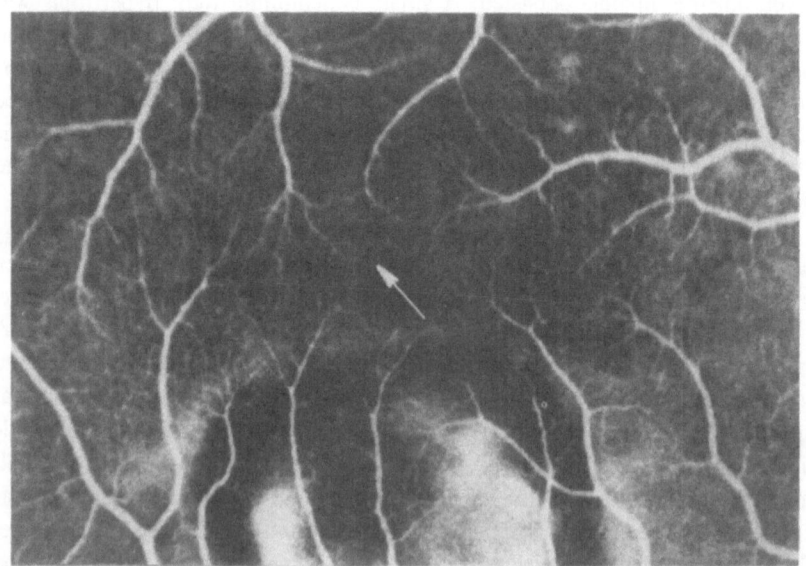

Fig. 2b

284

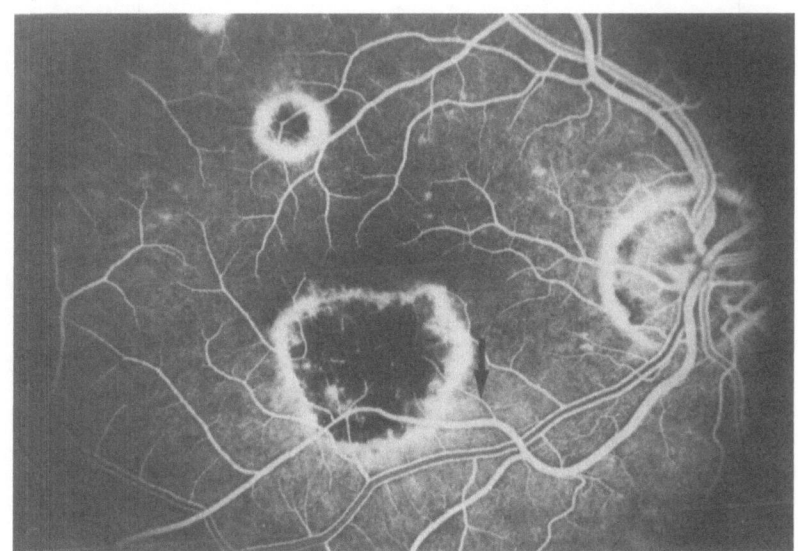

Fig. 2c

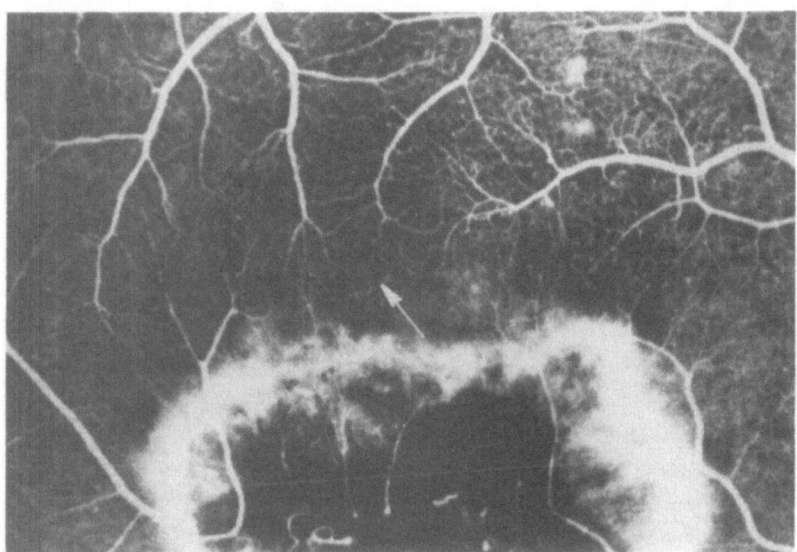

Fig. 2d

Fig. 2. Case 2, 38-year-old woman with presumed ocular histoplasmosis.
1. Presenting fluorescein angiogram of the right eye; vision 6/60 with diplopia. Arrow shows tortuous vessel for comparison with Fig. 2c.
b. Magnified view of Fig. 2a. Arrow indicates vessel for comparison with Fig. 2d.
c. Post-treatment fluorescein angiogram; vision 6/15 with persistant diplopia. Straightening of vessel compared with vessel in Fig. 2a (arrow).
d. Magnified view of Fig. 2c. Downward traction of vessel indicated in Fig. 2b (arrow).

Table 1. Summary of cases

Case	Age/Sex	Affected Eye	Lesion position relative to fovea	Lesion position relative to fixation	Ocular deviation *	Diplopia present preop./ postop.	Visual acuity before/after treatment	
1	49 yo F	Right	Inferior	Above	RHT	Yes/Yes	RE 6/9 LE 6/6	6/6
2	38 yo F	Right	Inferior	Above	RHT	Yes/Yes	RE 6/120 LE 6/5	6/15
3	26 yo M	Right	Inferotemporal	Above and left	RHT	Yes/Yes	RE 6/9 LE 6/5	6/6
4	36 yo M	Left	Superior	Below	RHT	Yes/Yes	RE 6/6 LE 6/6	6/6
5	53 yo F	Right	Inferior	Above and left	RHT c̄ X	Yes/Yes	RE 6/15 LE 6/6	6/7½
6	54 yo F	Right	Nasal	Right	RXT	Yes/Yes	RE 6/60 LE 6/5	6/7½ **
7	24 yo F	Right	Inferotemporal	Above and left	RHT c̄ RET	Yes/Yes	RE 6/6 LE 6/6	6/7½ **
8	31 yo M	Right	Inferotemporal	Above and left	RH c̄ E	Yes/Yes	RE 6/9 LE 6/6	6/7½
9	35 yo M	Left	Inferotemporal	Above and right	X c̄ LH	Yes/No	RE 6/6 LE 6/6	6/7½
10	20 yo F	Left	Inferior	Above	X c̄ LH	Yes/Yes	RE 6/6 LE 6/6	6/12
11	30 yo M	Left	Inferior	Above	X c̄ LH(T)	Yes/Yes	RE 6/5 LE 8/69	6/6

* RHT = Right Hypertropia.
RHT c̄ X = Right Hypertropia with Exophoria.
RXT = Right Exotropia.
RHT c̄ RET = Right Hypertropia with Right Esotropia.
RH c̄ E = Right Hyperphoria with Esophoria.
X c̄ LH = Exophoria with Left Hyperphoria.
X c̄ LH(T) = Exophoria with Intermittent Left Hypertropia.
** Subsequently lost central visual acuity secondary to a recurrence of the condition.

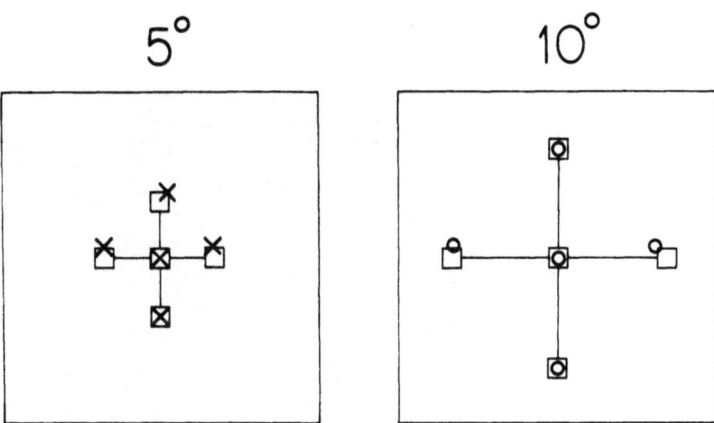

Fig. 3. Patient's impression (Case 2) of the experimental slides (Fig. 1) when superimposing the central targets on the synoptophore. Note the inexact superimposition of peripheral targets.

stating that the relief from her diplopia lasted only for a few seconds. At this point, the possibility of a retinal problem was considered; however, once again the fundus examination was within normal limits. On a subsequent visit the patient described the subjective sensation of seeing convection currents above every object of fixation, and in addition, that objects to the left of fixation appeared to be distorted and curved. Reexamination of the retina at this time revealed a small lesion inferior to the fovea (Fig. 4). Argon laser photocoagulation was performed with destruction of the membrane documented on fluorescein angiography, and the postoperative visual acuity was 6/9. Her symptom of diplopia persisted. The only relief that the patient obtained from her symptomatology was by the placing of a small circle of translucent hypoallergenic surgical tape (Blenderm) in the lower central portion of her spectacles, blocking the central vision of her affected eye.

DISCUSSION

Subretinal neovascular complexes with their associated hemorrhage and serous fluid elevate and distort the fovea. All of our patients reported metamorphopsia, a symptom presumed to be due to a relative change in the parallelism of the photoreceptor array. In addition, in these cases the subretinal neovascular membrane produced a shift of the foveal and parafoveal photoreceptor array toward the proliferating neovascular complex. Since the perceptual mechanisms of the human mind cannot deal with confusion (that is, the simultaneous appreciation of two different objects perceived in the same visual space as determined by the fovea) foveal suppression in the

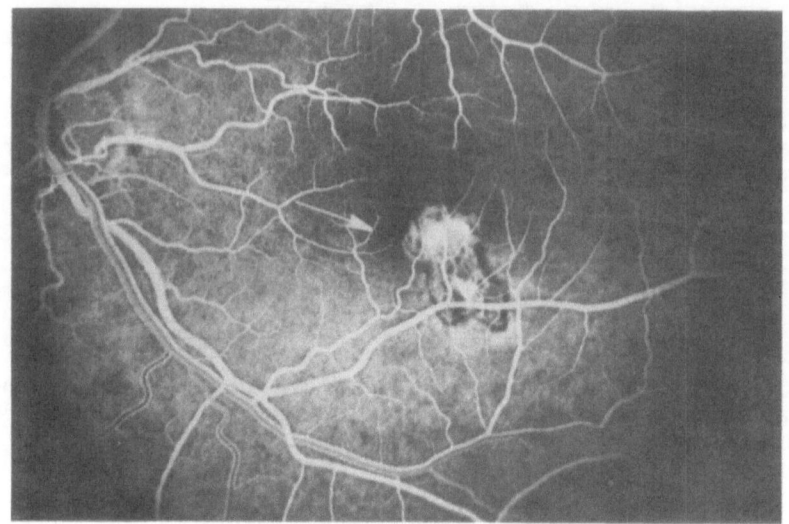

Fig. 4a.

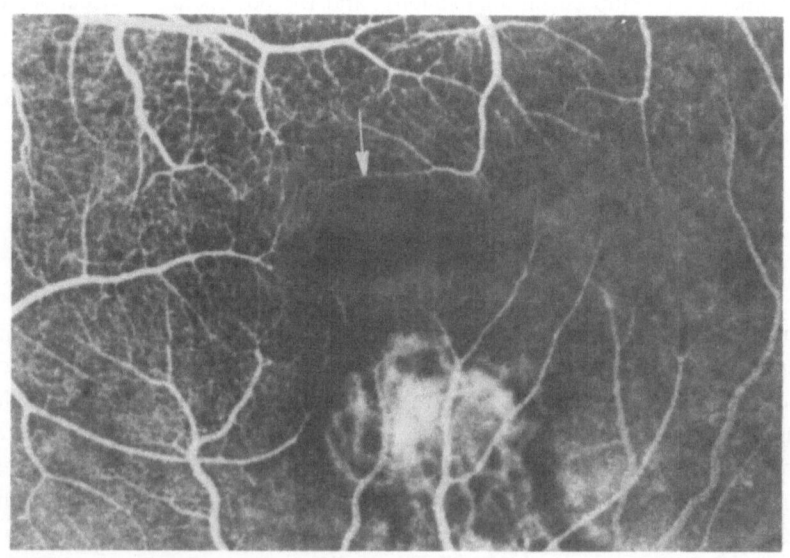

Fig. 4b.

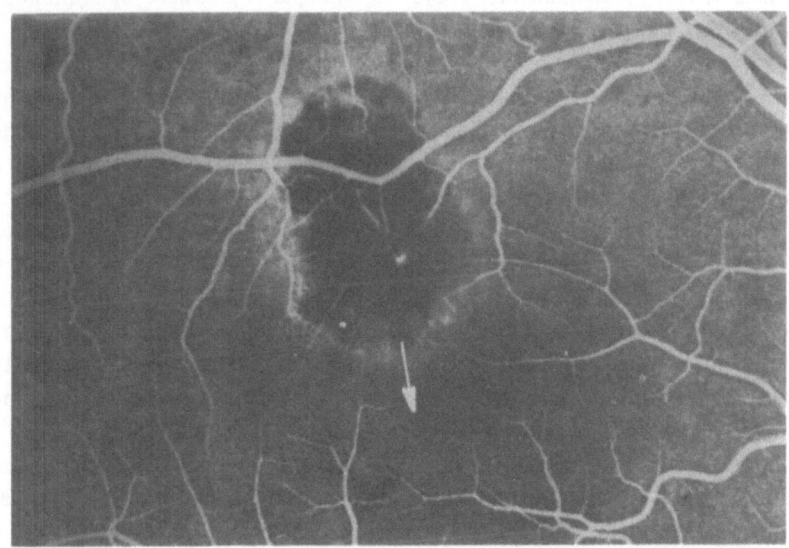

Fig. 4c.

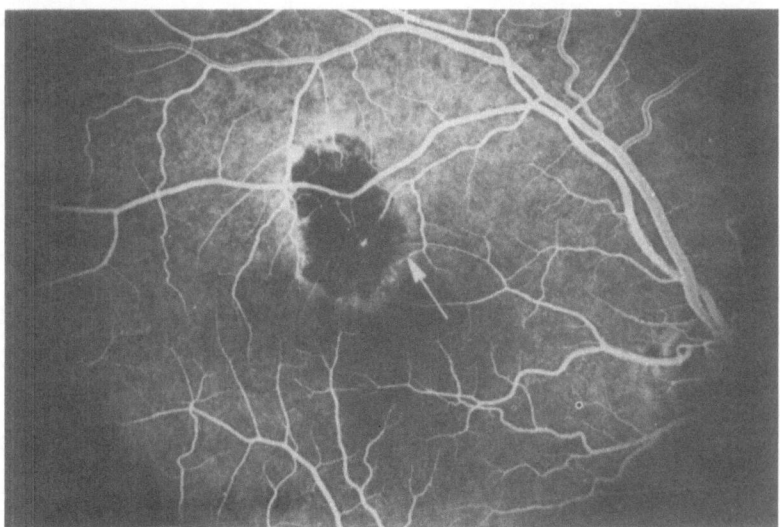

Fig. 4d.

Fig. 4. Case 10, 20-year-old woman with a subretinal neovascular membrane of undetermined etiology.

a. Presenting fluorescein angiogram with vision 6/7½ and marked diplopia. Arrow shows vessels for comparison with Fig. 7c.

b. Magnified view of Fig. 7a. Arrow indicates vessel for comparison with Fig. 7d.

c. Post-treatment fluorescein angiogram; vision 6/9. Temporal traction on large vessel (large arrow) compared with Fig. 7a. Straightening of vessel (small arrow) compared with Fig. 7a.

d. Magnified view of Fig 7c. Downward traction on parafoveal vessel (arrow) compared with Fig. 7b.

289

clinical sense is instantaneous. Therefore, diplopia is produced by stimulated extra-foveal receptors.

An example of this reasoning is that if the lesion is inferior to the fovea, foveal and parafoveal receptors will be shifted microscopically toward the subretinae neovascular membrane, and with both eyes open, superior retina relative to the fovea will be stimulated in the affected eye simulating a hypertropia (Fig. 5). If the non-affected eye is covered, superior retina will be stimulated in the affected eye. In order to foveally fixate the eye will move downward mimicking a true hypertropia. Similarly, the diplopic image which falls on superior retinal receptors will be projected inferiorly, again compatible with a true hypertropia (Table 2). All patients demonstrated the following consistent findings: a deviation (measured tropia) of the affected eye away from the position of the retinal lesion; the affected eye deviated toward the scotoma; and displacement of the diplopic image toward the lesion.

Since the work of Burian (1939, 1941) it has been known that peripheral retinal stimuli are strong enough to break fusion being held by macular targets. Crone has reported fusional disturbances in metamorphopsia in patients with parafoveal lesions (1973). His cases, which are mechanistically similar to ours, were unassociated with subretinal neovascular membranes. As would be expected from our experience, prism therapy failed to provide

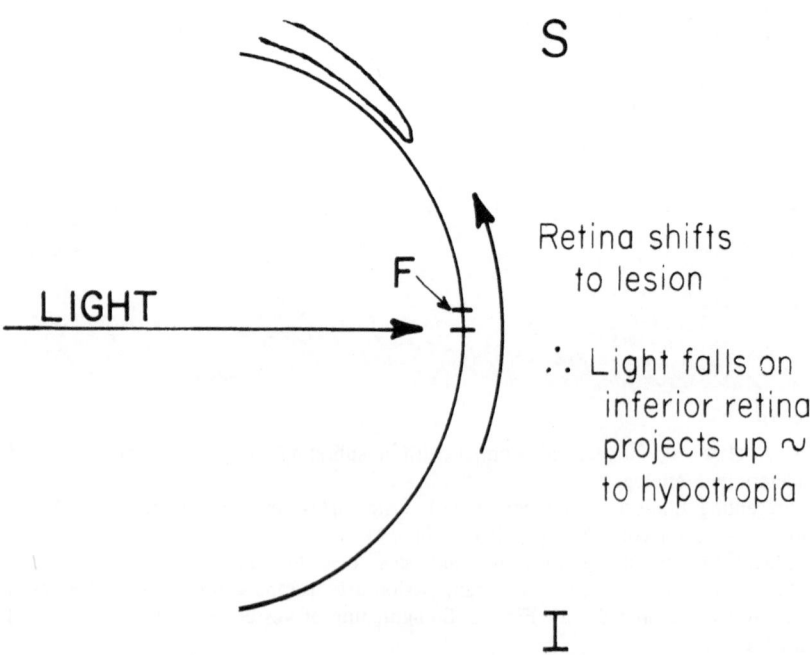

Fig. 5. Schematic representation of foveal shift.

relief in both Cases 2 and 10 because of the conflict between central and peripheral mechanisms. Constant binocular single vision is achieved and maintained by a delicate balance between motor and sensory fusional reflexes. These reflexes are dependent upon relatively normal anatomical substrates. The relative movement of the photoreceptor array in our patients can easily account for the presence of diplopia, and the persistence of diplopia is understood in terms of the dissociation of the fovea from its centric position with respect to its own physiologic periphery. This makes it impossible for corresponding central and peripheral areas to be stimulated simultaneously. Crone, in addition, has described two similar cases (Crone *et al.* 1970). None of these patients were helped by prism therapy, although eight patients note relief in the office with the use of appropriate prisms. Two patients have been relieved of their diplopic symptoms because they have lost central vision, but the remainder remain symptomatic, often not tolerating total Blenderm occlusion of their affected eyes. One patient so far has responded to Blenderm occlusion of the central portion of her glasses, thus allowing her full use of her peripheral mechanisms, and seems to be managing quite well.

The experimental synoptophore slides were designed to examine foveal and peripheral superimposition simultaneously. In six of the eight patients examined using this test, a discrepancy was found between central and peripheral superimposition, usually in the border region of the scar tissue, thus establishing the validity of the foveal peripheral rivalry. The symptomatic existence of this peculiar type of uniocular retinal rivalry lends credence to our assumption that there is a critical shift in the photoreceptor array toward the proliferating subretinal neovascular membrane. A similar situation can be produced by cicatricial changes induced by photocoagulation therapy. By understanding the presumed underlying pathophysiology, one can predict the position of a suspected lesion of this type based on the ocular deviation (Table 2).

Table 2.

Location of lesion	Induced deviation
Inferior	Hypertropia
Superior	Hypotropia
Nasal	Esotropia
Temporal	Exotropia

REFERENCES

Burian, H.M. Fusional movements. Role of peripheral fusion stimuli. Arch. Ophthalmol. 21: 486-491 (1939).

Burian, H.M. Fusional movements in permanent strabismus. A study of the role of central and peripheral retinal regions in the act of binocular vision in squint. Arch. Ophthalmol. 26: 626-650 (1941).

Crone, R.A. Diplopia. Amsterdam, 1973, Excerpta Medica, p. 410.

Crone, R.A., L. van de Gaer & E.L.M. Bonants. Spontaneous foveal diplopia with peripheral fusion. Arch. Ophthalmol. 84: 143-147 (1970).

Authors' addresses:

D. Burgess and G. Roper-Hall
Department of Ophthalmology and Neurology
Washington University School of Medicine
St. Louis, Missouri
U.S.A.

R.M. Burde (Requests for reprints)
Department of Ophthalmology
Box 8096
660 So. Euclid Avenue
St. Louis, Missouri 63110
U.S.A.

PARS PLANA VITRECTOMY IN THE TREATMENT OF VITREOGENIC APHAKIC CYSTOID MACULAR EDEMA

EDWARD OKUN & RICHARD F. ESCOFFERY

(*St. Louis, Missouri, U.S.A.*)

INTRODUCTION

Pars plana vitrectomy has been used effectively in the treatment of eight patients with vitreogenic aphakic cystoid macular edema. Follow-up is 3 to 18 months. The technique of surgery includes severance of all vitreous adhesions to the iris and corneal wound. In all cases treated, the cystoid edema either disappeared or was greatly reduced. In seven of eight cases, visual acuity improved. Documentation has been by fundus photography, fluorescein angiography, and slit lamp photography in certain cases.

Vitreous strands adherent to the pupillary margin of the iris, the cataract wound, the posterior surface of the iris, or possibly the ciliary processes can result in anterior uveitis or vitritis. The resulting inflammatory reaction may be an important factor in the pathogenesis of cystoid macular edema (Gass & Norton 1966). If this is the case, removal of the offending vitreous adhesions should improve the uveitis as well as the resultant cystoid macular edema. Such improvement has been reported by Aaberg (1977) and Michels *et al.* (1974). This report further supports this hypothesis.

MATERIALS AND METHOD

Eight patients with aphakic cystoid macular edema and mild vitritis secondary to vitreous adhesions to the pupil and the limbal scar were subjected to anterior pars plana vitrectomy after cystoid edema had been documented for 7 to 17 months. Cataract extraction had been performed one to four years prior to vitrectomy. Each patient had received topical or systemic steroids with either temporary or no significant visual improvement. All patients who underwent a pars plana vitrectomy had pre- and postoperative stereoscopic fundus photographs and fluorescein angiography. Anterior segment photographs were also taken in most cases.

The operative procedure consisted of removal of all adhesions to the iris, including those to the posterior surface. Iris adhesions could be detected

293

Docum. Ophthal. Proc. Series, Vol. 25, ed. by H. Zauberman
© *1981, Dr. W. Junk bv Publishers, The Hague*

Table 1. Pars plana vitrectomy for vitreogenic aphakic cystoid macular edema

Case		Interval Post-Cat. Extr.	Duration visual loss	Pre-op vision	Post-op vision	Follow-up
1	59 F	16 months	7 months	20/200	20/25	18 months
2	60 M	12 months	12 months	20/70	20/40	17 months
3	58 F	12 months	10 months	20/200	20/70	14 months
4	58F	4 years	7 months	20/200	20/70	8 months
5	62 M	13 months	13 months	20/70	20/20	9 months
6	59 M	4 years	17 months	20/70	20/70	6 months
7	61 M	3 years	12 months	20/100	20/30	5 months
8	54 M	2 years	12 months	20/400	20/200	3 months

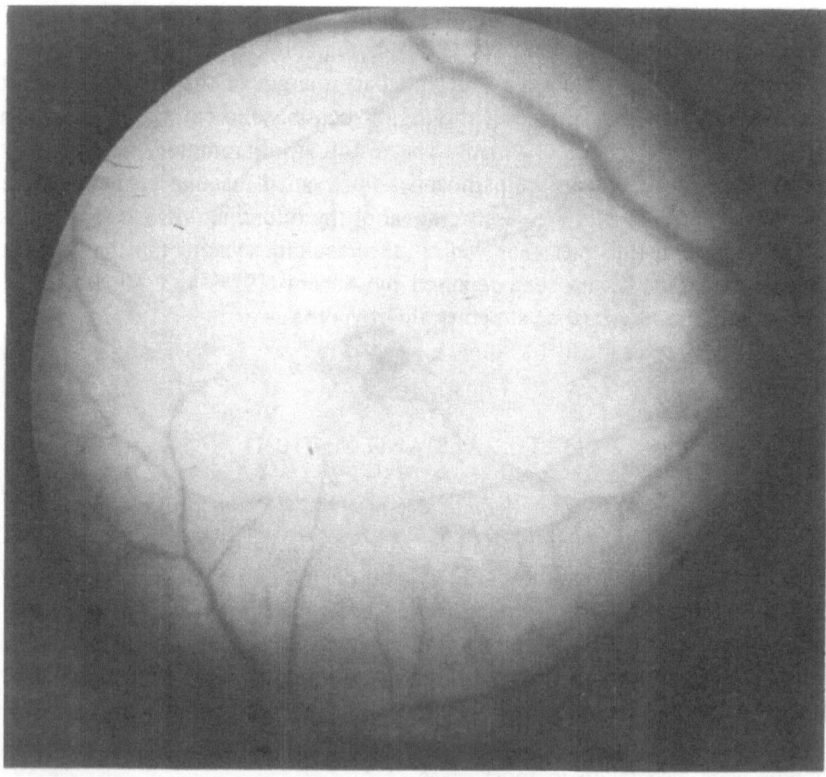

Fig. 1. Fundus photograph of Case 1, O.D. Ruptured inner wall macular cyst. V/A 20/400.

294

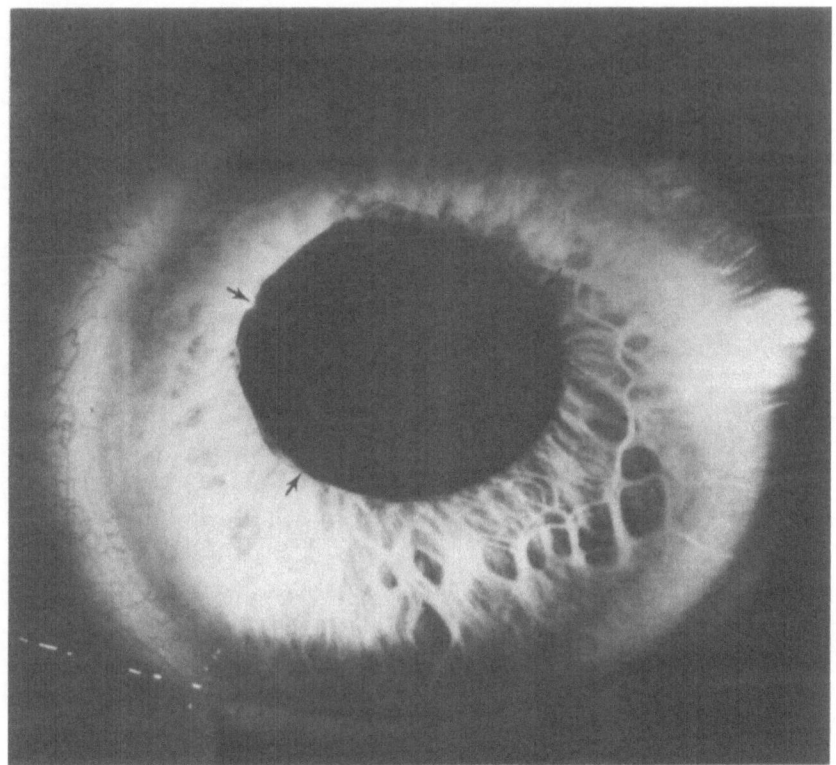

Fig. 2. Preoperative photograph of Case 1, O.S., anterior segment. Note vitreous adhesions to iris at 8 o'clock, 9 : 30 o'clock, and 12 : 30 to 2 o'clock (arrows).

easily by the displacement of the iris with mild suction of the surrounding vitreous. When all adhesions were free, the iris no longer moved when suction was applied nearby.

It was sometimes necessary to remove small amounts of the pupillary iris in order to insure the adequate removal of the adherent vitreous. If vitreous opacities were present, the vitrectomy was continued until a clear view of the posterior pole was obtained. If the vitreous was clear, the anterior vitrectomy was carried only as far posteriorly as the equatorial plane.

RESULTS

The results of pars plana vitrectomy for vitreogenic aphakic cystoid macular edema in eight consecutive patients are shown in Table 1. In each case, the cystoid edema was markedly improved following the vitrectomy. In seven of

295

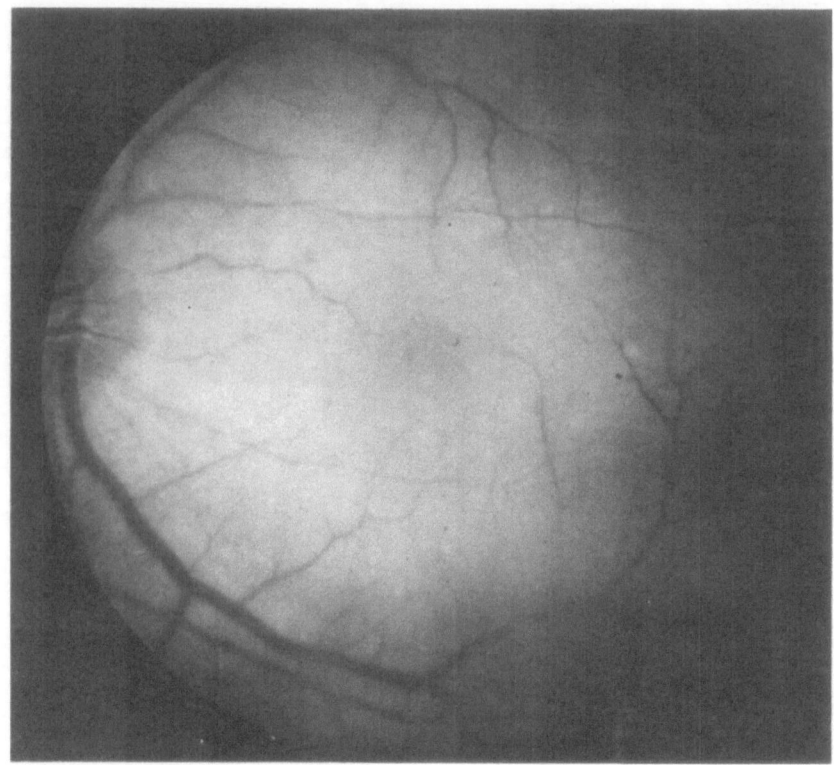

Fig. 3. Preoperative photograph of Case 1, O.S., showing cystoid macular edema. V/A 20/200.

the eight cases, the visual acuity was improved. In six eyes, the visual acuity was improved to 20/70 or better and in three eyes to 20/30 or better. The following case reports illustrates the effectiveness of pars plana vitrectomy in a patient with symmetrical vitreous adhesions to the iris and the limbal wound.

Case 1. This 59-year-old Caucasian female underwent an 'uncomplicated' intracapsular cataract extraction on her right eye. She had excellent vision for several months after which time she experienced a gradual decrease of vision. Cystoid macular edema was diagnosed in her right eye which showed vitreous adhesions to the iris and the limbal wound. Visual acuity gradually decreased to 20/400, at which time a defect was noted in the inner wall of one of the larger macular cystoid spaces (Fig. 1). Two years later, an intracapsular cataract extraction was performed on her left eye. This eye also experienced excellent postoperative vision for several months, after which time visual blurring occurred. The anterior segment was very similar to the

296

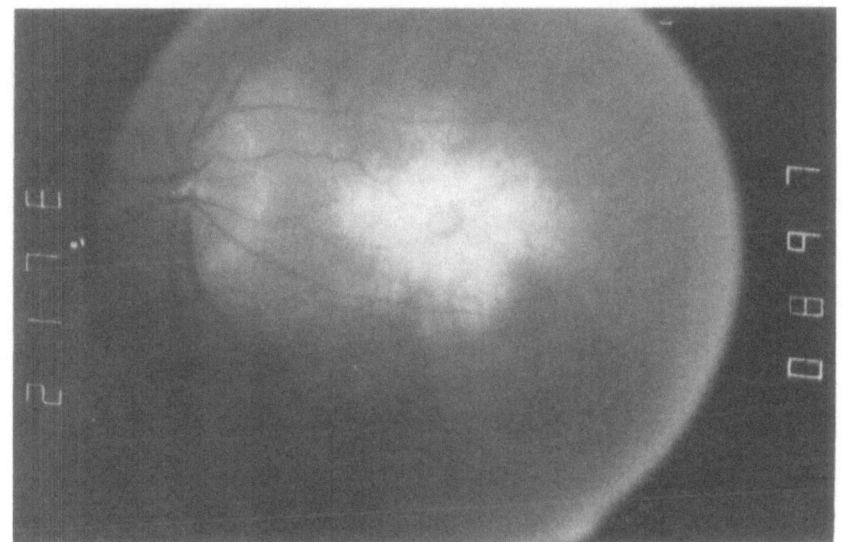

Fig. 4a. Preoperative fluorescein angiogram, Case 1, O.S., showing marked pooling of dye in cystoid spaces. V/A 20/200.

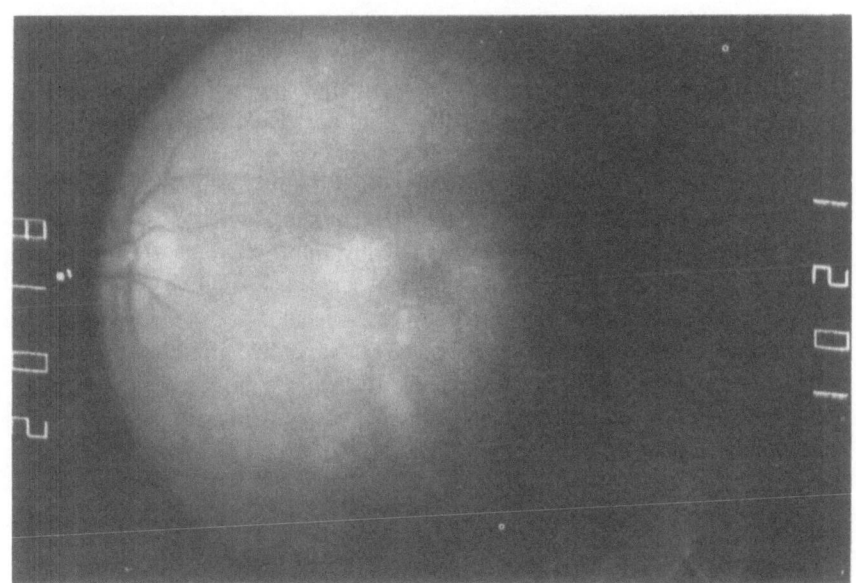

Fig. 4b. Two months postoperative. V/A 20/30-2.

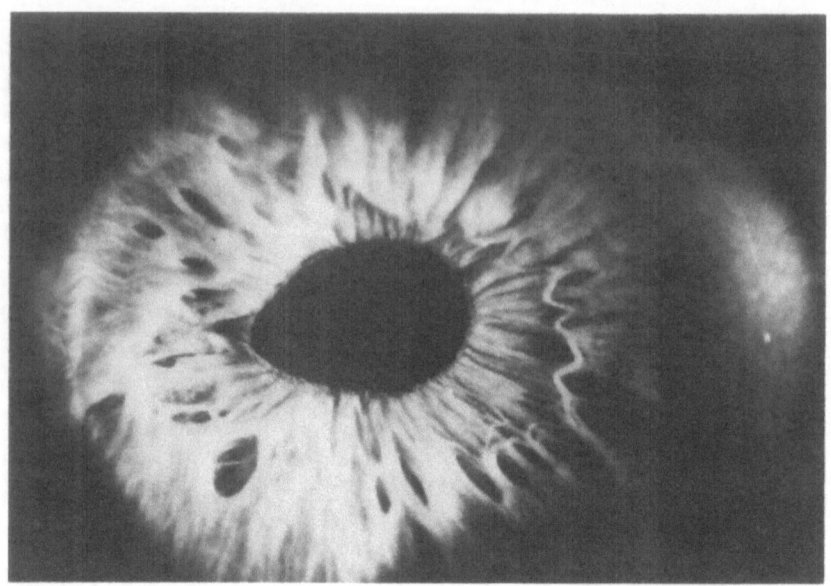

Fig. 5. Postoperative photograph, Case 1, O.S., anterior segment. Note pupil was clear of vitreous adhesions, slightly peaked toward 9 o'clock where pupillary margin has been nicked.

right eye with vitreous adhesions to the iris and cataract wound (Fig. 2). Cystoid macular edema was diagnosed eleven months post cataract extraction (Fig. 3). It was confirmed by fluorescein angiography one month prior to surgery (Fig. 4a). During the next three months, visual acuity dropped from 20/70 to 20/200. Seven months after cystoid was first noted, a pars plana vitrectomy was performed on the left eye. Vitreous adhesions were freed from the posterior iris surface, the pupillary margin, and the corneal wound (Fig. 5). Postoperative visual acuity gradually improved over the first three weeks from 20/200 to 20/50, and eight weeks postoperative, visual acuity was 20/30–2 (Fig. 4b). After six months, visual acuity had returned to 20/25, and the cystoid macular edema was markedly improved (Fig. 6). In this patient, as in each of the others, the vitritis and anterior chamber reaction gradually cleared and visual acuity has remained improved for the duration of follow-up.

Case 4. A 58-year-old Caucasian female had undergone cataract extraction three years prior to the onset of visual loss secondary to cystoid macular edema. After one year of progressive visual loss to the 20/200 level, pars plana vitrectomy was performed and all iris and corneal adhesions were

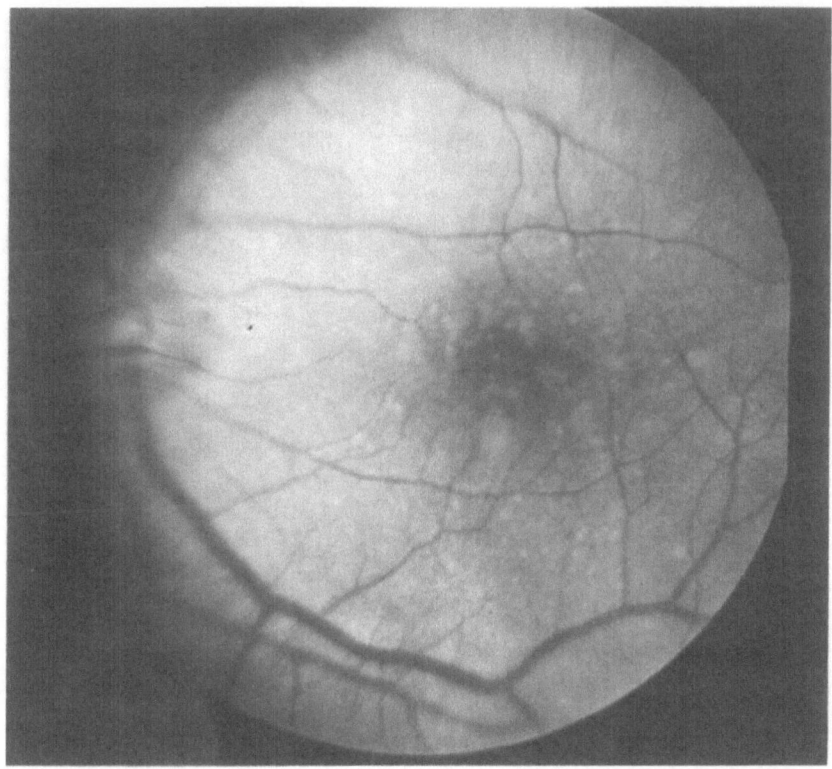

Fig. 6. Postoperative photograph, Case 1, O.S. Cystoid edema has resolved. Note pigmentary irregularity.

severed. Seven weeks following surgery, visual acuity had improved to 20/30. A vitreous hemorrhage occurred the next week and a retinal tear with subclinical retinal detachment was diagnosed (Fig. 7). This originated from a site of previous lattice degeneration. A successful scleral buckling procedure was followed by a reactivation of the cystoid macular edema which has been gradually clearing. The most recent visual acuity was 20/70.

COMMENT

Although aphakic cystoid macular edema with vitreous adhesions to the wound and iris has a poorer prognosis than that without vitreous adhesions, many cases will nevertheless clear spontaneously (Gass & Norton 1969). Since some cases take longer to clear, it is advisable to wait approximately

299

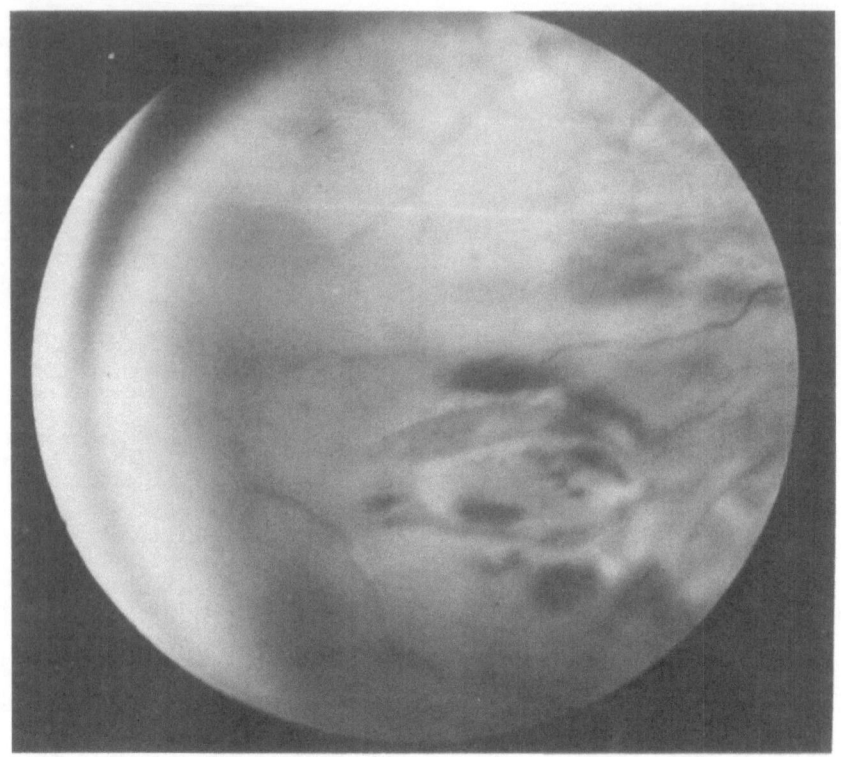

Fig. 7. Fundus photograph of retinal tear and limited retinal detachment.

one year before considering surgical intervention. If the course is rapidly and progressively downhill, or if the other eye has experienced cystoid edema which has failed to clear, surgical intervention might be advisable as early as six months after the onset of symptoms.

In general, the longer one waits, the lesser the chances for return of vision, although there will be some exceptions. The sudden reversal of the downhill course in several of these cases was so dramatic that it left little doubt concerning the effectiveness of the procedure. Whether or not the condition would have eventually cleared on its own will never be known. However, 40% of the eyes with vitreogenic aphakic cystoid macular edema followed by Gass and Norton were still chronically affected when last seen, most having been followed at least two years. If lattice degeneration is present in an eye with cystoid edema, it would be wise to treat this zone at least one month prior to vitrectomy.

REFERENCES

Aaberg, T. M. Pars plana vitrectomy for persistent aphakic cystoid macular edema secondary to vitreous incarceration in the cataract wound. In A. McPherson (ed.): New and controversial aspects of vitreoretinal surgery. St. Louis, C.V. Mosby Co., 1977.

Gass, J. D. M. & E. W. D. Norton. Cystoid macular edema and papilledema following cataract extraction: A fluorescein fundoscopic and angiographic study. Arch. Ophthalmol. 76: 646-661 (1966).

Gass, J. D. M & E. W. D. Norton. Follow-up study of cystoid macular edema following cataract extraction. Trans. Am. Acad. Ophthalmol. & Otol. 73: 665-682 (1969).

Michels, R. G., R. Machemer & K. Müller-Jensen. Vitreous surgery: History and current concepts. Ophthalmic Surg. 5 (4): 13-59 (1974).

Authors addresses:

4949 Barnes Hospital Plaza
Suite 17413/ East Pavilion
St. Louis, Mo. 63110
U.S.A.

REFERENCES

A SUMMARY OF THERAPEUTIC POSSIBILITIES IN THE CHRONIC RETINOPATHIES
Histological basis for hope

ISAAC C. MICHAELSON & L. YANKO

(*Jerusalem, Israel*)

ABSTRACT

In the group of cases classifiable as chronic arteriolar capillaropathies therapy may be directed towards a pre-retinopathy initiating general state, the arteriolar stage of the retinopathy with its diminished perfusion pressure, the capillaropathy stage with its leaking capillaries and to the reaction stage with neovascularisation. There are discussed the value of each approach, proven or theoretical, singly or in combination. There is stressed the need to bear in mind the individual arteriolar capillary unit, a number of which even in the severe cases may still be able to maintain some circulation as evidenced by the persistence of some vision however slight. A few pence to a poor person may be a gift.

There have been emphasized a number of chronic affections of the ocular fundus with a pathogenetic process characterised serially by an arteriolar stage in which there develops a diminished perfusion pressure of the blood, a sequential capillaropathy stage which often leads to the presence in the extravascular tissues of exudates of a seral or haemorrhagic nature, and as a consequence to this a reaction stage characterised by local capillary dilatation, aneurysmal formation, neovascularisation and macrophagic migration and activity. This sequence of events which can be recognised clinically and histologically is so regular among a group of conditions that they have been classified as the chronic arteriolar capillaropathies (Michaelson 1978, 1979, 1980). Fundal conditions possibly so classifiable include diabetic retinopathy, retinal vein occlusion, sickle-cell disease and other retinopathies of the anaemias, retrolental fibroplasia, hypertensive retinopathy, pulseless disease, ischaemic neuropathy, radiation retinopathy and disciform macular disease. All of these conditions are bilateral and most are initiated by a systemic disease.

There have been various therapeutic approaches to this group of disease, the efforts being variously directed to the initiating systemic condition, the diminished arteriolar perfusion pressure, capillary leakage, and the stage of reaction. The main forms of possible therapy are as follows:

I. Therapy directed to the prevention, improvement or cure of an initiating general state or states, for example, hypertension, diabetes, temporal arteritis, the blood dyscrasias, and prematurity. This is primary prevention

303

and its achievement is often not so much dependent on the ophthalmologist as on the internist, the genetecist and, as in the case of retrolental fibroplasia, on the neonatologist who is responsible for the management of the hyperbaric therapy of the premature infant.

II. Treatment directed towards the diminished arteriolar perfusion pressure. This can be considered to be the beginning of prevention of the secondary order. This consists of anti-occlusive therapy (A-OT) and anti-occlusive regime (A-OR) or both together (A-OTR) (Michaelson 1979, 1980). The management is similar to that prescribed for ischaemic conditions in general, cardiac, intracranial or those involving the peripheral circulation. The therapy consists of aspirin which decreases blood-platelet aggregation (Weiss et al. 1968; Mielke et al. 1973) and dipyridamole (persantin) which is a vasodilator and also an inhibitor of ADP-induced platelet aggregation (Mustard et al. 1972). The regime is directed towards control of diet, blood pressure, daily exercise, weight and smoking habits. Rigorous dietary restrictions specially with regard to unsaturated fats, may be imposed in order to prevent high serum cholesterol and its consequences which may include arteriosclerosis or atheroma.

III. Therapy directed towards leaking capillaries of the capillaropathy stage and towards new vessels of the reaction stage which commonly leak. Such vessels are often causes of macular oedema and severe intraocular haemorrhage which may lead to diminished vision and even to blindness. This therapy is commonly surgical consisting of photocoagulation by means of laser or xenon arc or of cryotherapy. The recent reports of BenEzra (1978) raise hopes that the use of inhibitors of Prostaglandin synthesis may furnish a medical approach to the problem of neovascularisation in these retinopathies.

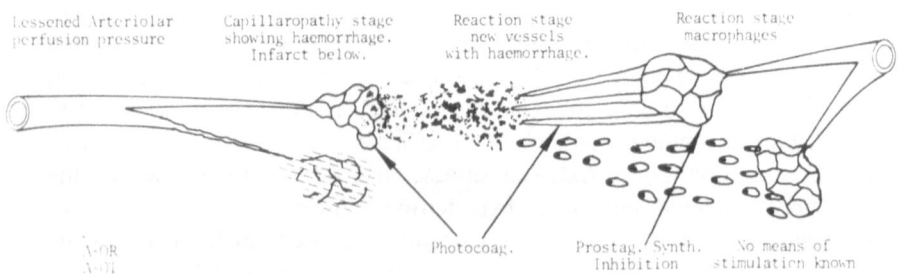

Fig. 1. Diagram illustrating relationship between the pathogenetic process and the corresponding therapeutic possibilities.

Management additional to that of main initiating factor, if any. The upper part of the diagram read from left to right indicates the progressive stages of the pathogenesis, the lower part indicates the corresponding therapy, stage by stage.

A-OR = Anti-occlusive regime

A-OT = Anti-occlusive therapy

in respect of multi-factorial causation.

IV. Therapy may be required for the stage of complications which chiefly includes vitreous haemorrhage and macular oedema. For the former there may be necessary vitreous removal and even vitrectomy.

It is not surprising that the retinopathies discussed have become within recent years the central focus of ophthalmic research both with regard to the better understanding of the pathogenetic process including its epidemiological aspects and the investigation of therapeutic possibilities. The majority of these retinopathies are age-related and in an ageing society it is well that all aspects of the pathogenesis be explored for their vulnerability to therapeutic measures (Kupfer 1975, Michaelson 1979, 1980). These measures are separately or in their combinations in many retinopathies still at the stage of requiring well organised controlled therapeutic trials.

The purpose of this report is to facilitate an integrated comprehension of the multiple, perhaps coincident, therapeutic possibilities. Their relation to each other and to the pathogenesis are illustrated in the diagram. The upper part of the diagram read from left to right indicates the progressive stages of the pathogenesis, the lower part indicates the corresponding therapy, stage by stage. It should be emphasised that each retinopathic fundus with its numerous arteriole cum capillary units is a kaleidoscopic mixture of such units. Each unit is at any one time at its own degree of local change within the different stages of the general retinal vascular process; arteriolar, capillary or reaction. One arteriole cum capillary unit might have given rise to oedema, one to haemorrhage, one to vascular dilatation or a by-pass, one to a microaneurysm and one to a new vessel. One unit may show a dot of hard exudate with. with its macrophages, while other units conglomerating together might stimulate a circinate exudate. If certain of these arteriolar-capillary units are by chance close to the fovea and if the blood flow in these particular units are still amenable to therapy, there may be grounds for hope despite the general unpromising appearance of the fundus. The therapy should be directed with the individual arteriole cum capillary units kept in mind and be continued as long as there are a number of such units in working order as indicated by the maintenance of some vision, however slight even if only sufficient as to maintain the perception of light and colours.

RELATIONSHIP BETWEEN BLOOD FLOW AND VISUAL FIELD CHANGES IN GLAUCOMA

The arteriolar flow diminution in the above retinal conditions may especially affect the neighbourhood of the optic nerve head and give rise to changes in visual field and disc as observed in diabetes mellitus and blood loss (Morgan and Drance 1975). It has been postulated that chronic ischaemia at the level of the optic nerve head is an important determinant of the glaucomatous process generally in open angle glaucoma (Ffytche et al. 1974). This relationship is even more marked in certain varieties of chronic simple glaucoma: in "low tension glaucoma" where the vascular system is affected by a normal intraocular pressure, and in ocular hypertension where the vascular system is not affected even by an increased intraocular pressure.

REFERENCES

BenEzra, D. Neovasculogenic ability of prostaglandins, growth factors and synthetic chemoatractants. Am. J. Ophthal. 86: 455 (1978).

Ffytche, t.J., C.J. Bulpitt, E.M. Kohner, D. Archer & C.T. Dollery. Effect of changes in intraocular pressure on the retinal circulation. Brit. J. Ophthal. 58: 514 (1974).

Kupfer, C. Cooperative clinical trials. The Second Ticho Memorial Lecture. Am. J. Ophthal. 79: 543 (1975).

Michaelson, I.C. Diabetic retinopathy as the prototype in the classification of certain retinopathies and the reaction stage in these conditions. Regnault, I. and Duhault, J. (eds.): Cellular and Biochemical Aspects in Diabetic Retinopathy. Amsterdam, Elsevier/North Holland. Biomedical Press. P. 257-275 (1978).

Michaelson, I.C. An examination of the possibilities of preventive therapy in arteriolar retinopathies. Am. J. Ophth. 88: 450-460 (1979).

Michaelson, I.C. Textbook of the Fundus of the Eye. Third Edition. Publishers: Churchill Livingston, Edinburgh and London. (In Press).

Mielke, C.H., J.C. Ramos & A.F.H. Britten. Aspirin as an antiplatelet agent: template bleeding time as a monitor of therapy. Am. J. Clin. Path. 59: 236 (1973).

Morgan, R.W. & S.M. Drance. Chronic open-angle glaucoma and ocular hypertension. Brit J. Ophthal. 59: 211 (1975).

Mustard, J.F., R.L. Kinlough-Rathbone, C.S.P. Jenkins & M.A. Packham. Modification of platelet function. Ann. N.Y. Acad. Sci. 201; 343 (1972).

Weiss, H.J., L.M. Aledort & S. Kochwa. The effect of solicylates on the hemostatic properties of platelets in man. J. Clin. Invest. 47: 2169 (1968).

Authors' address:
Hadassah University Hospital
Dept. of Ophthalmology
P.O. Box 12000
Jerusalem
Israel